MW01224319

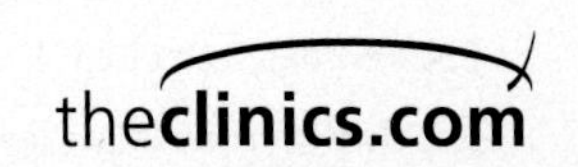

VETERINARY CLINICS OF NORTH AMERICA

Small Animal Practice

Current Topics in Clinical Pharmacology and Therapeutics

GUEST EDITOR
Dawn Merton Boothe, DVM, PhD

September 2006 • Volume 36 • Number 5

SAUNDERS
An Imprint of Elsevier, Inc.
PHILADELPHIA LONDON TORONTO MONTREAL SYDNEY TOKYO

W.B. SAUNDERS COMPANY
A Division of Elsevier Inc.

Elsevier, Inc., 1600 John F. Kennedy Blvd., Suite 1800, Philadelphia, PA 19103-2899

http://www.vetsmall.theclinics.com

VETERINARY CLINICS OF NORTH AMERICA: SMALL ANIMAL PRACTICE
September 2006
Editor: John Vassallo

Volume 36, Number 5
ISSN 0195-5616
ISBN 1-4160-3828-0

Veterinary Clinics of North America: Small Animal Practice (ISSN 0195-5616) is published bimonthly (For Post Office use only: volume 36 issue 5 of 6) by Elsevier Inc., 360 Park Avenue South, New York, NY 10010-1710. Months of issue are January, March, May, July, September, and November. Business and Editorial offices: 1600 John F. Kennedy Blvd., Suite 1800, Philadelphia, PA 19103-2899. Customer Service Office: 6277 Sea Harbor Drive, Orlando, FL 32887-4800. Periodicals postage paid at New York, NY and additional mailing offices. Subscription prices are $170.00 per year for US individuals, $275.00 per year for US institutions, $85.00 per year for US students and residents, $225.00 per year for Canadian individuals, $345.00 per year for Canadian institutions, $235.00 per year for international individuals, $345.00 per year for international institutions and $115.00 per year for Canadian and foreign students/residents. To receive student/resident rate, orders must be accompained by name of affiliated institution, date of term, and the *signature* of program/residency coordinator on institution letterhead. Orders will be billed at individual rate until proof of status is received. Foreign air speed delivery is included in all *Clinics* subscription prices. All prices are subject to change without notice. **POSTMASTER**: Send address changes to *Veterinary Clinics of North America: Small Animal Practice*, Elsevier Periodicals Customer Service, 6277 Sea Harbor Drive, Orlando, FL 32887-4800, USA; phone: 1-800-654-2452 [toll free number for US customers], or (+1)(407) 345-4000 [customers outside US]; fax: (+1)(407) 363-1354; email: usjcs@elsevier.com.

Veterinary Clinics of North America: Small Animal Practice is also published in Japanese by Inter Zoo Publishing Co., Ltd., Aoyama Crystal-Bldg 5F, 3-5-12 Kitaaoyama, Minato-ku, Tokyo 107-0061, Japan.

Reprints: For copies of 100 or more, of articles in this publication, please contact the Commercial Reprints Department, Elsevier Inc., 360 Park Avenue South, New York, New York 10010-1710. Tel. (212) 633-3813 Fax: (212) 462-1935, email: reprints@elsevier.com

Veterinary Clinics of North America: Small Animal Practice is covered in *Current Contents/Agriculture, Biology and Environmental Sciences, Science Citation Index, ASCA, Index Medicus, Excerpta Medica, and BIOSIS.*

Printed in the United States of America.

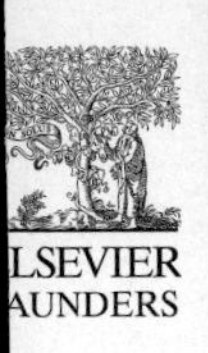

VETERINARY CLINICS
SMALL ANIMAL PRACTICE

Current Topics in Clinical Pharmacology and Therapeutics

GUEST EDITOR

DAWN MERTON BOOTHE, DVM, PhD, Diplomate, American College of Veterinary Internal Medicine; Diplomate, American College of Veterinary Clinical Pharmacology; Professor and Director of Clinical Pharmacology, Department of Anatomy, Physiology and Pharmacology, College of Veterinary Medicine, Auburn University, Auburn, Alabama

CONTRIBUTORS

ELLEN N. BEHREND, VMD, MS, PhD, Diplomate, American College of Veterinary Internal Medicine; Associate Professor, Department of Clinical Sciences, College of Veterinary Medicine, Auburn University, Auburn, Alabama

HARRY W. BOOTHE, JR, DVM, MS, Diplomate, American College of Veterinary Surgeons; Professor and Chief, Small Animal Surgery, Department of Clinical Sciences, College of Veterinary Medicine, Auburn University, Auburn, Alabama

DAWN MERTON BOOTHE, DVM, PhD, Diplomate, American College of Veterinary Internal Medicine; Diplomate, American College of Veterinary Clinical Pharmacology; Professor and Director of Clinical Pharmacology, Department of Anatomy, Physiology and Pharmacology, College of Veterinary Medicine, Auburn University, Auburn, Alabama

CYRIL R. CLARKE, BVSc, MS, PhD, Diplomate, American College of Veterinary Clinical Pharmacology; Professor and Associate Dean for Academic Affairs, Center for Veterinary Health Sciences, Oklahoma State University, Stillwater, Oklahoma

TERRENCE P. CLARK, DVM, PhD, Diplomate, American College of Veterinary Clinical Pharmacology; Principal Research Scientist, Department of Biology Research and Technology Acquisitions, Elanco Animal Health, A Division of Eli Lilly and Company, Greenfield, Indiana

CURTIS W. DEWEY, DVM, MS, Diplomate, American College of Veterinary Internal Medicine (Neurology); Diplomate, American College of Veterinary Surgeons; Associate Professor of Neurology/Neurosurgery, Department of Clinical Sciences, Cornell University College of Veterinary Medicine, Ithaca, New York

VIRGINIA FAJT, DVM, PhD, Diplomate, American College of Veterinary Clinical Pharmacology; Clinical Assistant Professor, Veterinary Physiology and

Pharmacology, College of Veterinary Medicine and Biomedical Sciences, Texas A&M University, College Station, Texas

LISA M. HOWE, DVM, PhD, Diplomate, American College of Veterinary Surgeons; Associate Professor and Co-Chief, Surgical Sciences Section, Department of Small Animal Clinical Sciences, College of Veterinary Medicine and Biomedical Sciences, Texas A&M University, College Station, Texas

DEBORAH T. KOCHEVAR, DVM, PhD, Diplomate, American College of Veterinary Clinical Pharmacology; Dean, Tufts Cummings School of Veterinary Medicine, North Grafton, Massachusetts; Formerly, Professor, Veterinary Physiology and Pharmacology and Associate Dean for Professional Programs, College of Veterinary Medicine and Biomedical Sciences, Texas A&M University, College Station, Texas

KATRINA L. MEALEY, DVM, PhD, Diplomate, American College of Veterinary Internal Medicine; Diplomate, American College of Veterinary Clinical Pharmacology; Department of Veterinary Clinical Sciences, College of Veterinary Medicine, Washington State University, Pullman, Washington

LAUREN A. TREPANIER, DVM, PhD, Diplomate, American College of Veterinary Internal Medicine; Diplomate, American College of Veterinary Clinical Pharmacology; Associate Professor, Department of Medical Sciences, University of Wisconsin-Madison, School of Veterinary Medicine, Madison, Wisconsin

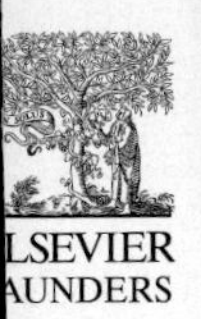
LSEVIER
AUNDERS

VETERINARY CLINICS
SMALL ANIMAL PRACTICE

Current Topics in Clinical Pharmacology and Therapeutics

CONTENTS VOLUME 36 • NUMBER 5 • SEPTEMBER 2006

Over the past decade, there have been several nonsteroidal anti-inflammatory drugs (NSAIDs) introduced in veterinary medicine with an increased gastrointestinal safety profile consistent with a cyclooxygenase (COX)-1–sparing effect. More recently, an NSAID with additional 5-lipoxygenase (5-LOX) activity has also been approved for use. Although it is tempting to equate in vitro COX-2/COX-1 and 5-LOX inhibition to overall in vivo safety, the data do not support this approach. The true overall safety for any individual compound is based on its evaluation in laboratory margin-of-safety studies, reproductive safety studies, and blind multicenter field studies in client-owned animals. Therefore, when choosing a COX-2–selective or dual-inhibitor NSAID for clinical use, all in vivo data must be taken into account to understand comparative safety, and continued use must be based on the drug's performance in the individual being treated. Until head-to-head trials in multicenter blind studies are published, comments on comparative safety and effectiveness must be reserved.

Drug therapy for the endocrine system is implemented to replace a hormone deficiency or to prevent or reduce the formation or effects of excess hormone. Treatment of endocrine disorders covers diseases of the pituitary, adrenal, parathyroid, and thyroid glands as well as the endocrine pancreas. This article focuses on new therapies currently available for specific diseases. Administration of trilostane for treatment of hyperadrenocorticism and use of insulin glargine, protamine zinc insulin (PZI), and porcine Lente insulin for diabetes mellitus are discussed. In addition, transdermal methimazole therapy for treatment of feline hyperthyroidism and administration of progestins for pituitary dwarfism are considered.

This article reviews anticonvulsant therapies in current use for dogs and cats and briefly describes new modes of anticonvulsant therapy that are being investigated or pending publication. Most of the information contained within the article is based on published information. Some of the information, however, is based on the author's clinical experience and is identified as such.

GOAL STATEMENT

The goal of the *Veterinary Clinics of North America: Small Animal Practice* is to keep practicing veterinarians up to date with current clinical practice in small animal medicine by providing timely articles reviewing the state of the art in small animal care.

ACCREDITATION

The *Veterinary Clinics of North America: Small Animal Practice* offers continuing education credits, awarded by Cummings School of Veterinary Medicine at Tufts University, Office of Continuing Education.

Cummings School of Veterinary Medicine at Tufts University is a designated provider of continuing veterinary medical education. Veterinarians participating in this learning activity may earn up to 6 credits per issue up to a maximum of 36 credits per year. Credits awarded may not apply toward license renewal in all states. It is the responsibility of each participant to verify the requirements of their state licensing board.

Credit can be earned by reading the text material, taking the examination online at ***http://www.theclinics.com/home/cme***, and completing the program evaluation. Following your completion of the test and program evaluation, and review of any and all incorrect answers, you may print your certificate.

TO ENROLL

To enroll in the *Veterinary Clinics of North America: Small Animal Practice* Continuing Veterinary Medical Education Program, call customer service at 1-800-654-2452 or sign up online at ***http://www.theclinics.com/home/cme***. The CVME program is now available at a special introductory rate of $99.95 for a year's subscription.

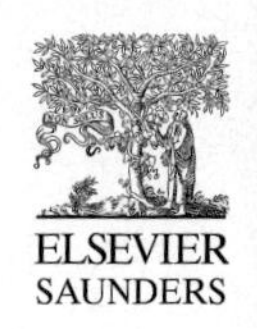

VETERINARY CLINICS
SMALL ANIMAL PRACTICE

FORTHCOMING ISSUES

November 2006

Dietary Management and Nutrition
Claudia A. Kirk, DVM, PhD
and Joseph W. Bartges, DVM, PhD
Guest Editors

January 2007

Effective Communication in Veterinary Practice
Karen Cornell, DVM, PhD
Jennifer Brandt, PhD, MSW
Kathleen A. Bonvicini, MPH
Guest Editors

March 2007

Clinical Pathology and Diagnostic Techniques
Robin W. Allison, DVM, PhD
and James Meinkoth, DVM, PhD
Guest Editors

RECENT ISSUES

July 2006

Wound Management
Steven F. Swaim, DVM, MS
D.J. Krahwinkel, DVM, MS
Guest Editors

May 2006

Pediatrics
Autumn P. Davidson, DVM, MS
Guest Editor

March 2006

Practice Management
David E. Lee, DVM, MBA
Guest Editor

Vet Clin Small Anim 36 (2006) xi–xiii

VETERINARY CLINICS
SMALL ANIMAL PRACTICE

ELSEVIER
SAUNDERS

Preface

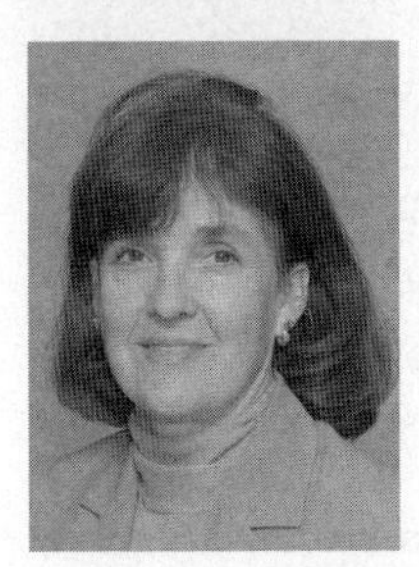

Dawn Merton Boothe, DVM, PhD
Guest Editor

It has been 8 years since the last issue of the *Veterinary Clinics of North America: Small Animal Practice* was dedicated to clinical pharmacology (March 1998). In the intervening years, the profession has enjoyed several advances in the discipline. Approximately 90 new drugs have been approved for either dogs or cats. Included is the reformulation of some tried-and-true drugs, as well as new members of diverse drug classes. The number of previously approved parasiticides, anesthetics, antimicrobials, analgesics, and hormones has increased, and new drug classes such as behavior-modifying drugs have been added. Several novel drug delivery systems also have been approved. The decade also has brought a relatively new paradigm: the availability of multiple products within the same drug class. Although competition has its attributes, practitioners must become increasingly more familiar with the clinical pharmacology, pharmacodynamics, and therapeutic use of each product, such that the basis for choice is rational. Advances in human pharmacology continue to "trickle down" to our small animal patients. Gratifyingly, veterinarians increasingly seek scientific support for extrapolation of the use of human drugs in their small animal patients. Not surprisingly, the literature has increased to incorporate several new scientific journals dedicated to veterinary therapeutics. However, availability of non–peer-reviewed information on the Internet often detracts from the science. Advances in molecular biology have made their mark–and promise to continue to do so–in veterinary clinical pharmacology. New understanding of drug actions, reactions, and species differences has benefited our patients. Unfortunately, however, not all changes have been beneficial. The decade has seen the advent of resistant microbes in response to decades of unfettered antimicrobial use.

0195-5616/06/$ – see front matter
doi:10.1016/j.cvsm.2006.08.004

vetsmall.theclinics.com

The topics chosen for this issue are intended to exemplify the changes that have occurred in the use of drugs in small animals. The lead article on evidenced-based medicine is perhaps the most important, because it is applicable to all aspects of pharmacology and therapeutics. Although seemingly a new concept, veterinarians have long embraced–perhaps unknowingly–this common sense approach to the practice of medicine. The article emphasizes the importance of critical scientific review of information and offers a hierarchy of import, as well as examples of credible resources. An article on pharmacogenomics has been included to demonstrate what can be anticipated in the future as we increase our understanding of the genetic basis for drug response in the individual patient. Already, collies have benefited following the elucidation of their basis for avermectin sensitivity. In the same context, molecular technology has helped us understand the role of cytochrome P450, a superfamily of drug metabolizing enzymes, in drug interactions.

Among the classes of drugs that have changed mechanistically in the last 10 years are the nonsteroidal anti-inflammatories. Six products have been approved in the intervening 8 years for use in either dogs or cats. Understandably, confusion exists regarding the importance of "COX-1 protection" and its impact on safety and efficacy. Accordingly, an article has been included in an attempt to offer guidance regarding the use of these exciting drugs in dogs and cats. Updates on endocrine and anticonvulsant therapy were chosen because of the lack of comprehensive and timely reviews elsewhere.

Perhaps no class of drugs has drawn as much attention in medical communities in the intervening years as has the antimicrobials. Their indiscriminant use increasingly is problematic. Public health considerations often elicit emotional responses that may not be scientifically justified. Yet bacterial resistance must be perceived as an insidious, unrelentless side effect of antimicrobial therapy. Antimicrobial resistance must be understood as both a global and local issue, hospital and community-based, impacting both populations and individuals. It is a side effect that will decline only with de-escalation and judicious use. Accordingly, three articles in this issue are dedicated to the use of antimicrobial therapy in dogs and cats. The first focuses on antimicrobial resistance and its advent in veterinary medicine. The second offers principles upon which the selection of an antimicrobial drug might be based. Guidelines are offered for the design of individual dosing regimens, such that therapeutic success can be achieved both in terms of eradicating infection and minimizing resistance. The third article addresses one of the more common uses of antimicrobial drugs: prophylaxis in the canine or feline surgical patient.

The rapid emergence of both internet and mortar and brick pharmacies specializing in veterinary compounding has been both a gain and bane to the advent of veterinary therapeutics. Compounding has always been a vital aspect of individual drug therapy to our veterinary patients and its presence in the forefront is associated with many sequelae that benefit our patients. However, in some respects the veterinary profession has come full circle, broadly embracing the use of therapeutic products for which little scientific evidence of efficacy or safety exists. Accordingly, this issue concludes by addressing a subject for which the application of evidence-based medicine is paramount: veterinary compounded drug products. The article is offered as a comprehensive review that addresses not only the long, rich history of veterinary compounding, but also the current (dynamic) regulations that must be understood in the context of both public health and veterinary patient considerations. The article concludes with a discussion of those aspects of compounding that may contribute to therapeutic failure due to quality assurance, safety, or efficacy concerns, with a particular focus on transdermal gels.

The intervening years since our last issue have been amazing. The increased standard of veterinary care has been astounding, surpassing what I had envisioned as a veterinary student many years ago. The discipline of clinical pharmacology has been the perfect venue within which to enjoy these changes. This preface would not be complete without recognition of the American College of Veterinary Clinical Pharmacology, whose members have dedicated their professional efforts to the advancement of knowledge and application in the field of clinical pharmacology and therapeutics. No one article in this issue could have been generated without the input provided by members of this College. It has been an honor to be among the members of this College and a privilege to contribute to its efforts through the editing of this issue.

Dawn Merton Boothe, DVM, PhD
Department of Anatomy, Physiology, and Pharmacology
College of Veterinary Medicine
Auburn University
109 Greene Hall
Auburn, AL 36849, USA

E-mail address: boothdm@auburn.edu

Vet Clin Small Anim 36 (2006) 943–959

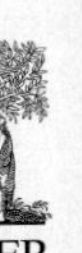

VETERINARY CLINICS
SMALL ANIMAL PRACTICE

Evidence-Based Decision Making in Small Animal Therapeutics

Deborah T. Kochevar, DVM, PhD[a,*], Virginia Fajt, DVM, PhD[b]

[a]Professional Programs, Dean's Office, College of Veterinary Medicine and Biomedical Sciences, 4461 Texas A&M University, College Station, TX 77843-4461, USA
[b]Veterinary Physiology and Pharmacology, College of Veterinary Medicine and Biomedical Sciences, 4466 Texas A&M University, College Station, TX 77843-4466, USA

The most modest goal of any therapeutic intervention is to "do no harm." We hope to achieve far more than that through rational therapies supported by sound clinical reasoning, scientific evidence, and an understanding of risk management. Evidence-based decision making (EBDM) has emerged in the health sciences as a means to advance these therapeutic best practices. Technology has greatly enhanced the ability of clinicians and patients to access the scientific literature and to become well informed. As a consequence, clinicians can and must stay current or risk making poor decisions that clients may challenge. This risk is greatest when it comes to therapeutic decisions that require administration or prescription of drugs. Unedited drug information readily available to clients via the Internet ensures that physicians and veterinarians are going to be faced with questions and suggestions about their therapeutic choices. Veterinary pharmacologists and clinicians must understand and be prepared to defend why recommended treatments are safe and effective.

At a time when outcomes assessment and accountability are increasingly required of self-regulated professions, health professionals should feel especially obligated to demonstrate the validity of their evidence-based clinical decision making. To do so, a number of skills must be in place. First, clinicians must be able to frame relevant answerable clinical questions. Although veterinarians are taught to define clinical problems to develop differential diagnoses, we often do not ask well-formulated questions about clinical outcomes. The necessary skills following on the first are the ability to identify and then critically appraise external evidence that informs the clinical question. It is here that the work of EBDM is largely accomplished. The validity and importance of information sources, the fundamentals of clinical trial and experimental design, and the application of statistics to evidence appraisal must be understood. In veterinary medicine, limited availability of high-quality clinical data confounds this critical appraisal

*Corresponding author. Tufts Cummings School of Veterinary Medicine, 200 Westboro Road, North Grafton, MA 01536, USA. *E-mail address:* deborah.kochevar@tufts.edu (D.T. Kochevar).

0195-5616/06/$ – see front matter
doi:10.1016/j.cvsm.2006.06.001

vetsmall.theclinics.com

process. Additionally, the critical appraisal process alone is insufficient to arrive at the best clinical decision for a given patient. The final therapeutic approach should be selected by integrating the critical appraisal with clinical expertise and an understanding of the unique biology and circumstances of individual patients and clients. Finally, it is important to assess the decision-making process and the therapeutic outcomes continually for effectiveness and efficiency so as to improve future appraisals and outcomes.

These fundamentals of the EBDM process, as classically defined by Sackett and colleagues [1], are summarized and described in more detail in Box 1. When applied appropriately, implementation of these steps shifts clinical decision making away from reliance on anecdotal clinical experience and pathophysiologic rationales and toward rational examination of best evidence from clinical research. In response to criticism that the original definition of EBDM devalued legitimate clinical experience, recent definitions have emphasized the need to integrate clinical expertise with assessment of best evidence.

PROCESS

Translating a therapeutic problem into an answerable question for which evidence can be found is the first step. The simplest approach is to ask, "Is this an effective treatment for this disease?" To refine this question into an answerable form, four elements should be considered: patient or problem, intervention, comparison, and outcome (PICO) [2]. By considering each of the PICO elements, a well-formulated clinical question should emerge. The primary goal with regard to the patient and problem is to use evidence derived from a population matching that of your patient (eg, large-breed dogs with degenerativc joint disease). Intervention in terms of therapeutics equates to what you plan to do for the patient and how you plan to do it (eg, medical management of degenerative joint disease by administration of a nonsteroidal anti-inflammatory drug or a glucosamine nutraceutic agent or prescription of a specialized diet). Comparison may be part of your question if there is a standard therapy with which the intervention you are planning can be compared (eg, administration of a nonspecific cyclooxygenase [COX] inhibitor

Box 1: Five steps for evidence-based decision making

1. Convert the need for information into an answerable question.
2. Locate the best evidence with which to answer the question.
3. Critically appraise that evidence for validity, impact, and applicability.
4. Integrate the critical appraisal with clinical expertise and with the patient's (and client's) unique biology, values, and circumstances.
5. Evaluate effectiveness and efficiency in executing the first four steps, and seek ways to improve them and the clinical outcomes.

Adapted from Sackett DL, Straus SE, Richardson SW, et al, editors. Evidence-based medicine: how to practice and teach EBM. Edinburgh (UK): Churchill Livingstone; 2001.

versus a COX2 inhibitor for management of pain associated with degenerative joint disease). Finally, what outcome is desirable to the patient and owner? Are there special characteristics of the outcome that are important (eg, occurs within a specified time frame, with minimal side effects, or within a defined cost range)? Risk management terms that may be required to determine if the outcome is likely to be positive include absolute risk reduction, relative risk reduction, and an understanding of the number of animals that must be studied to determine positive and negative effects (eg, number needed to harm; see Appendix).

Sources of information and how best to search these have been reviewed previously [3–5] and are noted only briefly here. The classic illustration for the hierarchy of evidence used in evidence-based medicine (EBM) is shown in Fig. 1. Many sources of veterinary information fall in the lower layers of the pyramid under ideas and opinions (eg, personal experience, colleague opinion, nonveterinary expertise, professional program or continuing education notes, textbook information, Internet-derived information). The frequently cited levels of evidence (1–5) for therapy and/or prevention as developed by the Oxford Center for Evidence-Based Medicine are shown in Table 1. These levels of evidence are translated into grades of recommendation (A–D), with A being the most desirable based on consistent availability of level 1 evidence (systematic reviews [SRs] or randomized control clinical trials [RCTs]) and D being the least desirable based on level 5 evidence or inconsistent or inconclusive studies of any level.

Understanding why certain types of evidence are more valuable than others and mastering vocabulary are important first steps for practitioners of evidence-based veterinary medicine (EBVM). An abbreviated glossary of selected definitions is provided in the Appendix, and more extensive glossaries are available at EBM resource sites, such as the Center for Evidence-Based Medicine at the University of

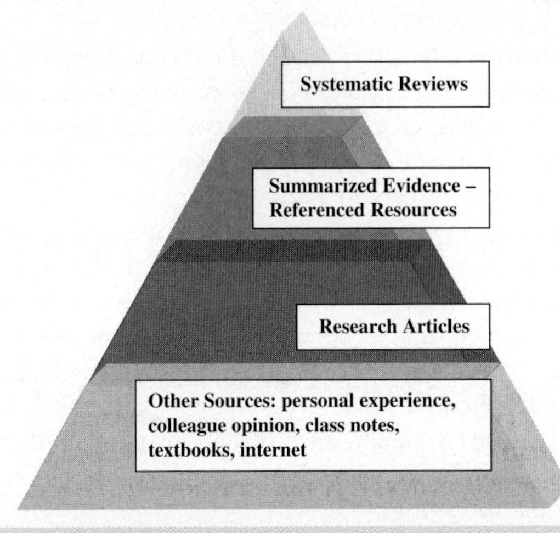

Fig. 1. Hierarchy of evidence used in evidence-based medicine. (*Modified from* Cockcroft P, Holmes M. Handbook of evidence-based veterinary medicine. Oxford (UK): Blackwell Publishing; 2003; with permission.)

Table 1
Oxford Centre for Evidence-Based Medicine levels of evidence (May 2001) and grades of recommendation based on evidence type

Level	Therapy/prevention
1a	Systematic reviews (SR) with homogeneity (limited variation in findings between individual studies) Randomized control clinical trials (RCTs)
1b	Individual RCTs with narrow confidence interval
1c	All or none; met when all patients died before the treatment became available but some now survive with the treatment or met when some patients died before the treatment became available and none now die as a result of treatment availability.
2a	SR with homogeneity of cohort studies
2b	Individual cohort study (including low-quality RCT [eg, <80% follow-up])
2c	"Outcomes" research; ecologic studies
3a	SR with homogeneity of case-control studies
3b	Individual case-control study
4	Case series and poor-quality cohort and case-control studies
5	Expert opinion without explicit critical appraisal or based on physiology, bench research, "first principles"
Grades of recommendation	**Evidence types**
A	Consistent level 1 studies
B	Consistent level 2 or 3 studies or extrapolations from level 1 studies
C	Level 4 studies or extrapolations from level 2 or 3 studies
D	Level 5 evidence or troublingly inconsistent or inconclusive studies of any level

Modified from Center for Evidence-Based Medicine, University of Toronto, Toronto, Ontario, Canada. Available at: http://www.cebm.net/levels_of_evidence.asp.

Toronto [6]. Some terms relate to mining of the literature (systematic review and meta-analysis), whereas others primarily address study design (eg, RCTs, cross-over design, cohort studies, cross-sectional survey, case-control studies, case reports). In either case, understanding the distinctions between these terms greatly improves the practitioner's ability to assess the evidence.

Assuming all preceding steps have gone well and that appropriate evidence has been identified and retrieved, careful appraisal of the evidence is then required. Understanding rudimentary statistics is essential for meaningful appraisal of articles on veterinary therapy. If a treatment effect is observed in a study, a number of questions should be considered before the validity of that finding is established. If these areas are not addressed, it is difficult to rule out bias and chance variation as explanations for the effect. As noted by Cockcroft and Holmes [2], key questions related to evaluation of therapeutic evidence include the following:

1. Was there a defined research question?
2. Were animals randomly assigned to treatment groups?
3. Were owners or clinicians blinded to the treatment assignments?

4. Were all patients accounted for when the study ended?
5. Was the study long enough to detect possible negative as well as positive outcomes?
6. If groups were being compared, were both populations treated equally throughout the study?

Ultimately, the risk of benefit or harm to the animal is what must be predicted as accurately as possible to increase the odds of therapeutic success and decrease the incidence of adverse reactions. Included in the glossary of terms are concepts that attempt to measure or describe the risk-to-benefit ratio.

RESOURCES FOR APPLYING EVIDENCE-BASED DECISION MAKING TO VETERINARY THERAPEUTICS

Medical

Many excellent resources are available that provide information about EBDM in the context of human medicine. These include centers and web sites, such as the Oxford Centre for Evidence-Based Medicine [7], the previously mentioned Center for Evidence-Based Medicine at the University of Toronto [6], and the American College of Physicians EBM Resource Center [8]. User guides like those published in the *Journal of the American Medical Association* [9–28] over a period of several years and a growing number of continuing education courses and books devoted to EBM are also available. The most important resources are those that allow EBDM to become an essential part of daily practice. These include well developed databases of critically appraised topics (CATs) created in response to specific clinical questions and presented in a user-friendly summary form. Tools for computer-assisted creation of CATs, such as CATmaker [29], and worksheets for construction of CATs related to therapeutics [30] are available without charge on the Internet. Summaries of the medical literature that use explicit methods for comprehensive literature searching and critical appraisal of individual studies are referred to as SRs. SRs use appropriate statistical techniques to combine studies that are deemed valid to arrive at defensible evidence-based conclusions. Through an effort known as the Cochrane Collaboration, a well-known library of medical SRs is maintained [31]. Specialty-specific SR databases also exist. Finally, secondary journals that publish summaries of best-quality evidence and current research findings on clinically useful topics have been established in an increasing number of specialty areas (eg, internal medicine, obstetrics and gynecology, public health, cardiovascular medicine). Several of these resources and terms associated with them have become part of the EBM vocabulary and are defined in the abbreviated glossary. Additionally, the National Library of Medicine (NLM) provides special search features termed *clinical queries* that improve identification of SRs and clinical trials for those engaged in the practice of EBM.

Veterinary

EBVM has a limited number of specific resources compared with evidence-based human medicine. No central database of veterinary CATs exists, SRs are only now beginning to appear in the veterinary literature, and no secondary EBVM journals are yet available. One of the best sources for biomedical data is freely available on the Internet, PubMed, as a service of the NLM [32]. Using the clinical queries feature of PubMed and searching using the clinical study category "therapy, human" in the "broad, sensitive search" mode, more than 1.6 million citations could be retrieved (as of May 2006). In the "narrow, specific search" mode, nearly 169,000 human therapy references were identified. By comparison, "therapy, dog" retrieved less than 1.4% of that number (broad, sensitive search) or 0.4% (narrow, specific search) as compared with human therapy. Using a second feature of PubMed's clinical queries designed to locate SRs, the numbers are no less discouraging. A search for SRs of "osteoarthritis therapy human" yielded 386 reviews, whereas the same search replacing human with dog yielded less than 1% of that number (3 reviews). More veterinary clinical studies, especially well-designed RCTs and SRs, are clearly needed. Additionally, a modified version of clinical queries should be designed that is capable of identifying a broader menu of clinical study types, in addition to RCTs, to facilitate veterinary search needs. Inherent in an expanded search capability for clinical trials is the need for veterinary clinicians to be able to evaluate diverse clinical study designs critically.

Not all the news is negative with regard to veterinary resources. Recent reviews [3–5] and a useful book by Cockcroft and Holmes [2] are good starting places to become familiar with EBVM terms and principles. There is a newly established (2006) Evidence-Based Veterinary Medicine Association (EBVMA) that maintains a web site [33] and has sponsored two symposia. This group plans to survey veterinary schools and colleges to determine the extent to which EBVM, epidemiology, and statistics are included in curricula and to assess availability of resources to support the practice and teaching of EBDM in veterinary programs. The EBVMA is also actively seeking resources from federal agencies and others to develop CATs and SRs. EBVMA-sponsored features entitled "What's the Evidence?" have been developed for the *Journal of the American Veterinary Medical Association*, and well-constructed veterinary SRs are beginning to appear in the literature [34,35].

The Veterinary Information Network (VIN) is a subscription veterinary resource that has the potential to advance evidence-based veterinary medical principles but may also promote non–evidence-based discussion based largely on anecdotal personal reports and expert opinion. VIN topic searches yield resources drawn from journal citations, conference proceedings, VIN message board postings and rounds discussions, and a variety of drug and clinical resources. Journal citations identified through VIN searches are useful, but the searches are not as comprehensive as what can be accomplished directly by using the NLM-based PubMed or similar comprehensive databases, such as CAB. Lower level evidence, such as veterinary conference proceedings, might be more readily obtained through a VIN search, because veterinary proceedings are often not available through other databases, such as PubMed. VIN message boards and rounds yield a mixture of expert opinion and anecdotal discussion, both of which are considered to be level 5, or the lowest level of evidence. Although these discussions provide appealing collegial exchange, they frequently lead to conclusions for which little, if any, evidence is presented. Such discussions may be useful to identify the range of approaches to a clinical problem, but further investigation using CATs and SRs of the literature is highly recommended.

As professionals in drug evaluation, veterinary clinical pharmacologists have long understood the need for critical evaluation of drug performance based on rigorous standards of evidence (eg, RCTs). The Veterinary Antimicrobial Decision Support (VADS) system is a web-based source of decision support developed by veterinary pharmacologists for the food animal practitioner who is designing antimicrobial regimens for cattle and swine (with sheep, goats, and poultry to be added in the future). It is an attempt to use all the available evidence to develop reasonable antimicrobial regimens that are likely to be effective. Although this effort has been focused on food animals, understanding the resource and how it is driven by evidence-based therapeutic principles is important for future development of evidence-based antimicrobial decision support systems for small animals.

The initial impetus for the development of the VADS system was the growing concern about antimicrobial resistance and the possible impact of antimicrobial use in animals on resistance in human bacterial pathogens. Multiple documents on prudent or judicious use of antimicrobials have been published and are not reiterated here, but one of the tenets of prudent use is to maximize efficacy by optimizing regimens using current pharmacologic information and principles. Often, however, the veterinary practitioner in the field is unlikely to have access to the latest pharmacologic information or may be unable to interpret that information. The goal of the VADS system is to provide the user with such an interpretation.

The VADS system provides the veterinary practitioner with the first three steps in the five-step EBVM sequence, with the specific therapeutic target being the construction of rational antimicrobial regimens. Steps 1 through 3 of a typical VADS inquiry are provided below. Steps 4 and 5 are the responsibility of the veterinarian in the field and are an integral part of the implementation of the evidence promulgated by the VADS system.

Step 1: answerable question(s)

There are actually multiple questions that are answered in the VADS system, but the most comprehensive and the most useful to the practitioner is: "What antimicrobial regimens can be expected to treat successfully (insert pathogen/disease/syndrome here)?" The multiple questions associated with that comprehensive question include the following. How should available antimicrobials be dosed to optimize the chance for successful treatment? What are the pharmacokinetics of available antimicrobials (ie, what is the concentration-time profile of each antimicrobial that might be selected for therapy)? A corollary question to the question about pharmacokinetics is: "Can we extrapolate reasonable doses of antimicrobials from the published data?" Is it reasonable to assume that if we double the dose of the antimicrobial, the serum concentrations are going to increase in a linear fashion? Are the mean pharmacokinetic data applicable to all the patients that are being treated, or is there a way to estimate what the pharmacokinetics look like in a population of animals?

Additionally, what are the pharmacodynamics of available antimicrobials (ie, what disposition profile maximizes efficacy)? What are the minimum inhibitory concentrations (MICs) of the pathogen(s) being treated? How long do we need to treat to reduce the population of bacteria to a level at which it can no longer replicate and can be eliminated from the patient?

Finally, which antimicrobials are legal for use in the animal(s) in question? If the antimicrobial must be used in an extralabel manner to be effective, is it legal? This question must ultimately be answered by the practitioner, who is responsible for making that determination. If an extralabel regimen is required, what withdrawal times are appropriate?

One question that the VADS system does not answer or provide help with answering is the diagnosis of bacterial disease. Once the user identifies a disease syndrome, however, he or she is presented with information about all the major potential organisms present. For example, for bovine respiratory disease, susceptibility data are presented for *Mannheimia haemolytica*, *Pasteurella multocida*, and *Histophilus somni*, and the practitioner is responsible for assessing the case in the context of the epidemiologically based profiles that are provided by the VADS system.

Step 2: tracking down the evidence

This step in the process of gathering evidence is often the most onerous for the practitioner, providing an opportunity for services like the VADS system to fulfill the need. Many literature databases are available, and knowing where to search is the first step in creating a good search strategy. An extensive search statement has been developed over time with the VADS system, which is used to search multiple databases, such as Current Contents, PubMed, and CAB abstracts. The evidence used in the construction of antimicrobial regimens falls into several major categories, and sources of evidence may thus differ slightly among those categories.

The first category, pharmacokinetic data, comes from literature reports of the study of antimicrobial drug disposition in the species of interest. Most reports are of single-dose studies, and, as discussed elsewhere in this article, require further manipulation to be useful in the system. Other sources of pharmacokinetic data are from investigators themselves (raw data associated with published reports) and from pharmaceutical companies.

Pharmacodynamics, the second data category, refers to the pharmacokinetic factors that are associated with clinical efficacy in the context of antimicrobial therapy. To develop criteria for pharmacodynamic parameters, the literature on retrospective and prospective studies in human beings and laboratory animals was reviewed. The first drugs modeled have been β-lactam antimicrobials, and the parameter that has been associated with efficacy is the percentage of the dosing interval for which the serum concentration of the antimicrobial remains above the MIC of the pathogen.

There are two important sources of the third major data category, susceptibility data. These sources are historical susceptibility data obtained from published reports or data obtained directly from diagnostic laboratories. Iowa State University and Kansas State University Diagnostic Laboratories have shared data, and the hope is that other laboratories may eventually agree to participate. The ultimate goal would be to have enough data that a practitioner could tailor the source of pathogen susceptibilities to a specific region if desired. Published data may become more useful for certain pathogens (eg, anaerobes that are commonly not subjected to susceptibility testing) but are not a large part of the VADS system at the moment. The best source of susceptibility data for the patient being treated is the isolate from that particular animal. The VADS system should help the practitioner to use patient-based susceptibility data to optimize therapy.

Step 3: critically appraising the evidence

This is the core of the VADS system's utility to the practitioner: all data are reviewed, and an interpretation is provided in the form of regimen recommendations. Interpretation of the data occurs in several steps:

a. Review the scientific literature on pharmacodynamics and establish a single criterion for each drug-pathogen combination (eg, time above MIC for 50% of the dosing interval for β-lactams).
b. Review the scientific literature on pharmacokinetics and select the reports that have usable data (many reports do not have sufficient detail in the methods or results to allow extrapolation to different dosages, frequencies, or duration of therapy).
c. Integrate the data from multiple sources for a single drug to derive an equation that relates bacterial susceptibility to dose. This is a multistep process that includes (1) superpositioning or other modeling of single-dose data to extrapolate multiple-dose serum concentrations, (2) computer simulations using information about the distribution in a population of serum concentrations to produce serum concentrations expected in 95% of the population of animals, and (3) linear regression of population concentration estimates from multiple sources to create one equation that relates MIC and dose.
d. Import susceptibility data from multiple diagnostic laboratories into the VADS database to allow for summarization of susceptibilities.
e. Future goals include critical appraisal of evidence of clinical success and using clinical trial data in the literature.

The information available up front to the practitioner is a table providing typically tested MIC concentrations with a dose recommendation for each and graphs summarizing all the available susceptibility data for the pathogens potentially involved in the disease in question.

Step 4: integrating the critical appraisals for application to patient circumstances and using clinical judgment

This step belongs to the practitioner and is not the purview of the VADS collaborators. The VADS system is a tool for decision support only, and all recommendations should then be filtered through the unique circumstances associated with the patient, client, and practitioner.

Step 5: evaluating Veterinary Antimicrobial Decision Support system success
Practitioner feedback to the VADS collaborators is sought. Because the system is implemented by veterinarians, its usefulness and validity are evaluated and the foregoing steps are reinterpreted and refined. All the steps taken and the reasoning behind the interpretation of all VADS data are available as hyperlinks from the dosage recommendation web pages. The VADS system seeks to be completely transparent so that every step in the process of appraisal and interpretation may be externally evaluated.

The VADS system provides an excellent example of the application of EBDM in veterinary pharmacology. Although the current system has been developed to promote safe and rational use of antimicrobials in food animals, creation of similar databases for companion animal therapeutics is appealing. Veterinary use of antimicrobial drugs also used in human medicine continues to be scrutinized in the context of antimicrobial resistance. Efforts like the VADS system support the contention that veterinarians can and do use antimicrobials judiciously. The VADS system was initially funded via small grants from multiple species specialty veterinary and producer organizations; the bulk of the funding came from a grant from the US Food and Drug Administration (FDA)-Center for Veterinary Medicine (CVM).

EVIDENCE-BASED VETERINARY MEDICINE EDUCATION

Preparing veterinarians to practice EBVM as described in the five-step process is not as straightforward as it might seem. Veterinary professional education has historically relied much more on establishing solid foundations in physiology and pathophysiology and providing venues for experiential learning than it has on rigorous analytic training. Problem solving and "learning how to learn" are critical skills that all veterinary medical students should (but sometimes do not) acquire before entering the profession. Veterinary medical curricula and veterinary pharmacology courses, in particular, often require processing of large amounts of data that tend to overshadow the more dynamic processes of thinking and problem solving. In our zeal to fill our students with important information, we often overlook the need to guide them in how to find, critically evaluate, and apply drug information. Veterinary pharmacologists must train their students to identify and prioritize clinical problems; be thorough in data collection from the patient, the client, and the literature; and be prepared to use evidence-based analysis to select and, ultimately, to defend a therapeutic regimen.

Assessing the quality of information is often difficult for experienced clinicians and is much harder for students in training. Veterinary pharmacology is frequently taught in the second or third preclinical year of the curriculum before students have had extensive clinical care responsibilities. Hence, it is important for veterinary pharmacology instructors to guide students in how to critically evaluate data sources as these relate to therapy.

Rx Educational Prescription

Patient's Name

Learner:

3-part Clinical Question

Target Disorder:

Intervention (+/- comparison):

Outcome:

Date and place to be filled:

Presentation will cover:

1. search strategy;
2. search results;
3. the validity of this evidence;
4. the importance of this valid evidence;
5. can this valid, important evidence be applied to your patient;
6. your evaluation of this process.

Fig. 2. Evidence-based learning prescription. (*From* Center for Evidence-Based Medicine, University of Toronto, Toronto, Ontario, Canada. Available at: http://www.cebm.utoronto.ca/practise/formulate/eduprescript.htm; with permission.)

The use of EBVM exercises that require students to assemble and evaluate information on their own first (eg, creation of their own CATs) before discussion as a class has potential for enhancing the learning process. Obstacles to the success of this approach include preconceived negative student biases, limitations on student time imposed by dense professional program curricula, and risk aversion on the part of veterinary instructors. Despite these potential obstacles, the use of EBVM can be an effective learning tool and offers engaging and highly relevant opportunities for critical thinking in the context of veterinary pharmacology and therapeutics.

Use of EBVM "prescriptions" for learning (Fig. 2) is one tangible way to encourage students and clinical trainees to define answerable questions carefully and then to use a deliberate process to identify valid evidence for critical appraisal. Educational prescriptions serve as tangible reminders of questions to be answered and allow the clinical instructor to task trainees with evidence-based investigations. "Filling" the prescription might occur individually or through a collaborative effort with other trainees or a medical librarian. Products that result from the filled prescription may be shared in a journal club, in rounds, in pharmacology teaching laboratories, or as web-based documents in the form of CATs.

Innovative approaches to incorporation of EBVM into curricula may be found in a variety of veterinary programs. The Accelerated Clinical Excellence (ACE) program at Tufts University [36] introduces the principles of EBVM and then provides opportunities for students to apply these principles to model cases. Formulation of answerable clinical questions, journal article review and evaluation, evaluation of the validity and origin of sources of information, statistical analysis, and application of information to clinical decision making are part of the program. Individual instructors at many schools use EBVM more informally in clinical rounds and as part of case discussions across the curriculum.

With a growing number of evidence-based resources being developed for use in veterinary medicine, the time is right for academicians, practitioners, and students to embrace the positive elements of EBVM. Clinical pharmacologists, more than most, have all the skills required to use an evidence-based approach effectively for the benefit of patients and the advancement of the profession.

Acknowledgments

Collaborators on the VADS system include Virginia Fajt (Texas A&M University), Michael Apley (Kansas State University College of Veterinary Medicine), Cory Langston (Mississippi State University College of Veterinary Medicine), and Jeff Wilcke (Virginia-Maryland Regional College of Veterinary Medicine).

APPENDIX: GLOSSARY OF EVIDENCE-BASED VETERINARY MEDICINE TERMS

A

Absolute benefit increase (ABI): the absolute arithmetic difference in rates of good outcomes between experimental and control patients in a trial, calculated as |EER − CER|, and accompanied by a 95% confidence interval (CI).

Absolute risk increase (ARI): the absolute arithmetic difference in rates of bad outcomes between experimental and control patients in a trial, calculated as |EER – CER|, and accompanied by a 95% CI; ARI is also used in assessing the impact of "risk factors" for disease.

Absolute risk reduction (ARR): the absolute arithmetic difference in rates of bad outcomes between experimental and control participants in a trial, calculated as |EER – CER|, and accompanied by a 95% CI; this is sometimes called the risk difference.

C

Case-control study: a study that involves identifying patients that have the outcome of interest (cases) and patients without the same outcome (controls) and looking back to see if they had the exposure of interest.

Case series: a report on a series of patients with an outcome of interest; no control group is involved.

Critically appraised topic (CAT): a document that you create yourself in response to a clinical question; it summarizes an individual item of evidence and presents the results in an easily digestible format.

Clinical practice guideline: a systematically developed statement designed to assist clinician and patient decisions about appropriate health care for specific clinical circumstances.

Cohort study: involves identification of two groups (cohorts) of patients, one that received the exposure of interest and one that did not, and following these cohorts forward for the outcome of interest.

Confidence interval (CI): quantifies the uncertainty in measurement; it is usually reported as a 95% CI, which is the range of values within which we can be 95% sure that the true value for the whole population lies. For example, for a number needed to treat (NNT) of 10 with a 95% CI of 5 to 15, we would have 95% confidence that the true NNT value lies between 5 and 15.

Control event rate (CER): the proportion of patients in the control group who are observed to experience the outcome of interest (see event rate).

Crossover study design: the administration of two or more experimental therapies one after the other in a specified or random order to the same group of patients.

Cross-sectional study: the observation of a defined population at a single point in time or time interval; exposure and outcome are determined simultaneously.

E

Event rate: the proportion of patients in a group in which the event is observed; thus, if of 100 patients, the event is observed in 27, the event rate is 0.27. The control event rate (CER) and experimental event rate (EER) are used to refer to this in control and experimental groups of patients, respectively. The patient expected event rate (PEER) refers to the rate of events we would expect in a patient that received no treatment or conventional treatment (see treatment effects).

Evidence-based medicine (EBM): the conscientious, explicit, and judicious use of current best evidence in making decisions about the care of individual patients; the practice of EBM requires the integration of individual clinical expertise with the best available external clinical evidence from systematic research and our patient's unique values and circumstances.

Experimental event rate (EER): the proportion of patients in the experimental treatment group who are observed to experience the outcome of interest (see event rate).

L

Likelihood ratio: the likelihood that a given test result would be expected in a patient with the target disorder compared with the likelihood that this same result would be expected in a patient without the target disorder.

M

Meta-analysis: a systematic review that uses quantitative methods to synthesize and summarize the results.

N

Number needed to harm (NNH): the number of patients who, if they received the experimental treatment, would result in one additional patient being harmed compared with patients who received the control treatment, calculated as 1/ARR and accompanied by a 95% CI.

Number needed to treat (NNT): the number of patients who need to be treated to prevent one bad outcome; calculated as the inverse of the ARR (1/ARR) and accompanied by a 95% CI.

O

Odds: a ratio of the number of animals incurring an event to the number of animals that do not have an event.

Odds ratio (OR): the ratio of the odds of having the target disorder in the experimental group relative to the odds in favor of having the target disorder in the control group (in cohort studies or systematic reviews) or the odds in favor of being exposed in subjects with the target disorder divided by the odds in favor of being exposed in control subjects (without the target disorder).

P

Patient expected event rate (PEER): refers to the rate of events we would expect in a patient who received no treatment or conventional treatment (see event rate).

R

Randomization (or random allocation): method analogous to tossing a coin to assign patients to treatment groups (the experimental treatment is assigned if the coin lands "heads," and a conventional, "control," or "placebo" treatment is given if the coin lands "tails").

Relative benefit increase (RBI): the proportional increase in rates of good outcomes between experimental and control patients in a trial, calculated as $|EER - CER|/CER$, and accompanied by a 95% CI.

Randomized control clinical trial (RCT): participants are randomly allocated into an experimental group or a control group and followed over time for the variables and/or outcomes of interest.

Relative risk increase (RRI): the proportional increase in rates of bad outcomes between experimental and control patients in a trial, calculated as |EER − CER|/CER, and accompanied by a 95% CI; RRI is also used in assessing the impact of "risk factors" for disease.

Relative risk reduction (RRR): the proportional reduction in rates of bad outcomes between experimental and control participants in a trial, calculated as |EER − CER|/CER, and accompanied by a 95% CI.

Risk ratio: the ratio of risk in the treated group (EER) to the risk in the control group (CER); this is used in randomized trials and cohort studies and is calculated as EER/CER (also called relative risk).

S

Systematic review: a summary of the medical literature that uses explicit methods to perform a comprehensive literature search and critical appraisal of individual studies and that uses appropriate statistical techniques to combine these valid studies.

Modified from Center for Evidence-Based Medicine, University of Toronto, Toronto, Ontario, Canada. Available at: http://www.cebm.utoronto.ca/glossary/; with permission.

References

[1] Sackett DL, Straus SE, Richardson SW, et al. Evidence-based medicine: how to practice and teach EBM. Edinburgh (UK): Churchill Livingstone; 2000.

[2] Cockcroft P, Holmes M. Handbook of evidence-based veterinary medicine. Oxford (UK): Blackwell Publishing; 2003.

[3] Holmes M, Cockcroft P. Evidence-based veterinary medicine. 1. Why is it important and what skills are needed? In Pract 2004;26(1):28–33.

[4] Cockcroft P, Holmes M. Evidence-based veterinary medicine. 2. Identifying information needs and finding the evidence. In Pract 2004;26(2):96–102.

[5] Holmes M, Cockcroft P. Evidence-based veterinary medicine. 3. Appraising the evidence. In Pract 2004;26(3):154–64.

[6] Center for Evidence-Based Medicine, University of Toronto, Toronto, Ontario, Canada. Available at: http://www.cebm.utoronto.ca, http://www.cebm.utoronto.ca/practise/formulate/eduprescript.htm, or http://www.cebm.utoronto.ca/glossary/. Accessed June 24, 2006.

[7] Oxford Centre for Evidence-Based Medicine. Available at: http://www.cebm.net/. Accessed June 24, 2006.

[8] American College of Physicians EBM Resource Center. Available at: http://www.ebmny.org/. Accessed June 24, 2006.

[9] Evidence-Based Medicine Working Group. Evidence-based medicine. A new approach to teaching the practice of medicine. JAMA 1992;268:2420–5.

[10] Oxman AD, Sackett DL, Guyatt GH. Users' guides to the medical literature. I. How to get started. Evidence-Based Medicine Working Group. JAMA 1993;270:2093–5.

[11] Guyatt GH, Sackett DL, Cook DJ. Users' guides to the medical literature. II. How to use an article about therapy or prevention. A. Are the results of the study valid? Evidence-Based Medicine Working Group. JAMA 1993;270:2598–601.

[12] Guyatt GH, Sackett DL, Cook DJ. Users' guides to the medical literature. II. How to use an article about therapy or prevention. B. What were the results and will they help me in caring for my patients? Evidence-Based Medicine Working Group. JAMA 1994;271:59–63.

[13] Jaeschke R, Guyatt G, Sackett DL. Users' guides to the medical literature. III. How to use an article about a diagnostic test. A. Are the results of the study valid? Evidence-Based Medicine Working Group. JAMA 1994;271:389–91.
[14] Jaeschke R, Guyatt GH, Sackett DL. Users' guides to the medical literature. III. How to use an article about a diagnostic test. B. What are the results and will they help me in caring for my patients? Evidence-Based Medicine Working Group. JAMA 1994;271:703–7.
[15] Levine M, Walter S, Lee H, et al. Users' guides to the medical literature. IV. How to use an article about harm. Evidence-Based Medicine Working Group. JAMA 1994;271:1615–9.
[16] Laupacis A, Wells G, Richardson WS, et al. Users' guides to the medical literature. V. How to use an article about prognosis. Evidence-Based Medicine Working Group. JAMA 1994;272:234–7.
[17] Oxman AD, Cook DJ, Guyatt GH. Users' guides to the medical literature. VI. How to use an overview. Evidence-Based Medicine Working Group. JAMA 1994;272:1367–71.
[18] Richardson WS, Detsky AS. Users' guides to the medical literature. VII. How to use a clinical decision analysis. A. Are the results of the study valid? Evidence-Based Medicine Working Group. JAMA 1995;273:1292–5.
[19] Richardson WS, Detsky AS. Users' guides to the medical literature. VII. How to use a clinical decision analysis. B. What are the results and will they help me in caring for my patients? Evidence Based Medicine Working Group. JAMA 1995;273:1610–3.
[20] Hayward RS, Wilson MC, Tunis SR, et al. Users' guides to the medical literature. VIII. How to use clinical practice guidelines. A. Are the recommendations valid? Evidence-Based Medicine Working Group. JAMA 1995;274:570–4.
[21] Wilson MC, Hayward RS, Tunis SR, et al. Users' guides to the medical literature. VIII. How to use clinical practice guidelines. B. What are the recommendations and will they help you in caring for your patients? Evidence-Based Medicine Working Group. JAMA 1995;274:1630–2.
[22] Guyatt GH, Sackett DL, Sinclair JC, et al. Users' guides to the medical literature. IX. A method for grading health care recommendations. Evidence-Based Medicine Working Group. JAMA 1995;274:1800–4.
[23] Naylor CD, Guyatt GH. Users' guides to the medical literature. X. How to use an article reporting variations in the outcomes of health services. Evidence-Based Medicine Working Group. JAMA 1996;275:554–8.
[24] Naylor CD, Guyatt GH. Users' guides to the medical literature. XI. How to use an article about a clinical utilization review. Evidence-Based Medicine Working Group. JAMA 1996;275:1435–9.
[25] Guyatt GH, Naylor CD, Juniper E, et al. Users' guides to the medical literature. XII. How to use articles about health-related quality of life. Evidence-Based Medicine Working Group. JAMA 1997;277:1232–7.
[26] Drummond MF, Richardson WS, O'Brien BJ, et al. Users' guides to the medical literature. XIII. How to use an article on economic analysis of clinical practice. A. Are the results of the study valid? Evidence-Based Medicine Working Group. JAMA 1997;277:1552–7.
[27] O'Brien BJ, Heyland D, Richardson WS, et al. Users' guides to the medical literature. XIII. How to use an article on economic analysis of clinical practice. B. What are the results and will they help me in caring for my patients? Evidence-Based Medicine Working Group. JAMA 1997;277:1802–6.
[28] Guyatt GH. Richardson WS for the Evidence-Based Medicine Working Group. Users' guides to the medical literature: XXV. Evidence-based medicine: principles for applying the users' guides to patient care. JAMA 2000;284:1290–6.
[29] Badenoch D, Sackett D, Straus S, et al. CATmaker. Available at: www.cebm.net/downloads.asp. Accessed July 23, 2006.
[30] Critically appraised topics related to therapeutics. Available at: http://www.cebm.utoronto.ca/teach/materials/therapy.htm. Accessed June 24, 2006.

[31] Cochrane Collaboration. Available at: http://www.cochrane.org/. Accessed June 24, 2006.
[32] National Library of Medicine. PubMed. Available at: http://www.nlm.nih.gov/. Accessed June 24, 2006.
[33] Evidence-Based Veterinary Medicine Association (EBVMA). Available at: www.ebvma.org/. Accessed June 24, 2006.
[34] Aragon CL, Budsberg SC, Applicati GH, et al. Applications of evidence-based medicine: cranial cruciate ligament repair in the dog. Vet Surg 2005;34:93–8.
[35] Olivry T, Mueller RS, the International Task Force on Canine Atopic Dermatitis. Evidence-based veterinary dermatology: a systematic review of the pharmacotherapy of canine atopic dermatitis. Vet Dermatol 2003;14:121–46.
[36] Accelerated clinical excellence (ACE) at Tufts University. Available at: http://www.tufts.edu/vet/ace/. Accessed June 24, 2006.

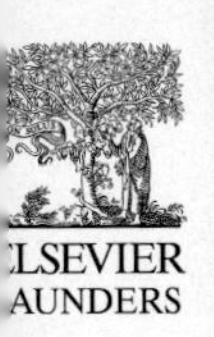

Vet Clin Small Anim 36 (2006) 961–973

VETERINARY CLINICS
SMALL ANIMAL PRACTICE

Pharmacogenetics

Katrina L. Mealey, DVM, PhD

Department of Veterinary Clinical Sciences, College of Veterinary Medicine, Washington State University, Pullman, WA 99164-6610, USA

Although the goal of drug therapy is to produce a specific pharmacologic effect without producing adverse effects, it is often difficult to predict how effective or how safe a medication may be for a particular patient. If the same drug were administered to 10 patients with a particular disease, each might respond differently with respect to drug efficacy and the likelihood of an adverse reaction. A number of factors may influence a patient's response to drug therapy, including the patient's age, health or disease status, concurrent medications, species, and others. Consideration of all these factors is often not sufficient to explain the degree of interpatient variation observed, however. The observed interpatient variability in drug response may result primarily from genetically determined differences in drug metabolism, drug distribution, and drug target proteins. Pharmacogenetics, the study of genetic determinants of response to drug therapy, is likely the ultimate way to establish the right drug and dose for each patient, thereby optimizing efficacy and minimizing toxicity. Despite the fact that this branch of pharmacology is still in its infancy as a science, a number of important discoveries have already contributed to improved pharmacotherapy in human and veterinary patients.

HISTORY OF PHARMACOGENETICS

The concept that inheritance might explain individual variation in drug efficacy and susceptibility to adverse drug interactions was proposed in 1957. The term *pharmacogenetics* was first introduced shortly afterward, in 1959. Interestingly, relatively little pharmacogenetic research occurred for the next 3 decades. A resurgence in pharmacogenetic research occurred coincidentally with the advent of the Human Genome Project in 1990. Research in pharmacogenetics has expanded at a remarkable rate since then. There are at least two journals exclusively devoted to pharmacogenetic/pharmacogenomic research and many other medical and pharmacologic journals encouraging submissions reporting results of pharmacogenetic research. After completion of the Human Genome

This work was supported by a grant from the Collie Health Foundation.

E-mail address: kmealey@vetmed.wsu.edu

0195-5616/06/$ – see front matter
doi:10.1016/j.cvsm.2006.05.006

Project (announced in 2003), the National Human Genome Research Institute challenged investigators to develop genome-based approaches to predict drug response. This certainly sets the stage for continued growth in the field of pharmacogenetics.

BASIC GENETIC CONCEPTS

The human genome contains approximately 3 billion nucleotide bases, which represent roughly 30,000 genes. When a gene is expressed, DNA is transcribed into RNA, which is then translated to make proteins. Three consecutive nucleotide bases form a specific codon, specifying a particular amino acid or amino acid chain termination (stop codons). The genetic code is said to have redundancy, which simply means that there may be two or more different codons for the same amino acid. In human beings, for example, GGA and GGC code for the amino acid glycine. A gene is simply the DNA sequence that represents a series of codons that specify a particular protein. The variation that occurs between individuals in a population is a result of mutations in specific genes.

A mutation alters the base sequence of DNA, which, in turn, alters the transcribed RNA and creates a different codon. Some mutations are silent, in that if the mutation results in a base change that leads to a codon for the same amino acid (ie, GGA to GGC) as in the original DNA sequence, there is no change in protein structure or function. If the mutation results in a different amino acid or the creation of a stop codon, however, the change in protein structure and function can be deleterious. At each gene locus, an individual carries two alleles, one from each parent. An allele is defined as the DNA sequence at a given gene's location on the chromosome. If an individual has two identical alleles, that individual is said to have a homozygous genotype. If an individual has two different alleles, that individual is said to have a heterozygous phenotype. The phenotype of each individual with regard to a specific gene is the outward physical manifestation of a given genotype. That outward physical manifestation might be something immediately obvious in a given individual, such as eye color, or it may not be apparent until a particular drug is given.

Genetic variations in a given gene may be present rarely in a population or in relatively large numbers in a population. Polymorphisms are defined as genetic variations occurring at a frequency of 1% or greater in the population (species of interest). In human beings, many of the genes encoding cytochrome P450 enzymes are polymorphic (specific mutations are present in greater than 1% of the population), whereas some inherited human diseases, such as cystic fibrosis, are caused by rare mutations occurring in less than 1% of the population. Identification of the specific mutation may be used to provide specific treatment regimens and, in the case of veterinary patients, to guide breeding decisions as well. Many common human diseases, such as diabetes mellitus or hypertension, are polygenic, however; more than one gene contributes to the disease. For diseases that are polygenic in nature, the pathophysiology of the disease is complex and specific treatments based on particular mutations are much more difficult to sort out. It is likely that many important diseases in veterinary medicine (ie, hip dysplasia, epilepsy, most types of cancer) are polygenic also; therefore, genes linked to disease susceptibility are not discussed in this article. Rather, this article focuses on genetic variations linked to responses to pharmacologic agents.

PHARMACOGENETICS

Genetic variation can affect the pharmacokinetics (ie, drug absorption, distribution, metabolism, excretion) and pharmacodynamics (ie, interaction with drug transporters and receptors) of pharmaceutic agents. Currently, the greatest body of knowledge with regard to pharmacogenetics involves genetic variation in drug metabolism. Indeed, the concept of pharmacogenetics originated in the 1950s as a result of the observation that the antimalarial drug primaquine caused hemolysis in a subpopulation of individuals [1]. These individuals were found to have decreased functional levels of the enzyme glucose 6-phosphate dehydrogenase compared with most of the population [1]. At the time, molecular biologic techniques had not yet been discovered; thus, the field of pharmacogenetics was initially based purely on phenotypic observations (measurement of enzyme function). Discovery of the specific gene mutation would occur a few decades later.

With the rapid advancement of molecular techniques, modern pharmacogenetic research is quite different from those initial phenotypic observations. It currently involves identifying the phenotype and the genetic variation responsible for it. Researchers perform systematic searches to identify functionally significant variations in DNA sequences in genes that affect drug disposition. In many instances, the genetic variation in a gene is identified before the phenotypic consequence is known. Sequencing of the human genome, and now the canine genome, should speed the progress of pharmacogenetic discoveries, facilitating the ultimate goal of pharmacogenetics, which is individualization of drug therapy.

It is important to note that individualization of drug therapy encompasses two distinct yet equally important clinical implications. First is the ability to predict those patients at high risk for developing drug toxicity. These patients may have a mutation in a drug-metabolizing enzyme that results in low clearance rates for the drug. For such patients, a lower drug dose or alternate drug should be administered. Second is the ability to predict those patients that are most likely to benefit from a particular drug because of appropriate receptor interactions. Patients with mutations in drug receptors may be poor responders to certain pharmaceutic agents. Rather than using a trial and error approach to drug therapy, a veterinarian could select the drug most likely to produce the desired pharmacologic response in a particular patient, decreasing the amount of time in which the patient's disease state is poorly controlled.

Several recent discoveries in veterinary pharmacogenetics are described in this article, and examples of pharmacogenetically based differences in drug absorption, distribution, metabolism, excretion, and drug-receptor interactions are provided. The role of these discoveries in clinical veterinary medicine is also presented. To date, most of the clinically relevant pharmacogenetic discoveries involve dogs. When applicable, information about other species is also included.

PHARMACOGENETICS OF ORAL DRUG ABSORPTION

Until recently, systemic bioavailability of orally administered drugs has been considered to be a function of physicochemical characteristics of the drug and subsequent hepatic metabolism. A number of other factors have recently been shown to have an impact on the ability of a drug to be absorbed into the systemic circulation after oral administration. Intestinal phase I drug metabolism and active drug extrusion by efflux transporters are now considered to be among the most important determinants of oral drug bioavailability. Consequently, genetic variation in intestinal drug-metabolizing enzymes and drug transporters should dramatically affect oral drug absorption.

In people, CYP3A is expressed at higher levels in mature villus tip enterocytes than in hepatocytes [2]. Because intestinal villi comprise such a large surface area, there is a high likelihood of absorbed drug interacting with intestinal CYP3A enzyme, facilitating substantial first-pass metabolism. Interpatient variability in intestinal CYP3A levels has been studied in a small sample of human patients. Eleven-fold variations in CYP3A protein content and sixfold variations in enzymatic activity were identified, suggesting that CYP3A polymorphisms exist in the human population [3]. Although intestinal drug metabolism is also thought to be important in veterinary patients, relatively little is known with regard to interpatient variability in enzyme activity.

Drug transporters are also known to play an important role in drug absorption. Many drug transporters have been identified in people, but the most well-characterized drug transporter is P-glycoprotein (P-gp), the product of the MDR1 (also known as the *ABCB1*) gene. The potential impact of transporter pharmacogenetics on drug pharmacokinetics is dramatically illustrated by P-gp. P-gp is a transmembrane protein that was first described in highly resistant tumor cell lines [4]. Tumor cells expressing P-gp were cross-resistant to various anticancer agents (anthracyclines, vinca alkaloids, taxanes, and others). P-gp has since been shown to act as an ATP-dependent pump that exports drugs from nonneoplastic cells as well. In normal mammalian tissues, P-gp seems to function in a protective capacity. P-gp is expressed on bile canaliculi, renal tubular epithelial cells, the placenta, brain capillary endothelial cells, and at the luminal border of intestinal epithelial cells [5]. At these locations, P-gp pumps selected drugs out of the body (into the bile, urine, or intestinal lumen) or away from protected sites (eg, brain tissue, fetus).

The significant role that intestinal P-gp can play in determining oral drug bioavailability has been demonstrated in rodent studies. In mdr1(−/−) knockout mice, oral bioavailability of many P-gp substrate drugs (vinblastine, paclitaxel, digoxin, loperamide, ivermectin, cyclosporine A, and others) is substantially greater than in wild-type mice [6,7]. Similarly, MDR1 polymorphisms in people have been shown to result in altered oral bioavailability of P-gp substrate drugs.

Studies have shown that oral bioavailability of digoxin, a P-gp substrate, is greater in subjects with the MDR1 3435TT genotype compared with those with the MDR1 3435CC genotype [8]. Similarly, the P-gp substrate phenytoin has been shown to have lower oral bioavailability in subjects with the MDR1 3435CC genotype [9].

P-gp has been fairly well characterized in dogs. The tissue distribution of P-gp in dogs is similar to that in people [10], and it has been shown to contribute to chemotherapeutic drug resistance in vitro and in vivo [11–13]. Although its role in determining oral drug bioavailability is not well characterized, there is some evidence that P-gp is important. Bioavailability of the anticancer agent (and P-gp substrate) docetaxel was increased 17-fold when coadministered with a P-gp inhibitor. A polymorphism of the MDR1 gene has also been described in dogs, but results of studies investigating the effect of this polymorphism on oral drug bioavailability are not yet available.

The MDR1 polymorphism in dogs consists of a four base-pair deletion mutation. This deletion results in a shift of the reading frame that generates several premature stop codons [14]. Because protein synthesis is terminated before even 10% of the protein product is synthesized, dogs with two mutant alleles exhibit a P-gp null phenotype, similar to mdr1 (–/–) knockout mice. Affected dogs include many herding breeds. For example, roughly 75% of Collies in the United States, France, and Australia have at least one mutant allele [15]. Other affected herding breeds, albeit at a lower frequency, include Old English Sheepdogs, Australian Shepherds, Shelties, English Shepherds, Border Collies, German Shepherds, Silken Windhounds, McNabs, and Long-Haired Whippets [16]. Studies investigating the effect of the MDR1 deletion mutation on oral drug bioavailability in herding breeds are ongoing in the author's laboratory.

PHARMACOGENETICS OF DRUG DISTRIBUTION

Drug distribution, the delivery of drugs from the systemic circulation to tissues, can be dramatically affected by pharmacogenetics. The drug transporter P-gp serves as an important barrier to the distribution of substrate drugs to selected tissues. For example, P-gp is a component of the blood-brain barrier, the blood-testes barrier, and the placenta. Therefore, distribution of P-gp substrate drugs to these tissues is greatly enhanced in dogs with the MDR1 deletion mutation. Dogs homozygous for the deletion (MDR1 [mutant/mutant]) experience adverse neurologic effects after a single dose of ivermectin (120 μg/kg). Heterozygous (MDR1 [wild-type/mutant]) or homozygous wild-type dogs are not sensitive to ivermectin neurotoxicity at the 120-μg/kg dose, but heterozygote animals may experience neurotoxicity at ivermectin doses greater than 300 μg/kg, particularly if daily doses are administered (ie, protocols for treatment of demodectic mange). Dogs homozygous for the normal MDR1 allele (normal/normal) can receive 2000 μg/kg in a single dose without signs of toxicity and can receive 600 μg/kg/d for months without signs of toxicity. Affected Collies also seem to have increased susceptibility to neurologic adverse effects of other avermectins, including milbemycin, selamectin, and moxidectin [17].

Interestingly, a retrospective study conducted by a national veterinary poison center reported that Collies were overrepresented in canine cases of loperamide-induced neurotoxicity [18]. Many Collies displayed signs of neurologic toxicity after administration of routinely recommended doses of the antidiarrheal agent loperamide. Loperamide is an opioid that is generally devoid of central nervous system (CNS) activity because it is excluded from the brain by P-gp [19,20]. Loperamide neurotoxicity was recently reported in a Collie that had received a routine dose (0.14 mg/kg administered orally) [21]. The dog in this report had the MDR1 (mutant/mutant) genotype. Homozygous wild-type (normal/normal) dogs do not exhibit neurologic signs after receiving even higher doses of loperamide, indicating that P-gp plays a key role in modulating distribution of substrates like loperamide to canine brain tissue. Less information is available regarding P-gp and the blood-brain barrier in cats. The author has received anecdotal reports of ivermectin toxicity in cats after standard doses, but whether or not the underlying cause is a result of altered P-gp expression or function is not currently known.

Distribution of some drugs to the testes and fetus may also be limited by P-gp. In human patients, this creates a problem for treating certain diseases. For example, the testes and brain are considered to be sanctuary sites for HIV [22]. Because HIV-1 protease inhibitors are substrates for P-gp, the virus can remain viable in these sanctuary sites, hampering effective therapy. Similarly, therapeutic concentrations of certain chemotherapeutic agents may not be achievable for testicular cancers because of active efflux by P-gp [23]. The effect of placental P-gp on distribution of drugs to the fetus is an area of active research in human medicine [24]. Understanding the role of pregnancy-related hormones in regulating P-gp expression and function is one possible key in developing strategies to deliver drugs to the mother with minimal fetal risk.

PHARMACOGENETICS OF DRUG METABOLISM

Pharmacogenetic variation can affect phase I and phase II metabolic enzyme activity. A mutation in the pseudocholinesterase enzyme serves as an example of how pharmacogenetic variation can result in dramatic differences in drug response between patients. Patients with a normal pseudocholinesterase genotype metabolize succinylcholine and recover from neuromuscular blockade rapidly, whereas those with the mutant genotype undergo sustained neuromuscular blockade that can result in prolonged apnea and the necessity for mechanical ventilation. [25] A number of polymorphisms have been described in human cytochrome P450 enzymes, with many of these resulting in profound variations in clinical response. For example, CYP2D6 is a highly variable P450 pathway in people, with individuals ranging from undetectable activity (found in 6%–10% of whites) to "ultrarapid" activity (found in 3%–10% of Europeans and 30% of one black population) [26]. The ultrarapid phenotype is attributable to a highly unusual gene duplication. Drugs that are substrates for CY2D6 in people include β-receptor antagonists (eg, propranolol, timolol, metoprolol), antiarrhythmics (eg, quinidine, flecainide), antidepressants (eg, amitriptyline, clomipramine, fluoxetine, imipramine), neuroleptics, and certain opioid derivatives. Depending on the patient's CYP2D6 genotype, the "typical" dose of a substrate drug may need to be decreased (poor metabolizers require one tenth of the standard dose of nortriptyline to avoid toxicity) or increased (ultrarapid metabolizers require five times the standard dose to achieve therapeutic concentrations).

Relatively few polymorphisms in drug-metabolizing enzymes have been described in veterinary patients, although this is likely to change because research in this area is currently in progress. Nevertheless, variation in the metabolism of some drugs has been documented in dogs. CYP2B11 has been shown to have at least a 14-fold variation in activity in mixed-breed dogs [27]. Greyhounds have been shown to have particularly low CYP2B11 activity, which results in sustained plasma concentrations of propofol and delayed recovery compared with mixed-breed dogs [28]. The specific genetic alteration responsible for reduced CYP2B11 in Greyhounds as compared with other canine breeds has not been determined. There is some evidence to suggest that CYP2D15 may also be polymorphic in dogs. The nonsteroidal anti-inflammatory drug (NSAID) celecoxib is metabolized to a large degree by CYP2D15. Clearance of celecoxib in Beagles is polymorphic, with approximately half of the population being extensive metabolizers and the remainder being poor metabolizers [29]. Celecoxib has a 1.5- to 2-hour half-life in extensive metabolizers and a 5-hour half-life in poor metabolizers. One pharmacogenetic variant that has been identified in the canine CYP2D15 gene, a deletion of exon 3, results in undetectable celecoxib metabolism. The frequency and breed distribution of this polymorphism have not yet been determined. It is likely to have clinical significance for other drugs that are CYP2D15 substrates, however, including dextromethorphan, imipramine, and others.

A number of other mutations in drug-metabolizing enzymes have been described in animals, but the clinical relevance of these mutations, if any, has yet to be determined. For example, 10% of Beagles in one study were deficient in CYP1A2 because of a mutation that resulted in premature termination of protein synthesis [30]. CYP1A2 does not seem to be responsible for metabolizing clinically used drugs in veterinary medicine, but CYP1A2 is studied frequently in people with regard to susceptibility to certain types of cancers. A feline hepatic CYP2E polymorphism has been identified, but the clinical relevance of this polymorphism has not been described [31]. Similarly, polymorphisms have been described in several drug-metabolizing enzymes in cattle [32], but these single nucleotide polymorphisms are used as molecular markers available in cattle for linkage analysis, testing of parentage, and distinction of breeds rather than for predicting response to drug therapy.

With respect to phase II metabolic enzymes, a panspecies defect in uridine diphosphate (UDP)-glucuronyl transferase exists in cats. Although this is not a true example of pharmacogenetics, it serves as an example of genetic variation between species rather than within a species that significantly affects drug disposition. Cats have a pseudogene rather than a functional glucuronyltransferase gene; therefore, acetaminophen and other drugs are not conjugated with glucuronide as they are in other species. Another panspecies phase II metabolic defect occurs in dogs. *N*-acetyltransferase is the enzyme responsible for metabolizing sulfonamides, procainamide, hydralazine, and other drugs. Both *N*-acetyltransferase genes are absent in dogs, increasing the risk for hypersensitivity reactions and adverse effects from these drugs relative to other species [33].

A true pharmacogenetic variation exists for the thiopurine methyltransferase (TPMT) enzyme. TPMT is a phase II enzyme that is responsible for metabolizing azathioprine and its active metabolites to their inactive forms. A ninefold range in TMPT activity exists in dogs, and enzyme activity level seems to be related to breed. Giant Schnauzers had lower TPMT activity, whereas Alaskan Malamutes had high TMPT activity [34]. Decreased TPMT activity has been documented to be associated with increased susceptibility to azathioprine-induced bone marrow suppression.

PHARMACOGENETICS OF DRUG EXCRETION

Drugs are eliminated from the body unchanged or as metabolites. Renal excretion and biliary excretion are the most important pathways of drug elimination, but excretion may occur by other routes as well. As noted previously, P-gp is expressed on renal tubular cells and biliary canalicular cells, suggesting that it may play a role in drug excretion. Concurrent administration of a P-gp inhibitor decreases the biliary and renal clearance of doxorubicin in rats [35]. In a separate study, biliary and renal excretion of digoxin and vincristine were increased in rats after treatment with a P-gp inhibitor [36]. Further research is necessary to define the role of P-gp in regulating renal and biliary drug excretion fully in veterinary patients. Altered biliary or renal excretion may play a role in the apparent increased sensitivity of herding breeds to chemotherapeutic drugs that are P-gp substrates, however. For example, a Collie with lymphoma developed myelosuppression and gastrointestinal (GI) toxicity after treatments with vincristine or doxorubicin, even at lowered doses, but tolerated cyclophosphamide at the full dose. The patient was subsequently genotyped and was determined have one mutant MDR1 allele and one normal MDR1 allele [37]. It is possible that deficient P-gp in this patient resulted in delayed renal or biliary excretion and subsequent toxicity. Other reports of severe doxorubicin or vincristine sensitivity in Collies and other herding breeds have surfaced on Internet veterinary discussion groups. The MDR1 mutation may be a reasonable explanation for this apparent breed predilection to chemotherapeutic (eg, vinca alkaloids, anthracyclines) drug sensitivity.

PHARMACOGENETICS OF DRUG RECEPTORS

A relatively new and important area of pharmacogenetics research involves polymorphisms in genes encoding drug receptors and effector proteins. In human patients, polymorphisms have been described in angiotensin converting enzyme, β_2-adrenergic receptors, the dopamine receptor, the estrogen receptor, and others [38]. In vitro functional studies suggest that these polymorphisms have functional significance, but reports regarding clinical effects are not available. A polymorphism in the canine dopamine receptor D4 gene has been described, but its clinical implications, if any, are not yet understood [39].

PHARMACOGENETICS AND HYPERSENSITIVITY REACTIONS

Pharmacogenetic differences in metabolic pathways cannot only affect type A adverse drug reactions (ie, predictable, generally correlating with plasma drug concentration) but can also affect type B adverse drug reactions (idiosyncratic). Idiosyncratic toxicity to sulfonamides is similar in dogs and people and can be characterized by fever, arthropathy, blood dyscrasias (neutropenia, thrombocytopenia, or hemolytic anemia), hepatopathy consisting of cholestasis or necrosis, skin eruptions, uveitis, or keratoconjunctivitis sicca [40]. In people, slow acetylation by NAT2 has been shown to be a risk factor for sulfonamide hypersensitivity reactions. It has been proposed that the alternative metabolic pathway in these individuals produces reactive metabolites [41]. Covalent binding of reactive metabolites of these drugs to cell macromolecules results in cytotoxicity and immune response to neoantigens. Ongoing research in one veterinary pharmacology laboratory (Department of Medical Sciences, School of Veterinary Medicine, University of Wisconsin-Madison, Madison, Wisconsin; available at: latrepanier@svm.vetmed.wisc.edu) is underway to characterize dogs with possible idiosyncratic sulfonamide reactions, using several methodologies, including ELISA for antidrug antibodies, immunoblotting for antibodies directed against liver proteins, flow cytometry for drug-dependent antiplatelet antibodies, and in vitro cytotoxicity assays.

PHARMACOGENETICS IN CLINICAL PRACTICE

Scientific interest in the field of human pharmacogenetics has increased each year in parallel with the knowledge of the human genome. Interest in this field by physicians has lagged significantly behind, however, presumably because relatively few significant clinical consequences can be correlated to the vast number of pharmacogenetic mutations described in the literature. There are two main reasons for this discrepancy. Up to this point, polymorphisms described in human patients have had low allelic frequencies or the clinical relevance of a particular polymorphism was not significant. For example, a highly clinically relevant polymorphism in the human TPMT gene has been described. TMPT metabolic activity in affected patients is essentially absent; thus, these patients experience severe neutropenia after a "normal" dose of azathioprine. Because this TPMT polymorphism affects approximately 0.3% of the white population, pharmacogenetic testing is not routinely performed in clinical practice [42]. Conversely, the allelic frequency of a genetic polymorphism of the human MDR1 gene has been shown to be associated with lower levels of P-gp expression in the duodenum and other tissues. Although the allelic frequency of this particular MDR1 polymorphism is relatively high (>10%), it does not seem to have an important and predictable clinical impact on drug disposition. Most pharmacogenetic research in human medicine has not extended to clinical medical practice.

Box 1: Selected P-glycoprotein substrates

Anticancer agents
- Doxorubicin
- Docetaxel[a]
- Vincristine[a]
- Vinblastine[a]
- Etoposide[a]
- Mitoxantrone
- Actinomycin D

Steroid hormones
- Aldosterone
- Cortisol[a]
- Dexamethasone[a]
- Methylprednisolone

Antimicrobial agents
- Erythromycin[a]
- Ketoconazole
- Itraconazole[a]
- Tetracycline
- Doxycycline
- Levofloxacin
- Sparfloxacin

Opioids
- Loperamide
- Morphine

Cardiac drugs
- Digoxin
- Diltiazem[a]
- Verapamil[a]
- Talinolol

Immunosuppressants
- Cyclosporine[a]
- Tacrolimus[a]

Box 1 (*continued*)

Miscellaneous
- Ivermectin
- Amitriptyline
- Terfenadine[a]
- Ondansetron
- Domperidone
- Phenothiazines
- Vecuronium

[a]Substrate of CYP3A.

In veterinary medicine, however, a commercial veterinary pharmacogenetics laboratory (Veterinary Clinical Pharmacology Laboratory, Washington State University, Pullman, Washington; available at www.vetmed.wsu.edu/vcpl) is performing canine MDR1 genotyping for veterinarians, dog breeders, and owners. Important reasons why commercial pharmacogenetic testing is readily available for canine patients and not for human patients are because the MDR1 mutation in dogs has a high allelic frequency (55% in Collies, 42% in Long-Haired Whippets, and roughly 20% in Australian Shepherds) and because the polymorphism is highly predictive for serious adverse drug events not just for one drug class but for several drug classes. A partial list of drugs that are substrates for P-gp is listed in Box 1 [43–47].

FUTURE DIRECTIONS

The field of pharmacogenetics, particularly in veterinary medicine, is still in its infancy. We have an ever-increasing arsenal of molecular tools that can be used to expand our knowledge of pharmacogenetics, however. Furthermore, with the recent completion of the canine genome project and the ongoing elucidation of its data, we may soon know the sequences of virtually all genes encoding drug-metabolizing enzymes, drug transporters, receptors, and other drug targets. With this information, the traditional pharmacogenetics approach (phenotype-to-genotype) is likely to give way to a pharmacogenomics approach (genotype-to-phenotype). In other words, genetic variation identified in a specific gene can be investigated to determine if it alters pharmacologic response. Although the ultimate goal of modern pharmacogenomics, individualization of drug therapy, may not be achieved for all drugs, it certainly has the potential to increase the safety and efficacy of many drugs.

References

[1] Hochstein P. Glucose-6-phosphate dehydrogenase deficiency: mechanisms of drug-induced hemolysis. Exp Eye Res 1971;11(3):389–95.

[2] Patel J, Mitra AK. Strategies to overcome simultaneous P-glycoprotein mediated efflux and CYP3A4 mediated metabolism of drugs. Pharmacogenomics 2001;2(4):401–15.
[3] Scordo MG, Spina E. Cytochrome P450 polymorphisms and response to antipsychotic therapy. Pharmacogenomics 2002;3(2):201–18.
[4] Roninson IB. The role of the MDR1 (P-glycoprotein) gene in multidrug resistance in vitro and in vivo. Biochem Pharmacol 1992;43(1):95–102.
[5] Thiebaut F, Tsuruo T, Hamada H, et al. Cellular localization of the multidrug-resistance gene product P-glycoprotein in normal human tissues. Proc Natl Acad Sci USA 1987;84(21): 7735–8.
[6] Schinkel AH, Wagenaar E, van Deemter L, et al. Absence of the Mdr1a P-glycoprotein in mice affects tissue distribution and pharmacokinetics of dexamethasone, digoxin, and cyclosporin A. J Clin Invest 1995;96(4):1698–705.
[7] Sills GJ, Kwan P, Butler E, et al. P-glycoprotein-mediated efflux of antiepileptic drugs: preliminary studies in Mdr1a knockout mice 2002;3(5):427–32.
[8] Verstuyft C, Schwab M, Schaeffeler E, et al. Digoxin pharmacokinetics and MDR1 genetic polymorphisms. Eur J Clin Pharmacol 2003;58(12):809–12.
[9] Kerb R, Aynacioglu AS, Brockmoller J, et al. The predictive value of MDR1, CYP2C9, and CYP2C19 polymorphisms for phenytoin plasma levels. Pharmacogenomics J 2001;1(3): 204–10.
[10] Ginn PE. Immunohistochemical detection of P-glycoprotein in formalin-fixed and paraffin-embedded normal and neoplastic canine tissues. Vet Pathol 1996;33(5):533–41.
[11] Mealey KL, Barhoumi R, Rogers K, et al. Doxorubicin induced expression of P-glycoprotein in a canine osteosarcoma cell line. Cancer Lett 1998;126(2):187–92.
[12] Page RL, Hughes CS, Huyan S, et al. Modulation of P-glycoprotein-mediated doxorubicin resistance in canine cell lines. Anticancer Res 2000;20(5B):3533–8.
[13] McEntee M, Silverman JA, Rassnick K, et al. Enhanced bioavailability of oral docetaxel by co-administration of cyclosporin A in dogs and rats. Vet Comp Oncol 2003;2(1):105–12.
[14] Mealey KL, Bentjen SA, Gay JM, et al. Ivermectin sensitivity in collies is associated with a deletion mutation of the Mdr1 gene. Pharmacogenetics 2001;11(8):727–33.
[15] Mealey KL, Bentjen SA, Waiting DK. Frequency of the mutant MDR1 Allele associated with ivermectin sensitivity in a sample population of collies from the northwestern United States. Am J Vet Res 2002;63(4):479–81.
[16] Neff MW, Robertson KR, Wong AK, et al. Breed distribution and history of canine Mdr1–1Δ, a pharmacogenetic mutation that marks the emergence of breeds from the collie lineage. Proc Natl Acad Sci USA 2004;101:11725–30.
[17] Tranquilli WJ, Paul AJ, Todd KS. Assessment of toxicosis induced by high-dose administration of milbemycin oxime in collies. Am J Vet Res 1991;52(7):1170–2.
[18] Hugnet C, Cadore JL, Buronfosse F, et al. Loperamide poisoning in the dog. Vet Hum Toxicol 1996;38(1):31–3.
[19] Ericsson CD, Johnson PC. Safety and efficacy of loperamide. Am J Med 1990;88(6A): 10S–4S.
[20] Wandel C, Kim R, Wood M, et al. Interaction of morphine, fentanyl, sufentanil, alfentanil, and loperamide with the efflux drug transporter P-glycoprotein. Anesthesiology 2002;96(4):913–20.
[21] Sartor LL, Bentjen SA, Trepanier L, et al. Loperamide toxicity in a collie with the MDR1 mutation associated with ivermectin sensitivity. J Vet Intern Med 2004;18(1):117–8.
[22] Choo EF, Leake B, Wandel C, et al. Pharmacological inhibition of P-glycoprotein transport enhances the distribution of HIV-1 protease inhibitors into brain and testes. Drug Metab Dispos 2000;28(6):655–60.
[23] Katagiri A, Tomita Y, Nishiyama T, et al. Immunohistochemical detection of P-glycoprotein and GSTP1–1 in testis cancer. Br J Cancer 1993;68(1):125–9.
[24] Young AM, Allen CE, Audus KL. Efflux transporters of the human placenta. Adv Drug Deliv Rev 2003;55(1):125–32.

[25] Wing JP. Blood protein polymorphisms in Jewish populations. Hum Hered 1974;24(4): 323–44.
[26] Cascorbi I. Pharmacogenetics of cytochrome P4502D6. Genetic background and clinical implication. Eur J Clin Invest 2003;33(Suppl 2):17–22.
[27] Hay Kraus BL, Greenblatt DJ, Venkatakrishnan K, et al. Evidence for propofol hydroxylation by cytochrome P4502B11 in canine liver microsomes: breed and gender differences. Xenobiotica 2000;30(6):575–88.
[28] Court MH, Hay-Kraus BL, Hill DW, et al. Propofol hydroxylation by dog liver microsomes. Assay development and dog breed differences. Drug Metab Dispos 1999;27(11):1293–9.
[29] Paulson SK, Engel L, Reitz B, et al. Evidence for polymorphism in the canine metabolism of the cyclooxygenase 2 inhibitor celecoxib. Drug Metab Dispos 1999;27(10):1133–42.
[30] Tenmizu D, Endo Y, Noguchi K, et al. Identification of the novel canine CYP1A2 1117 C > T SNP causing protein deletion. Xenobiotica 2004;34(9):835–46.
[31] Tanaka N, Shinkyo R, Sakaki T, et al. Cytochrome P450 2E polymorphism in feline liver. Biochim Biophys Acta 2005;1726:194–205.
[32] Theilmann JL, Skow LC, Baker JF, et al. Restriction fragment length polymorphisms for growth hormone, prolactin, osteonectin, alpha crystallin, gamma crystallin, fibronectin and 21-steroid hydroxylase in cattle. Anim Genet 1989;20(3):257–66.
[33] Collins JM. Inter-species differences in drug properties. Chem Biol Interact 2001;134(3): 237–42.
[34] Kidd LB, Salavaggione OE, Szumlanski CL, et al. Thiopurine methyltransferase activity in red blood cells of dogs. J Vet Intern Med 2004;18(2):214–8.
[35] Kiso S, Cai SH, Kitaichi K, et al. Inhibitory effect of erythromycin on P-glycoprotein-mediated biliary excretion of doxorubicin in rats. Anticancer Res 2000;20(5A):2827–34.
[36] Song S, Suzuki H, Kawai R, et al. Effect of PSC 833, a P-glycoprotein modulator, on the disposition of vincristine and digoxin in rats. Drug Metab Dispos 1999;27(6):689–94.
[37] Mealey KL, Northrup NC, Bentjen SA. Increased toxicity of P-glycoprotein-substrate chemotherapeutic agents in a dog with the MDR1 deletion mutation associated with ivermectin sensitivity. J Am Vet Med Assoc 2003;223(10):1453–5, 1434.
[38] Tribut O, Lessard Y, Reymann JM, et al. Pharmacogenomics. Med Sci Monit 2002;8(7): RA152–63.
[39] Ito H, Nara H, Inoue-Murayama M, et al. Allele frequency distribution of the canine dopamine receptor D4 gene exon III and I in 23 breeds. J Vet Med Sci 2004;66(7):815–20.
[40] Trepanier LA. Idiosyncratic toxicity associated with potentiated sulfonamides in the dog. J Vet Pharmacol Ther 2004;27(3):129–38.
[41] Spielberg SP. N-acetyltransferases: pharmacogenetics and clinical consequences of polymorphic drug metabolism. J Pharmacokinet Biopharm 1996;24(5):509–19.
[42] Becquemont L. Clinical relevance of pharmacogenetics. Drug Metab Rev 2003;35(4): 277–85.
[43] Schwab M, Eichelbaum M, Fromm MF. Genetic polymorphisms of the human MDR1 drug transporter. Annu Rev Pharmacol Toxicol 2003;43:285–307.
[44] Fromm MF. Genetically determined differences in P-glycoprotein function: implications for disease risk. Toxicology 2002;181/182:299–303.
[45] Sakaeda T, Nakamura T, Okumura K. MDR1 genotype-related pharmacokinetics and pharmacodynamics. Biol Pharm Bull 2002;25(11):1391–400.
[46] Sakaeda T, Nakamura T, Okumura K. Pharmacogenetics of MDR1 and its impact on the pharmacokinetics and pharmacodynamics of drugs. Pharmacogenomics 2003;4(4): 397–410.
[47] Marzolini C, Paus E, Buclin T, et al. Polymorphisms in human MDR1 (P-glycoprotein). Recent advances and clinical relevance. Clin Pharmacol Ther 2004;75(1):13–33.

ELSEVIER
SAUNDERS
Vet Clin Small Anim 36 (2006) 975–985
VETERINARY CLINICS
SMALL ANIMAL PRACTICE

Cytochrome P450 and Its Role in Veterinary Drug Interactions

Lauren A. Trepanier, DVM, PhD
Department of Medical Sciences, University of Wisconsin–Madison, School of Veterinary Medicine, 2015 Linden Drive, Madison, WI 53706-1102, USA

OVERVIEW OF CYTOCHROME P450'S

Cytochrome P450's (CYPs) are heme-containing enzymes involved in the metabolism of drugs, hormones, and environmental chemicals. These membrane-bound enzymes are expressed in the endoplasmic reticulum of the liver, intestine, kidney, brain, adrenal, and other organs. There are hundreds of CYPs recognized; CYP enzymes are categorized within and between different species using a family/subfamily/individual enzyme nomenclature [1]. For example, CYP3A4, an abundant P450 in human liver, is a member of the CYP3 family and CYP3A subfamily and represents a unique enzyme (3A4) in human beings. The ortholog (comparable enzyme) in dogs is CYP3A12. Orthologs among species are evolutionarily related, share high amino acid identity, and may share similar substrate ranges. There can also be unexpected differences in substrate specificity among orthologous P450 enzymes between species, however. This has important implications for attempts to extrapolate known drug interactions from people to veterinary patients.

CYPs in dogs are not as completely characterized as they are in human beings, and little work has been done in cats. There is recent interest, however, in learning more about the differences between human and canine CYPs because of the use of dogs by pharmaceutical companies for preclinical drug testing. Most of the major CYP subfamilies have been identified in dogs, but substrate specificities (from which we derive clinical information for predicting drug interactions) are not well established. The canine P450's characterized to date are shown in Table 1, along with known substrates in human beings and dogs.

MECHANISMS OF CYTOCHROME P450–MEDIATED DRUG INTERACTIONS

CYPs perform oxidation or reduction reactions on xenobiotics; the overall function of this system is to inactivate chemicals and render them more polar (water soluble) to promote renal or biliary excretion. CYPs may convert drugs

E-mail address: latrepanier@svm.vetmed.wisc.edu

0195-5616/06/$ – see front matter
doi:10.1016/j.cvsm.2006.05.003

vetsmall.theclinics.com

Table 1
Human and canine cytochrome P450 substrates

Cytochrome P450 in people	Human substrates	Cytochrome P450 in dogs	Known canine substrates [19]
CYP1A1	Dioxin, other environmental chemicals	CYP1A	Induced by environmental toxins (eg, polychlorinated biphenyls)
CYP1A2	Caffeine, theophylline Inhibited by ciprofloxacin	Canine ortholog of CYP1A2	Fluoroquinolones (?) Theophylline (?) Induced by omeprazole [4]
CYP2B6	Propofol	CYP2B11 Second gene?	Propofol, diazepam Progesterone, androstenedione [72] Testosterone (16-α-hydroxylation) Diclofenac Cyclophosphamide Induced by phenobarbital [69,73] Inhibited by chloramphenicol [63,64]
CYP2E1	Ethanol, chlorzoxazone Bioactivation of acetaminophen Inhibited by cimetidine	CYP2E ortholog	Chlorzoxazone [74]
CYP2C9	Phenytoin, fluconazole, warfarin, glipizide, flubiprofen, piroxicam, ibuprofen, celecoxib, naproxen, meloxicam	CYP2C21	Testosterone (16-α-hydroxylation) Diclofenac Modest induction by phenobarbital [73]
	Bioactivation of cyclophosphamide Inhibited by cimetidine, fluconazole, some NSAIDs	CYP2C41	Substrates not established
CYP2D6	Codeine, tramadol, propranolol and other beta-blockers, phenothiazines, quinidine, dextromethorphan, chlorpheniramine, imipramine, fluoxetine, amitriptyline, chlorpromazine, metoclopramide Inhibited by quinidine [75]	CYP2D15	Celecoxib, dextromethorphan, imipramine, metoprolol, propranolol [25] Inhibited by quinidine [76]

(*continued on next page*)

Table 1
(continued)

Cytochrome P450 in people	Human substrates	Cytochrome P450 in dogs	Known canine substrates [19]
CYP3A4	Ketoconazole, itraconazole, cyclosporine, tacrolimus, erythromycin, clindamycin, clarithromycin, cisapride, diazepam, midazolam, diltiazem, digoxin, quinidine, verapamil, aflatoxin, budesonide Induced by rifampin [77] Inhibited by grapefruit juice (bergamottin), ketoconazole, itraconazole	CYP3A12 CYP3A26	Erythromycin, tacrolimus cyclosporine, midazolam, diazepam, nordiazepam progesterone, testosterone (6-β-hydroxylation) Induced by phenobarbital, rifampin [2,3] Inhibited by grapefruit juice (bergamottin) Inhibited by ketoconazole, itraconazole not evaluated

Abbreviation: NSAID, nonsteroidal anti-inflammatory drug.

into inactive metabolites (eg, warfarin, phenytoin), bioactivate prodrugs into active drugs (eg, codeine, tramadol, enalapril), or generate reactive toxic metabolites (eg, acetaminophen). When two drugs have affinity for the same CYP, drug interactions can result. An interacting compound may compete for the same catalytic site (competitive inhibition) or may bind to another site on the enzyme that alters the protein's structure, and thus its ability to bind other drugs at the active site (noncompetitive inhibition). Alternatively, an inhibitor may generate a reactive metabolite that binds irreversibly to a CYP and terminates its function (mechanism-based or suicide inhibition).

Drugs and other chemicals can also affect CYPs through enzyme induction. CYP inducers bind to specific nuclear receptors, which then associate with xenobiotic response elements in the promoter regions of specific CYP genes. This leads to transcriptional activation of the gene, resulting in increased enzyme synthesis and higher overall activity. Examples of known CYP inducers in dogs are phenobarbital, rifampin, and omeprazole (see Table 1) [2–4].

CYTOCHROME P450'S AND DRUG INTERACTIONS IN HUMAN BEINGS

The CYPs most commonly involved in drug interactions in human beings are CYP1A2, CYP2C9, CYP2D6, and CYP3A4. CYP1A2 metabolizes theophylline, aminophylline, theobromine (found in chocolate), and other methylxanthines (see Table 1). This enzyme is inhibited by ciprofloxacin [5], leading to decreased theophylline clearance [6,7] and clinical signs of theophylline toxicity in some human patients cotreated with ciprofloxacin [8,9]. In dogs, enrofloxacin and marbofloxacin have been shown to decrease theophylline clearance (Table 2) [10,11], but reports documenting a clinical interaction between theophylline and fluoroquinolones in dogs are still lacking.

Human CYP2C9 substrates include warfarin, phenytoin, glipizide, and several nonsteroidal anti-inflammatory agents, including piroxicam, naproxen, celecoxib, meloxicam, and ibuprofen (see Table 1) [12]. Naproxen, ibuprofen, and diclofenac seem to inhibit CYP2C9-mediated clearance of warfarin in that they are associated with exaggerated anticoagulation (international normalized ratio) in patients also treated with warfarin [12,13]. Fluconazole, another inhibitor of CYP2C9 [14], has a similar interaction with warfarin that can lead to clinical bleeding [15–17].

In dogs, two CYP2C isoforms have been identified: CYP2C21 and CYP2C41 [18]. CYP2C21 is the predominant CYP characterized to date in canine liver [3]. This CYP is known to metabolize testosterone and diclofenac [19] and is modestly induced by phenobarbital [3]. CYP2C41 is only present in some dogs [18,20], which may well have implications for clinically used drugs. Unfortunately, the substrate ranges of each of these enzymes are as yet poorly characterized.

A large number of clinically important drugs are metabolized by human CYP2D6, including beta-blockers (eg, propranolol, timolol, metoprolol), antiarrhythmics (eg, quinidine, flecainide), antidepressants (eg, amitriptyline, clomipramine, fluoxetine, imipramine), antiemetics (eg, chlorpromazine, metoclopramide) [21], and opioid derivatives (eg, codeine, dextromethorphan, tramadol) (see Table 1) [22]. This wide substrate range leads to a number of clinically relevant drug interactions. For example, codeine exerts its effects via bioactivation into morphine; this CYP2D6 reaction is inhibited by quinidine, leading to decreased analgesic efficacy of codeine with quinidine coadministration in human beings [23]. Quinidine's potent CYP2D6 inhibition has even been exploited to pharmaceutic advantage. Dextromethorphan, a traditional cough suppressant, is being developed for the treatment of mood disorders and neuropathic pain in people; for this application, dextromethorphan is formulated along with quinidine, which inhibits CYP2D6-mediated dextromethorphan metabolism and prolongs its duration of action [24].

The canine ortholog of CYP2D6 is CYP2D15. Drugs metabolized by CYP2D15 include propranolol [25], dextromethorphan [19], and imipramine [25]. Celecoxib is a CYP2D15 substrate in dogs, although another CYP may also be involved [26]. As an example of the difficulties in extrapolating CYP substrates across species, celecoxib clearance is mediated by the CYP2C family in human beings rather than by CYP2D.

Compared with other P450's, the human CYP3A4 pathway mediates the clearance of the largest number of drugs in people (see Table 1). Drug interactions are a common cause of drug toxicity for CYP3A substrates. For example, ketoconazole is a potent inhibitor of CYP3A4 metabolism and has led to cardiac arrhythmias secondary to impaired metabolism of cisapride in human beings [21,27] and sedation attributable to high plasma concentrations of

Table 2
Presumptive cytochrome P450-based drug interactions in the dog

Effector drug	Affected drug	Effects/Mechanism	Strength of evidence in the dog
Fluoroquinolones	Theophylline	Increased serum theophylline concentrations Inhibition of theophylline clearance (presumably through CYP1A2 inhibition)	In vivo studies in dogs with enrofloxacin and marbofloxacin [10,11]
Chloramphenicol	Phenobarbital, phenytoin, pentobarbital	Prolonged elimination half-lives and prolonged sedation Likely CYP2B11 inhibition	In vivo studies in dogs [67,68] In vivo study in cats [66]
	Propofol	Prolonged elimination half-life and prolonged recovery Likely CYP2B11 inhibition	In vivo study in dogs [65]
Ketoconazole	Cyclosporine: increased whole blood concentrations for a given dose	Presumably CYP3A inhibition and/or contribution of P-glycoprotein	In vivo study in dogs [40] In vivo study in cats [41]
	Midazolam	Prolonged midazolam elimination half-life CYP3A12 inhibition	In vivo study in dogs [37]
	Nifedipine	Decreased nifedipine clearance	In vivo study in dogs [78]
Cimetidine	Verapamil	Decreased clearance of verapamil	In vivo study in dogs [60]
	Theophylline	Trend toward prolonged elimination half-life and decreased clearance	In vivo study in dogs [61]
	Cyclosporine	Cimetidine may delay cyclosporine absorption but overall clearance is not affected	In vivo study in dogs [59]
Phenobarbital	Digoxin	Decreased digoxin elimination half-life acutely No significant effect with chronic co-administration CYP3A12 induction?	In vivo study in dogs [79,80]
	Propranolol	Decreased propranolol bioavailability and decreased elimination half-life Target CYP not identified	In vivo study in dogs [81]

midazolam [28]. Itraconazole is also a CYP3A4 inhibitor [29], leading to increased systemic exposure to budesonide in people [30]; this interaction has even led to clinical signs of hyperadrenocorticism in patients cotreated with itraconazole and budesonide [31]. Constituents of grapefruit juice (bergamottin) are potent suicide inhibitors of CYP3A4 [32] and can lead to toxicity in association with amlodipine, cyclosporine, diazepam, and several other 3A4 substrates [33].

Substrates of CYP3A12, the CYP3A ortholog in dogs, include midazolam [4], diazepam, nordiazepam, and testosterone [19]. CYP3A12 in dogs is induced by phenobarbital and rifampin [4,34,35] and is inhibited by ketoconazole [36,37]. In addition, another isoform, CYP3A26, is present in dogs, which has lower activity for testosterone and other steroid substrates compared with CYP3A12 [19,38,39]. The biochemical and clinical implications of these two 3A variants in dogs are not yet known.

Inhibition of CYP3A by ketoconazole has been exploited clinically to yield higher cyclosporine concentrations in dogs treated for perianal fistulas [40] and in cats given cyclosporine after renal transplantation [41]. Ketoconazole has also been shown to prolong the elimination half-life of midazolam in dogs [37]. Like ketoconazole, itraconazole is a CYP3A inhibitor in vivo in dogs, although studies have used high doses of itraconazole (eg, 100 mg/kg) [42]; the drug interaction potential of therapeutic dosages of itraconazole remains to be determined in dogs and cats.

The grapefruit derivative bergamottin is a potent CYP3A12 inhibitor in dogs [43] and increases plasma concentrations of cyclosporine [44] and diazepam in dogs in vivo [43]. Whether grapefruit extract would be clinically useful in increasing plasma concentrations of drugs, such as cyclosporine or itraconazole, in dogs remains to be determined.

The interpretation of drug interactions that seem to involve CYP3A is complicated by the fact that many CYP3A substrates are also substrates of P-glycoprotein. P-glycoprotein is a transmembrane efflux pump that is expressed along with CYP3A4 in human intestine and contributes to first-pass clearance (and diminished bioavailability) of some oral drugs. P-glycoprotein also contributes to drug elimination in the biliary epithelium, renal tubular epithelium, central nervous system, and other sites. Known p-glycoprotein substrates include ketoconazole, itraconazole, erythromycin, cortisol, digoxin, diltiazem, cyclosporine, and ondansetron [45]. Some of these substrates can compete for drug efflux, leading to impaired elimination of a second compound. For example, in human beings, the well-described interaction between quinidine and digoxin may be attributable not (only) to CYP3A4 interactions but to inhibition of P-glycoprotein–mediated digoxin efflux [46]. Examples of known and likely P-glycoprotein substrates in dogs include ivermectin, loperamide, ondansetron, vincristine, vinblastine, digoxin, and doxorubicin [45,47–49]. Central nervous system toxicity from the combination of ketoconazole and ivermectin has been observed anecdotally in dogs (Katrina Mealey, DVM, PhD, DACVIM, DACVCP, personal communication, 2005). Additional work is needed to characterize clinically significant drug interactions among P-glycoprotein substrates in dogs and cats.

INHIBITORS OF MULTIPLE CYTOCHROME P450'S

Cimetidine inhibits several CYPs, including CYP1A2 [50], CYP2C9, CYP2D6, and CYP3A4 [51]. Cimetidine decreases the clearance of the CYP1A2 substrate theophylline [52–54], but this effect may be clinically significant in only a subset of human patients [52,55]. Cimetidine also increases the risk of bleeding from warfarin [56] and of hypoglycemia from glipizide in people [57]. Cimetidine has even been shown to interact with topical ophthalmic timolol drops used to treat glaucoma, leading to enhanced systemic beta-blockade (eg, decreased heart rate, lowered exercise tolerance) [58].

In dogs, cimetidine delays the absorption of cyclosporine but does not significantly increase cyclosporine blood concentrations [59]. Cimetidine reduces the clearance of verapamil in dogs [60], and high intravenous doses (300 mg/kg) of cimetidine modestly impair theophylline elimination [61]. There are also anecdotal reports of an interaction between metronidazole and cimetidine in dogs (secondary neurologic toxicity from metronidazole; author's unpublished observations), which may be CYP-mediated but require further characterization.

OTHER CYTOCHROME P450 INTERACTIONS IN DOGS

In dogs, CYP2B11 catalyzes the bioactivation of cyclophosphamide [62], the biotransformation of diazepam (along with CYP3A12) [19], and the clearance of propofol (see Table 1) [63]. CYP2B11 is inhibited selectively by chloramphenicol [63,64], which is consistent with the finding that chloramphenicol dramatically prolongs recovery times in propofol-anesthetized dogs (see Table 2) [65]. Chloramphenicol also leads to prolonged elimination half-lives of pentobarbital, phenobarbital, and phenytoin in dogs (see Table 2) [66–68], likely because of a CYP2B11 interaction. CYP2B11 activity is also induced by phenobarbital [34,69].

CYTOCHROME P450'S IN CATS

Virtually no work has been done to characterize feline CYPs, their substrate ranges, and their potential for drug interactions. Only CYP2E has been identified in the cat [70]; no orthologs of CYP2C, CYP2D, or CYP3A have been characterized. Ketoconazole is known to interact with cyclosporine in the cat as it does in human beings and dogs, however, leading to increased cyclosporine levels compared with cyclosporine alone [41]. This is presumably via an interaction at the feline CYP3A ortholog and/or an interaction at the P-glycoprotein, but the mechanism has not been confirmed. Interestingly, phenobarbital is not a CYP inducer in the cat [71], although the reasons for this difference from dogs have not been pursued.

SUMMARY

There are many opportunities for clinically relevant research on the likelihood of drug interactions in veterinary patients. We have a long way to go to reach the same degree of understanding of CYPs and drug interactions in veterinary patients that has been established in human patients. Luckily, there are many substrate similarities among human and canine CYPs that can help us to make reasonable predictions about possible or likely interactions in dogs. Although comparative work on human and canine CYPs is underway at many pharmaceutical companies, work on CYP-mediated biotransformation and drug-drug interactions in cats is sorely needed.

References

[1] Nelson DR, Zeldin DC, Hoffman SM, et al. Comparison of cytochrome P450 (CYP) genes from the mouse and human genomes, including nomenclature recommendations for genes, pseudogenes and alternative-splice variants. Pharmacogenetics 2004;14(1):1–18.

[2] Graham RA, Downey A, Mudra D, et al. In vivo and in vitro induction of cytochrome P450 enzymes in beagle dogs. Drug Metab Dispos 2002;30(11):1206–13.

[3] Eguchi K, Nishibe Y, Baba T, et al. Quantification of cytochrome P450 enzymes (CYP1A1/2, 2B11, 2C21, and 3A12) in dog liver microsomes by enzyme-linked immunosorbent assay. Xenobiotica 1996;26(7):755–63.

[4] Lu C, Li A. Species comparison in P450 induction: effects of dexamethasone, omeprazole, and rifampin on P450 isoforms 1A and 3A in primary cultured hepatocytes from man, Sprague-Dawley rat, minipig, and beagle dog. Chem Biol Interact 2001;134:271–81.

[5] Fuhr U, Anders EM, Mahr G, et al. Inhibitory potency of quinolone antibacterial agents against cytochrome P450IA2 activity in vivo and in vitro. Antimicrob Agents Chemother 1992;36(5):942–8.

[6] Thomson AH, Thomson GD, Hepburn M, et al. A clinically significant interaction between ciprofloxacin and theophylline. Eur J Clin Pharmacol 1987;33(4):435–6.

[7] Nix DE, DeVito JM, Whitbread MA, et al. Effect of multiple dose oral ciprofloxacin on the pharmacokinetics of theophylline and indocyanine green. J Antimicrob Chemother 1987;19(2):263–9.

[8] Wijnands WJ, Vree TB. Interaction between the fluoroquinolones and the bronchodilator theophylline. J Antimicrob Chemother 1988;22(Suppl C):109–14.

[9] Spivey JM, Laughlin PH, Goss TF, et al. Theophylline toxicity secondary to ciprofloxacin administration. Ann Emerg Med 1991;20(10):1131–4.

[10] Hirt RA, Teinfalt M, Dederichs D, et al. The effect of orally administered marbofloxacin on the pharmacokinetics of theophylline. J Vet Med A Physiol Pathol Clin Med 2003;50(5):246–50.

[11] Intorre L, Mengozzi G, Maccheroni M, et al. Enrofloxacin-theophylline interaction: influence of enrofloxacin on theophylline steady-state pharmacokinetics in the beagle dog. J Vet Pharmacol Ther 1995;18(5):352–6.

[12] Visser LE, van Schaik RH, van Vliet M, et al. Allelic variants of cytochrome P450 2C9 modify the interaction between nonsteroidal anti-inflammatory drugs and coumarin anticoagulants. Clin Pharmacol Ther 2005;77(6):479–85.

[13] van Dijk KN, Plat AW, van Dijk AA, et al. Potential interaction between acenocoumarol and diclofenac, naproxen and ibuprofen and role of CYP2C9 genotype. Thromb Haemost 2004;91(1):95–101.

[14] Niwa T, Shiraga T, Takagi A. Effect of antifungal drugs on cytochrome P450 (CYP) 2C9, CYP2C19, and CYP3A4 activities in human liver microsomes. Biol Pharm Bull 2005;28(9):1805–8.

[15] Black DJ, Kunze KL, Wienkers LC, et al. Warfarin-fluconazole. II. A metabolically based drug interaction: in vivo studies. Drug Metab Dispos 1996;24(4):422–8.

[16] Allison EJ Jr, McKinney TJ, Langenberg JN. Spinal epidural haematoma as a result of warfarin/fluconazole drug interaction. Eur J Emerg Med 2002;9(2):175–7.

[17] Mootha VV, Schluter ML, Das A. Intraocular hemorrhages due to warfarin fluconazole drug interaction in a patient with presumed Candida endophthalmitis. Arch Ophthalmol 2002;120(1):94–5.

[18] Blaisdell J, Goldstein J, Bai S. Isolation of a new canine cytochrome P450 cDNA from the cytochrome P450 2C subfamily (CYP2C41) and evidence for polymorphic differences in its expression. Drug Metab Dispos 1998;26:278–83.
[19] Shou M, Norcross R, Sandig G, et al. Substrate specificity and kinetic properties of seven heterologously expressed dog cytochromes P450. Drug Metab Dispos 2003;31(9):1161–9.
[20] Graham MJ, Bell AR, Crewe HK, et al. mRNA and protein expression of dog liver cytochromes P450 in relation to the metabolism of human CYP2C substrates. Xenobiotica 2003;33(3):225–37.
[21] Desta Z, Wu GM, Morocho AM, et al. The gastroprokinetic and antiemetic drug metoclopramide is a substrate and inhibitor of cytochrome P450 2D6. Drug Metab Dispos 2002;30(3):336–43.
[22] Pedersen RS, Damkier P, Brosen K. Tramadol as a new probe for cytochrome P450 2D6 phenotyping: a population study. Clin Pharmacol Ther 2005;77(6):458–67.
[23] Caraco Y, Sheller J, Wood AJ. Impact of ethnic origin and quinidine coadministration on codeine's disposition and pharmacodynamic effects. J Pharmacol Exp Ther 1999;290(1): 413–22.
[24] Dextromethorphan/quinidine: AVP 923, dextromethorphan/cytochrome P450-2D6 inhibitor, quinidine/dextromethorphan. Drugs R D 2005;6(3):174–7.
[25] Tasaki T, Nakamura A, Itoh S, et al. Expression and characterization of dog CYP2D15 using baculovirus expression system. J Biochem (Tokyo) 1998;123(1):162–8.
[26] Paulson SK, Engel L, Reitz B, et al. Evidence for polymorphism in the canine metabolism of the cyclooxygenase 2 inhibitor, celecoxib. Drug Metab Dispos 1999;27(10):1133–42.
[27] Dresser GK, Spence JD, Bailey DG. Pharmacokinetic-pharmacodynamic consequences and clinical relevance of cytochrome P450 3A4 inhibition. Clin Pharmacokinet 2000;38(1): 41–57.
[28] Lam YW, Alfaro CL, Ereshefsky L, et al. Pharmacokinetic and pharmacodynamic interactions of oral midazolam with ketoconazole, fluoxetine, fluvoxamine, and nefazodone. J Clin Pharmacol 2003;43(11):1274–82.
[29] Sakaeda T, Iwaki K, Kakumoto M, et al. Effect of micafungin on cytochrome P450 3A4 and multidrug resistance protein 1 activities, and its comparison with azole antifungal drugs. J Pharm Pharmacol 2005;57(6):759–64.
[30] Raaska K, Niemi M, Neuvonen M, et al. Plasma concentrations of inhaled budesonide and its effects on plasma cortisol are increased by the cytochrome P4503A4 inhibitor itraconazole. Clin Pharmacol Ther 2002;72(4):362–9.
[31] Bolland MJ, Bagg W, Thomas MG, et al. Cushing's syndrome due to interaction between inhaled corticosteroids and itraconazole. Ann Pharmacother 2004;38(1):46–9.
[32] Zhou S, Chan E, Lim LY, et al. Therapeutic drugs that behave as mechanism-based inhibitors of cytochrome P450 3A4. Curr Drug Metab 2004;5(5):415–42.
[33] Maskalyk J. Grapefruit juice: potential drug interactions. CMAJ 2002;167(3):279–80.
[34] Jayyosi Z, Muc M, Erick J, et al. Catalytic and immunochemical characterization of cytochrome P450 enzyme induction in dog liver. Fundam Appl Toxicol 1996;31:95–102.
[35] Nishibe Y, Wakabayashi M, Harauchi T, et al. Characterization of cytochrome P450 (CYP3A12) induction by rifampicin in dog liver. Xenobiotica 1998;28:549–57.
[36] Lu P, Singh SB, Carr BA, et al. Selective inhibition of dog hepatic CYP2B11 and CYP3A12. J Pharmacol Exp Ther 2005;313(2):518–28.
[37] Kuroha M, Azumano A, Kuze Y, et al. Effect of multiple dosing of ketoconazole on pharmacokinetics of midazolam, a cytochrome P450 3A substrate in beagle dogs. Drug Metab Dispos 2002;30:63–8.
[38] He Y, Roussel F, Halpert J. Importance of amino acid residue 474 for substrate specificity of canine and human cytochrome P450 3A enzymes. Arch Biochem Biophys 2001;389(2):264–70.
[39] Fraser D, Feyereisen R, Harlow G, et al. Isolation, heterologous expression, and functional characterization of a novel cytochrome P450 3A enzyme from a canine liver cDNA library. J Pharmacol Exp Ther 1997;283:1425–32.

[40] Patricelli AJ, Hardie RJ, McAnulty JE. Cyclosporine and ketoconazole for the treatment of perianal fistulas in dogs. J Am Vet Med Assoc 2002;220(7):1009–16.
[41] McAnulty JF, Lensmeyer GL. The effects of ketoconazole on the pharmacokinetics of cyclosporine A in cats. Vet Surg 1999;28(6):448–55.
[42] Kim EJ, Seo JW, Hwang JY, et al. Effects of combined treatment with sildenafil and itraconazole on the cardiovascular system in telemetered conscious dogs. Drug Chem Toxicol 2005;28(2):177–86.
[43] Sahi J, Reyner EL, Bauman JN, et al. The effect of bergamottin on diazepam plasma levels and P450 enzymes in beagle dogs. Drug Metab Dispos 2002;30(2):135–40.
[44] Amatori FM, Meucci V, Giusiani M, et al. Effect of grapefruit juice on the pharmacokinetics of cyclosporine in dogs. Vet Rec 2004;154(6):180–1.
[45] Mealey KL. Therapeutic implications of the MDR-1 gene. J Vet Pharmacol Ther 2004;27(5): 257–64.
[46] Collett A, Tanianis-Hughes J, Carlson GL, et al. Comparison of P-glycoprotein-mediated drug-digoxin interactions in Caco-2 with human and rodent intestine: relevance to in vivo prediction. Eur J Pharm Sci 2005;26(5):386–93.
[47] Sartor LL, Bentjen SA, Trepanier L, et al. Loperamide toxicity in a collie with the MDR1 mutation associated with ivermectin sensitivity. J Vet Intern Med 2004;18(1):117–8.
[48] Mealey KL, Bentjen SA, Gay JM, et al. Ivermectin sensitivity in collies is associated with a deletion mutation of the mdr1 gene. Pharmacogenetics 2001;11(8):727–33.
[49] Mealey KL, Northrup NC, Bentjen SA. Increased toxicity of P-glycoprotein-substrate chemotherapeutic agents in a dog with the MDR1 deletion mutation associated with ivermectin sensitivity. J Am Vet Med Assoc. 2003;223(10):1434, 1453–5.
[50] Martinez C, Albet C, Agundez JA, et al. Comparative in vitro and in vivo inhibition of cytochrome P450 CYP1A2, CYP2D6, and CYP3A by H2-receptor antagonists. Clin Pharmacol Ther 1999;65(4):369–76.
[51] Furuta S, Kamada E, Suzuki T, et al. Inhibition of drug metabolism in human liver microsomes by nizatidine, cimetidine and omeprazole. Xenobiotica 2001;31(1):1–10.
[52] Fraser IM, Buttoo KM, Walker SE, et al. Effects of cimetidine and ranitidine on the pharmacokinetics of a chronotherapeutically formulated once-daily theophylline preparation (Uniphyl). Clin Ther 1993;15(2):383–93.
[53] Loi CM, Parker BM, Cusack BJ, et al. Aging and drug interactions. III. Individual and combined effects of cimetidine and cimetidine and ciprofloxacin on theophylline metabolism in healthy male and female nonsmokers. J Pharmacol Exp Ther 1997;280(2):627–37.
[54] Ohashi K, Sakamoto K, Sudo T, et al. Effects of diltiazem and cimetidine on theophylline oxidative metabolism. J Clin Pharmacol 1993;33(12):1233–7.
[55] Nix DE, Di Cicco RA, Miller AK, et al. The effect of low-dose cimetidine (200 mg twice daily) on the pharmacokinetics of theophylline. J Clin Pharmacol 1999;39(8):855–65.
[56] Choonara IA, Cholerton S, Haynes BP, et al. Stereoselective interaction between the R enantiomer of warfarin and cimetidine. Br J Clin Pharmacol 1986;21(3):271–7.
[57] Feely J, Collins WC, Cullen M, et al. Potentiation of the hypoglycaemic response to glipizide in diabetic patients by histamine H2-receptor antagonists. Br J Clin Pharmacol 1993;35(3): 321–3.
[58] Ishii Y, Nakamura K, Tsutsumi K, et al. Drug interaction between cimetidine and timolol ophthalmic solution: effect on heart rate and intraocular pressure in healthy Japanese volunteers. J Clin Pharmacol 2000;40(2):193–9.
[59] Daigle JC, Hosgood G, Foil CS, et al. Effect of cimetidine on pharmacokinetics of orally administered cyclosporine in healthy dogs. Am J Vet Res 2001;62(7):1046–50.
[60] Johnson LM, Lankford SM, Bai SA. The influence of cimetidine on the pharmacokinetics of the enantiomers of verapamil in the dog during multiple oral dosing. J Vet Pharmacol Ther 1995;18(2):117–23.
[61] Ritschel WA, Banerjee PS, Cacini W, et al. Animal model for theophylline-cimetidine drug interaction. Methods Find Exp Clin Pharmacol 1985;7(12):627–9.

[62] Chen CS, Lin JT, Goss KA, et al. Activation of the anticancer prodrugs cyclophosphamide and ifosfamide: identification of cytochrome P450 2B enzymes and site-specific mutants with improved enzyme kinetics. Mol Pharmacol 2004;65(5):1278–85.
[63] Hay-Kraus B, Greenblatt D, Venkatakrishnan K, et al. Evidence of propofol hydroxylation by cytochrome P4502B11 in canine liver microsomes: breed and gender differences. Xenobiotica 2000;30(6):575–88.
[64] Ciaccio P, Duignan D, Halpert J. Selective inactivation by chloramphenicol of the major phenobarbital-inducible isozyme of dog liver cytochrome P450. Drug Metab Dispos 1987;15(6):852–6.
[65] Mandsager R, Clarke C, Shawley R, et al. Effects of chloramphenicol on infusion pharmacokinetics of propofol in Greyhounds. Am J Vet Res 1995;56(1):95–9.
[66] Adams HR, Dixit BN. Prolongation of pentobarbital anesthesia by chloramphenicol in dogs and cats. J Am Vet Med Assoc 1970;156(7):902–5.
[67] Sanders JE, Yeary RA, Fenner WR, et al. Interaction of phenytoin with chloramphenicol or pentobarbital in the dog. J Am Vet Med Assoc 1979;175(2):177–80.
[68] Teske RH, Carter GG. Effect of chloramphenicol on pentobarbital-induced anesthesia in dogs. J Am Vet Med Assoc 1971;159(6):777–80.
[69] Graham R, Downey A, Mudra D, et al. In vivo and in vitro induction of cytochrome P450 enzymes in beagle dogs. Drug Metab Dispos 2002;30:1206–13.
[70] Tanaka N, Shinkyo R, Sakaki T, et al. Cytochrome P450 2E polymorphism in feline liver. Biochim Biophys Acta 2005;1726(2):194–205.
[71] Truhaut R, Ferrando R, Graillot C, et al. [Induction of cytochrome P 450 by phenobarbital in cats.] C R Acad Sci Hebd Seances Acad Sci D 1978;286(4):371–3 [in French].
[72] Born S, Fraser D, Harlow G, et al. Escherichia coli expression and substrate specificities of canine cytochrome P450 3A12 and rabbit cytochrome P450 3A6. J Pharmacol Exp Ther 1996;278:957–63.
[73] Eguchi K, Nishibe Y, Baba T, et al. Quantitation of cytochrome P450 enzymes (CYP1A1/2, 2B11, 2C21 and 3A12) in dog liver microsomes by enzyme-linked immunosorbent assay. Xenobiotica 1996;26(7):755–63.
[74] Lankford S, Bai S, Goldstein J. Cloning of canine cytochrome P450 2E1 cDNA: identification and characterization of two variant alleles. Drug Metab Dispos 2000;28:981–6.
[75] McLaughlin LA, Paine MJ, Kemp CA, et al. Why is quinidine an inhibitor of cytochrome P450 2D6? The role of key active-site residues in quinidine binding. J Biol Chem 2005;280(46):38617–24.
[76] Roussel F, Duignan D, Lawton M, et al. Expression and characterization of canine cytochrome P450 2D15. Arch Biochem Biophys 1998;357(1):27–36.
[77] Glaeser H, Drescher S, Eichelbaum M, et al. Influence of rifampicin on the expression and function of human intestinal cytochrome P450 enzymes. Br J Clin Pharmacol 2005;59(2):199–206.
[78] Kuroha M, Kayaba H, Kishimoto S, et al. Effect of oral ketoconazole on first-pass effect of nifedipine after oral administration in dogs. J Pharm Sci 2002;91(3):868–73.
[79] Ravis WR, Pedersoli WM, Turco JD. Pharmacokinetics and interactions of digoxin with phenobarbital in dogs. Am J Vet Res 1987;48(8):1244–9.
[80] Breznock EM. Effects of phenobarbital on digitoxin and digoxin elimination in the dog. Am J Vet Res 1975;36(4 Pt 1):371–3.
[81] Vu VT, Bai SA, Abramson FP. Interactions of phenobarbital with propranolol in the dog. 2. Bioavailability, metabolism and pharmacokinetics. J Pharmacol Exp Ther 1983;224(1):55–61.

Vet Clin Small Anim 36 (2006) 987–1001

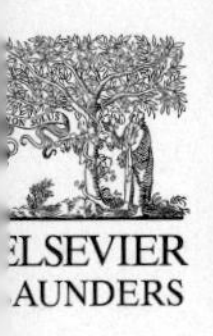

VETERINARY CLINICS
SMALL ANIMAL PRACTICE

Antimicrobial Resistance

Cyril R. Clarke, BVSc, MS, PhD
Center for Veterinary Health Sciences, Oklahoma State University, Stillwater, OK 74078, USA

Development of antimicrobial resistance by microbial pathogens and commensals represents a major threat to animal and public health. In the United States, resistant bacterial infections are estimated to increase human health care costs by approximately $6000 to $30,000 per patient [1] and by at least $4 billion [2] annually. Although the economic impact of antimicrobial resistance in small companion animals is unknown, it is clear that the decreased efficacy of commonly used antibacterial agents and the need to use more expensive drugs not only limit therapeutic options but inflate the expense of treating infectious diseases. In several instances, the armamentarium of antibacterial drugs available to treat infections caused by certain resistant bacteria, such as methicillin-resistant *Staphylococcus aureus* (MRSA), may be so restricted that the ability to cure an infection without producing toxicity is compromised.

Microbes are ubiquitous in the environment, including on the skin and mucous membranes as well as in the gastrointestinal tracts of animals. The ecologic success of microorganisms is largely attributable to their ability to survive hostile conditions and adapt to changes in the environment. Therefore, development of antimicrobial resistance is not a recent phenomenon but an inevitable consequence of microbial cell evolution. Indeed, the ability of bacteria to develop resistance was described soon after the introduction of the pioneer antibacterial agents [3,4]. Current concerns relating to antimicrobial resistance arise principally from the rapid rate of development of resistance relative to the slow rate at which new mechanistic groups of antibiotics are introduced and the conviction that development of resistance is accelerated by overuse of antibiotics. Furthermore, the ability of bacteria to acquire and transfer multiple resistance genes to other bacteria is alarming. The ease with which these genes are transferred between bacteria accelerates the emergence of antibacterial resistance in a particular animal species and increases the risk of spread of resistance to other species, including human beings. The latter is particularly relevant to concerns that use of antibacterial agents in food animals increases the occurrence of resistant infections in human consumers of food animal products. Recently, concerns have also been expressed that contact with small animal pets may serve as a source of infection for people, especially with regard to resistant

E-mail address: cyril.clarke@okstate.edu

0195-5616/06/$ – see front matter
doi:10.1016/j.cvsm.2006.05.002

vetsmall.theclinics.com

Staphylococcus spp. Clearly, if the development and spread of resistance are to be retarded, it is necessary that veterinarians understand the mechanisms that bacteria use to resist antibacterial agents and the processes whereby this capacity is acquired and transferred.

MECHANISMS OF ANTIMICROBIAL RESISTANCE

Microorganisms generally resist the actions of antimicrobial agents by (1) interfering with the stereospecific requirements necessary for binding of the drug to its target site, (2) destroying or altering the conformational integrity of the drug, or (3) preventing the drug from attaining an effective concentration at its site of action. The stereospecific requirements that must be met for antibacterial agents to interact with target receptors can be disrupted by mutations that produce structural changes to ribosomal binding sites (relevant to aminoglycosides, chloramphenicol, tetracyclines, macrolides, and lincosamides), enzymes responsible for nucleic acid synthesis and function (relevant to fluoroquinolones and rifampin), and enzymes responsible for synthesis of bacterial cell walls (relevant to β-lactams). This mechanism of resistance often results in large increases in minimal inhibitory concentration (MIC) values, as is encountered with the structural changes in DNA gyrase that cause substantial decreases in binding affinities to fluoroquinolones.

Examples of mechanisms involving destruction of antibacterial agents or changes in conformational integrity are hydrolysis of the β-lactam ring of penicillins and cephalosporins by β-lactamases and conjugation of aminoglycosides, thus preventing transport of drug into the bacterial cell. Initially identified as being produced by gram-positive staphylococci, β-lactamases are now recognized to be produced in multiple forms by many pathogenically important gram-positive and gram-negative bacterial genera, such as *Staphylococcus*, *Bacillus*, *Pseudomonas*, *Proteus*, *Klebsiella*, *Escherichia*, *Salmonella*, *Shigella*, *Bacteroides*, and *Haemophilus*. The genes encoding production of β-lactamase enzymes may be located on the bacterial chromosome or extrachromosomally on plasmids. Gram-negative bacteria generally produce smaller amounts of β-lactamases than gram-positive bacteria, but this difference has little functional relevance, because gram-negative bacteria usually secrete these enzymes strategically in the periplasmic space, which is where the penicillin or cephalosporin binding proteins are located.

Resistant bacteria can impede attainment of an effective concentration of an antibacterial agent at the site of action by preventing transport across the cell membranes or by active efflux of drug [5] from the bacterial cytoplasm. Impermeability of the cell wall or cell membranes of gram-negative bacteria frequently is a consequence of a reduction in the number of outer membrane porins [6]. Porins are transmembrane protein structures that provide access to relatively water-soluble antibacterial agents. Efflux pumps actively transport drugs from the inner phospholipid layer of the inner cytoplasmic membrane, a site that is sequestered from the aqueous cytoplasm, and therefore is accessible primarily to relatively lipid-soluble drugs. In contrast to mutational changes in the structure of antibacterial target sites, which confer resistance to similar drugs that meet stringent stereospecific characteristics, changes in porin expression and the action of efflux pumps generally are less specific for individual antimicrobial agents. For example, multidrug-resistant efflux pumps exist that have wide substrate activities across a variety of different chemical groups of antibacterial agents.

Surveys of antimicrobial susceptibility trends indicate increasing resistance to multiple antibacterial agents, which greatly complicates selection of effective antimicrobial therapies. As described previously, a single gene operon encoding for a single mechanism, such as expression of outer membrane porins or an efflux pump, may confer multiple drug resistance because these mechanisms are not specific for particular classes of drugs but discriminate only on the basis of general physicochemical characteristics, such as lipid solubility. Multiple drug resistance may also arise from the accumulation of multiple gene operons, each encoding for a different mechanism of resistance. Accumulation of resistance-encoding genes is promoted by a variety of genetic processes that greatly facilitate transfer of nucleic acids between bacteria.

ACQUISITION AND TRANSFER OF RESISTANCE GENES

De novo acquisition of resistance-encoding genes occurs by mutations arising from random errors in nucleic acid sequence resulting from polymerase-mediated replication of DNA. Mutation rates for antimicrobial-resistant phenotypes may range from 1 in 10^9 to 1 in 10^6 cell divisions. Although this rate may seem to be low, the likelihood of resistant mutants arising is actually quite high because of the high replication rate of bacteria. Indeed, resistant mutants generally can be produced after only a few sequential isolations and cultures on media containing a gradient of antibacterial agent concentration.

Once resistance has been acquired by mutation, it can be transferred by several processes, including conjugation, transduction, and transformation. Although transduction and transformation may be important in specific circumstances, such as transfer of resistance by transduction between staphylococci, conjugation presents the greatest risk for transfer of resistance genes among gram-negative bacteria. Conjugation involves transfer of a plasmid or circular extrachromosomal DNA via an intercellular bridge from a donor to a recipient bacterium [7]. The entire process, including formation of the intercellular bridge, known as a pilus, is encoded by genes on the plasmid (Fig. 1). Once the mating pair of bacteria is linked by the pilus, a single strand of the plasmid is cut and transferred to the recipient cell. Replication of the recipient and donor nucleic acid strands restores the resistance-encoding potential of the separated bacteria. In this manner, resistance genes can be transferred between bacteria of different strains, species, and possibly even genera.

Although resistance genes can be expressed from plasmids acquired by conjugation, the stability of such expression may be enhanced by insertion of these genes in the bacterial chromosome. This often involves a recombination event

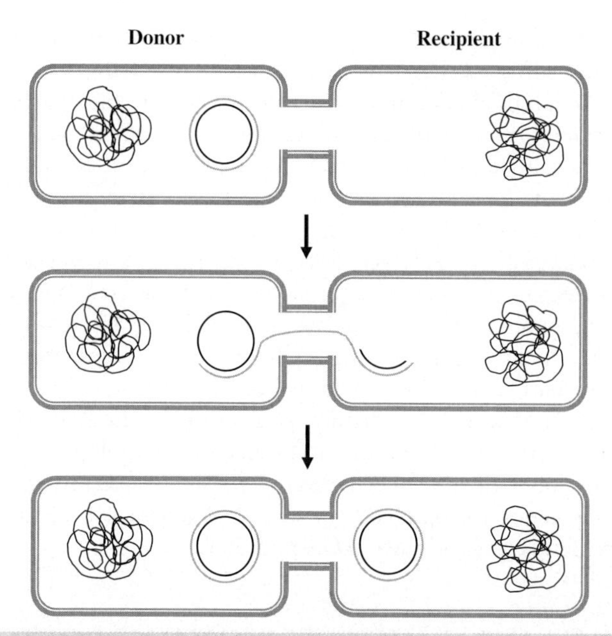

Fig. 1. Acquisition of antimicrobial resistance gene(s) by conjugation. After production of a pilus, a single strand of plasmid DNA is transferred to the recipient. During transfer, the remaining DNA strand in the donor and the newly acquired strand in the recipient undergo replication to produce functional double-stranded plasmids.

referred to as transposition [8]. Transposons are DNA elements that can move from one DNA location to another, including between plasmids and chromosomes. Transposases, encoded by the transposon, cut out donor DNA and insert this into the recipient, without regard to a stringent requirement that the DNA sequences have complementary base pairing. Such nonhomologous recombinations provide considerable mobility to antimicrobial resistance genes.

Conjugation and transposition may collaborate with integrases to facilitate transfer and accumulation of multiple genes encoding for antimicrobial resistance (Fig. 2). Integrases are site-specific recombinases encoded by integrons, which are genetic units that provide for assembly of multiple resistance gene cassettes in a single DNA location, including within a transposon or plasmid. Each gene cassette may contain an antimicrobial resistance gene and an integrase-specific recombination site. Under the influence of integrases, multiple gene cassettes may be sequentially inserted in the integron at a cassette receptor site. Expression of these genes can be regulated collectively by a single promoter, thus providing for coordinated defense against many different antimicrobial agents. Therefore, once acquired by random mutation, the collaborative function of conjugation, transposons, and integrons can greatly facilitate transfer and expression of multiple drug resistance, thus demonstrating that bacteria have a phenomenal adaptive ability to survive antibacterial therapy.

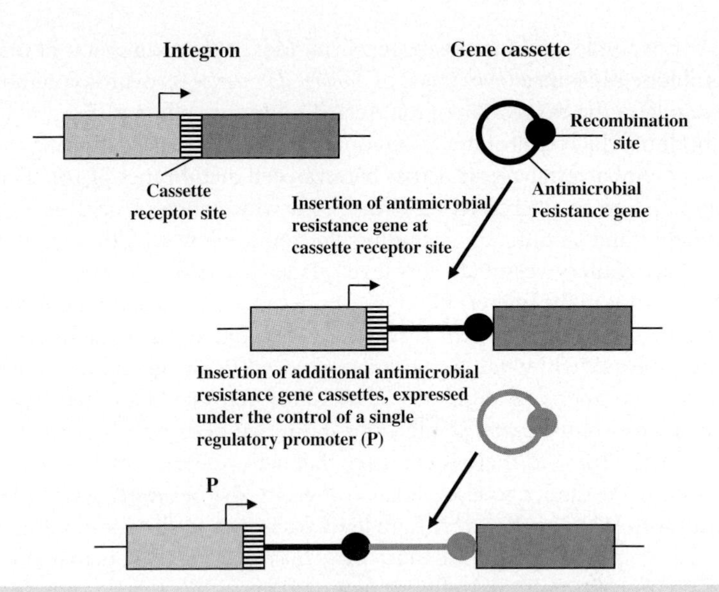

Fig. 2. Accumulation of mobile antimicrobial resistance gene cassettes in an integron.

SELECTION AND EXPRESSION OF RESISTANCE RESULTING FROM EXPOSURE TO ANTIBACTERIAL AGENTS

Generally, antibiotic exposure does not cause a susceptible strain to mutate to a resistant one. Nevertheless, exposure to antimicrobial agents promotes emergence of resistance by facilitating the survival of resistant strains or inducing the expression of existing antimicrobial resistance genes. Classically, resistance in a bacterial population can be identified by the existence of at least two distinct subpopulations separated on the basis of MIC values. Survival of the relatively resistant subpopulation is promoted by exposure to concentrations of antibiotics that inhibit only the susceptible subpopulation. As a result of this differential effect, resistant strains increase in number until they represent a larger proportion of the population as a whole, thus increasing the likelihood that they cause infectious diseases. Within environments that are subject to frequent and consistent antibacterial use patterns, such as intensive care units, the emergence of predominant populations of resistant strains is accelerated, particularly when little care is taken to prevent transfer of resistant strains between patients. Antibiotic exposure not only promotes the survival of drug-resistant pathogenic bacteria but increases the population of drug-resistant nonpathogenic bystanders, many of which are commensals in the upper respiratory and gastrointestinal tracts, thus increasing the reservoir of resistance in the bacterial population as a whole and increasing the opportunity for resistance to be transferred to pathogenic bacteria by processes like conjugation and transposition.

Aside from the effect of antimicrobial exposure on survival of resistant mutants, antimicrobial agents may also induce the expression of existing resistance genes. For example, antimicrobial agents can induce the expression of the multiple antibiotic resistance (*mar*) locus in *Salmonella enterica* serovar Typhimurium, which regulates the expression of the AcrAB multidrug efflux pump and OmpF porin, both of which contribute to multiple drug resistance by affecting the permeation of antibacterial agents across bacterial cell membranes [9,10]. The Mar phenotype possesses increased resistance to a wide range of organic solvents, disinfectants, and antibiotics, including fluoroquinolones. Although the *marRAB* system confers relatively low-level resistance (MIC values are usually only two to four times higher) [9], it is considered to be clinically important because expression of this system serves as a stepping stone to higher levels of resistance, particularly when bacteria are exposed to marginal and/or subtherapeutic concentrations of antibiotics. The Mar phenotype has been implicated in antibiotic-resistant *Salmonella* infections in human beings and a variety of domestic animals [10], and there is evidence that active efflux may be the primary mechanism of resistance to ciprofloxacin used by the *Salmonella enterica* serovar Typhimurium [11]. Furthermore high-level resistance to fluoroquinolones, mediated primarily by DNA gyrase mutations, may depend on concurrent expression of the AcrAB multidrug efflux pump [12].

Another example of an inducible mechanism of resistance is the protection conferred by the *erm* genes of staphylococci. Under the influence of macrolides and lincosamides, expression of *erm* genes encodes for a change in the bacterial ribosomal binding site targeted by these antibacterial agents. A recent study conducted in the United Kingdom indicated a high incidence of inducible *erm*-mediated resistance to clindamycin in MRSA and recommended routine screening of these isolates for inducible resistance [13].

EMERGENCE OF RESISTANCE IN SMALL COMPANION ANIMALS

In comparison with people and food animals, relatively few studies have addressed the emergence of resistance in small companion animals and the relationships between the use of antibacterial agents and development of resistance. The small number of investigations that have tracked changes in resistance over time generally indicate that resistance of notable bacteria, such as *Escherichia coli* and *Staphylococcus* spp, to newer antibacterial therapies is increasing. For example, a review of antimicrobial drug use and resistance in dogs based on 15 years of records (1984–1998) from a teaching hospital in Canada concluded that the incidence of resistant coagulase-positive *Staphylococcus* spp varied according to concurrent use patterns for individual antibacterial agents [14]. There was a significant decrease in resistance to penicillin G and ampicillin, which correlated with a decline in the use of these antibacterial agents over a similar period, whereas resistance to cephalothin and enrofloxacin increased concurrently with increased use of these newer antibacterial agents. During the same period, isolation of multidrug-resistant *Enterococcus* spp and *Pseudomonas aeruginosa* from urinary tract infections increased relative to other causes of infection, again suggesting that exposure to antibacterial agents promoted emergence of resistant bacterial genera and strains. A more recent study conducted in the United States indicated that ciprofloxacin and enrofloxacin resistance of bacteria isolated from the urinary tracts of dogs had increased, although more than 80% of isolates were still susceptible to these fluoroquinolones [15]. The bacteria most commonly isolated were *E coli*, *Proteus mirabilis*, and *Staphylococcus intermedius*. In the United Kingdom, a retrospective study of resistance of *E coli* and *Staphylococcus* spp to antimicrobials used in a small animal referral hospital revealed significantly increasing trends only with respect to resistance of *E coli* to amoxicillin, enrofloxacin, and streptomycin [16]. No changes in resistance were identified for most bacterial-drug interactions; neither were there any significant differences in prevalences of multiple drug-resistant *E coli*, *Proteus* spp, *Pseudomonas* spp, staphylococci, or streptococci. Analysis of resistance of *E coli* to antimicrobials used in a companion animal community practice revealed significant rising trends of resistance to clavulanate-amoxicillin and streptomycin and in multiple drug resistance of *E coli*, *Proteus* spp, and *Pseudomonas* spp, whereas resistance of *Staphylococcus* spp to ampicillin and penicillin G was observed to decrease [17]. In contrast to the results of these studies, the introduction of marbofloxacin in Europe was not associated with any significant increase in resistance over a 7-year period (1994–2001) [18].

Irrespective of whether trends have been identified whereby increases in resistance are correlated with the use of specific antibacterial agents, it is clear that resistance of certain small animal pathogens is high enough to justify concern. This is particularly true of *Staphylococcus* spp, which is the subject of much attention in the human health domain, especially with regard to methicillin and vancomycin resistance. An analysis of canine *S intermedius* isolated in France in 2002 revealed that more than 60% of strains produced β-lactamases against penicillin G [19]. Lower levels of resistance were measured for alternative non-β-lactam antibacterial agents, such as oxytetracycline (46%), chloramphenicol (30%), erythromycin (28%), clindamycin (22%), doxycycline (6%), gentamicin (2%), and fluoroquinolones (2%). No resistance was observed to the combination of clavulanate and amoxicillin, cephalosporins, the combination of sulfonamide-trimethoprim, and oxacillin, which serves as a reliable indicator of methicillin resistance. These observations are consistent with those of studies conducted in the United States, United Kingdom, Denmark, and Germany between 1986 and 1995, in which resistance of *S intermedius* to penicillin and tetracycline was relatively high but resistance to the sulfonamide-trimethoprim combination and enrofloxacin was either low or nonexistent [20].

More recent studies published in 2005 indicate that higher levels of methicillin resistance exist among small animal isolates than were described in earlier reports, however. A survey of seven veterinary teaching hospitals in the United States revealed that 11% of *S aureus* isolated from dogs was methicillin resistant [21]. Studies conducted in the United Kingdom and Ireland also confirm the recent emergence of MRSA, often associated with postoperative and wound infections [22,23]. In addition to methicillin resistance, these isolates may be resistant to other antibacterial agents, such as macrolides, lincosamides, and fluoroquinolones, thus presenting few alternatives for successful therapy [22].

Although resistance of gram-negative bacteria seems to vary according to geographic origin, there is evidence that resistance to newer antibacterial agents, including those with important human therapeutic value, may be emerging. Results of a study conducted in Sweden during 2002 and 2003 indicate that resistance of *E coli* derived from urogenital infections was generally low and no different from levels of resistance reported approximately 10 years earlier [24]. The highest proportion of resistance observed (26%) in this study was for strains isolated from urine of dogs in hospitals during 1991 through 1993. Similarly, resistance of *E coli* isolated from dogs in Finland, irrespective of prior antimicrobial therapy, was reported to be low [25]. Nevertheless, a study conducted in Italy over the period 2001 through 2003 reported that 45% of *E coli* strains were resistant to tetracycline, 34% to the combination of sulfamethoxazole and trimethoprim, 15% to enrofloxacin, and 7% to cefotaxime [26]. Likewise, in Trinidad, more than one third of all *Salmonella* spp isolated from dogs were resistant to cephalothin [27], thus suggesting that resistance of Enterobacteriaceae to cephalosporins may present a therapeutic concern, especially considering the importance of this group of antibacterial agents in the treatment of gastrointestinal infections in human patients.

In summary, antimicrobial resistance of small animal pathogens varies considerably depending on geographic location, the history of exposure to antibacterial agents, and the specific microorganism of interest. Although resistance of microorganisms affecting small animals may be less widespread than in human beings and food animals, probably because of differences in antibacterial exposure, there are nevertheless sufficient data to conclude that the prevalence of resistance in dogs and cats is high enough to pose therapeutic challenges and to justify development and implementation of strategies to retard further development of resistance.

HUMAN HEALTH IMPLICATIONS OF ANTIBACTERIAL RESISTANCE IN SMALL ANIMALS

Emergence of antibiotic-resistant bacteria in food animals and the risk posed to human consumers when these resistant bacteria contaminate food products have been subjects of considerable concern in the veterinary and human health communities. Indeed, the use of newer drugs, such as fluoroquinolones, to control animal diseases has been the target of much criticism by the human health community because of the possibility that selection of resistant bacteria and subsequent bacterial contamination of food products may lead to an increase in resistant infections in people [28,29]. Until recently, less attention has been directed at the possibility of direct transfer of resistant microorganisms between small animal pets and people, despite their close physical contact in home environments and use of the same antibacterial agents in human and veterinary practices. In their excellent review of the role of pet animals as reservoirs of antimicrobial-resistant bacteria, Guardabassi and colleagues [30] noted that veterinarians frequently use first-line antibacterials, such as amoxicillin-clavulanate, cephalosporins, and fluoroquinolones, in pet animals and that the ensuing resistance in pathogenic bacteria as well as commensals presents a significant risk for zoonotic transfer between pets and people. Resistance phenotypes of particular clinical interest include MRSA (including strains producing the highly pathogenic Panton-Valentine leukocidin toxin [31]), vancomycin-resistant enterococci (VRE), and multidrug-resistant *Salmonella* spp.

Antimicrobial-resistant strains isolated from small animals often are indistinguishable from strains isolated from people caring for these animals [23]. For example, using pulsed-field gel electrophoresis, investigators in Ireland observed that the most frequently occurring pattern of MRSA from veterinary sources was the same as the most prevalent strain found in the human population [22]. Based on the epidemiologic analyses of disease outbreaks, transfer of a variety of resistant infections between pets and people has been reported, including multiple drug-resistant *S typhimurium* [30]. In most instances, however, transfer seems to be from people to their pets [32], as is probably true for the transfer of most MRSA strains [33,34] and VRE. Nevertheless, such transfer still poses a risk to human health, because pets can then serve as reservoirs of these microorganisms and as a source of infection for other susceptible people and animals living in the same household.

NEW ANTIMICROBIAL DRUGS ON THE HORIZON

Historically, the principal strategy used against antimicrobial resistance has been the introduction of new antibacterial agents with novel mechanisms of action to which previously resistant microorganisms are susceptible. For example, initial β-lactamase–mediated resistance to natural penicillins was addressed by the development of the antistaphylococcal penicillins, such as methicillin and cloxacillin. When multidrug-resistant bacteria subsequently developed resistance to methicillin, veterinarians and physicians turned to vancomycin as a drug of last resort, thus severely limiting therapeutic options. Although newer products, such as teicoplanin and linezolid, may be used systemically to treat vancomycin-resistant staphylococcus, the pace at which new drugs are being introduced is clearly insufficient to keep up with the rate at which resistance currently develops. Indeed, the number of new antibacterial agents approved by the US Food and Drug Administration in recent years has declined by more than 50% relative to the approval rate 20 years ago [35]. Challenges involved in antimicrobial drug development as well as economic incentives in favor of developing other drugs used to treat chronic medical conditions in elderly people, such as hypercholesterolemia, hypertension, psychologic and/or psychiatric disorders, and arthritis, have discouraged pharmaceutical companies from developing new molecular entities with activity against microorganisms. During the period 1998 through 2002, nine new antibacterial agents were approved for use in human beings, and only two of these (linezolid and daptomycin) exert their antibacterial activity via novel mechanisms [35]. Based on public disclosures of the world's 15 largest pharmaceutical companies, five new antibacterial molecular entities were estimated to be under development in 2004, whereas the numbers of new molecular entities being developed to treat erectile dysfunction, bladder hyperactivity, and anxiety were four, eight, and nine, respectively [35]. None of the antibacterial agents currently under development seem to have novel mechanisms of action.

Clearly, concerted efforts need to be directed at improving the prospects for development of new antibacterial agents, including modification of existing drugs and discovery of novel bacterial target mechanisms [36]. Irrespective of any successes in this regard, however, it is imperative that currently available agents be used in such a manner that the inevitable development of resistance is retarded and their efficacy is prolonged as much as possible.

STRATEGIES TO AVOID DEVELOPMENT OF ANTIMICROBIAL RESISTANCE

Strategies considered effective in delaying development of resistance involve minimizing the use of antimicrobial agents and using dosage regimens to achieve drug concentrations at the site of infection that eliminate pathogenic organisms without promoting survival of more resistant microbial subpopulations. In support of these strategies, a plethora of antimicrobial prudent use guidelines have been published by a variety of agencies, including the American Veterinary Medical Association [37], the American Animal Hospital Association [38], and the American Association of Feline Practitioners [39]. Generally, these guidelines adhere to the following principles:

1. Antibacterial agents should only be used when bacterial infection is confirmed or strongly suspected to exist. Obviously, patients that have viral, mycotic, neoplastic, or parasitic diseases do not respond to antibacterial therapy. Furthermore, increased body temperature does not necessarily indicate the presence of a bacterial infection but can also be caused by immune-mediated diseases, neoplasia, drug reactions, exercise, excitement, and increased environmental temperature. In particular, antibacterial agents should be avoided in the treatment of viral upper respiratory tract infections unless secondary bacterial infection is confirmed. Studies conducted in children have demonstrated that antibacterial treatment of these uncomplicated infections does not enhance resolution of the disease, even in the presence of purulent exudates from the nares or throat [40]. Similarly, antibacterial agents are seldom indicated in the treatment of feline lower urinary tract infections, which generally do not have a bacterial cause.

Use of antimicrobial agents should also be minimized by using sound patient care management practices, such as vaccination and isolation of infected animals. The effectiveness of strategies designed to prevent the spread of resistant microorganisms between infected individuals is best illustrated by the success of containing the spread of MRSA in human hospitals by diagnostic screening of patients, followed by isolation, use of disposable gloves and gowns by medical personnel, and washing of hands with antiseptic soaps [41,42].

2. When possible, in vitro sensitivity testing and pharmacokinetic data should be used to ensure attainment of an efficacious concentration of antibacterial drug at the site of infection. It is essential that an effective concentration of antimicrobial agent be attained at the site of infection for a duration sufficient to achieve elimination of the infection and minimize development of resistance. Therefore, pharmacodynamic as well as pharmacokinetic factors need to be considered in the selection of specific antibacterial agents and appropriate dosage regimens. The former involves use of in vitro sensitivity testing, especially for microbial isolates that have an unpredictable response to antibacterial therapy, such as Enterobacteriaceae, *Staphylococcus* spp, and *Pseudomonas* spp. The latter involves consideration of such factors as lipid solubility of the drug and whether there are diffusional barriers that impede distribution of the drug between the vascular system and the site of infection, such as the blood-brain barrier and infectious lesions that become sequestered by accumulation of exudates and fibrous tissue. Doses used should always be high enough to inhibit growth and survival of more resistant subpopulations of microorganisms, irrespective of whether the antibacterial agent is used prophylactically or to treat existing infection.

An approach developed by Drlica and his coworkers [43,44] to promote administration of doses that are high enough to minimize survival of relatively resistant strains of bacteria involves the use of MIC and mutant prevention concentration (MPC) values. The latter is defined as the lowest drug concentration at which growth of the least susceptible single-step mutant strain is inhibited (Fig. 3). Drug doses that achieve concentrations at the site of infection that are higher than the MIC_{90} but lower than the MPC can be expected to promote emergence of resistant subpopulations of bacteria because of the competitive advantage resulting from the inhibitory effects of the antibacterial agent on more susceptible strains. Doses that result in concentrations that exceed the MPC limit the selection of resistant mutants, however. When the difference between the MIC_{90} and MPC (termed the *mutant selection window*) is wide and no single drug can be identified that can be used safely to produce concentrations higher that the MPC for a particular pathogen, consideration should be given to combining antibacterial agents with different mechanisms of action. Estimates of MPC values for particular drug-pathogen combinations can be generated by culturing large numbers of bacteria on media containing a range of antibacterial drug concentrations. Considering that the frequency of single-step mutations conferring resistant phenotypes can be lower than 10^{-7}, at least 10^{10} bacteria are needed to ensure the presence of resistant subpopulations in the test culture. Using this approach, mutant selection windows have been estimated for a variety of drug-pathogen combinations [45]. Although there clearly are several challenges in using these data to predict in vivo activity, such as differences in efficacy requirements for concentration-dependent (eg, aminoglycosides, fluoroquinolones) versus time-dependent (eg, β-lactams, macrolides) antibacterial agents, using mutant selection windows offers a quantitative approach to designing drug doses that are less likely to promote emergence of antibacterial resistance.

3. Avoid prolonged use of antibacterial agents. Although it is important that the use of antibacterial agents be minimized, treatment should not be discontinued before the infection is eliminated. Premature termination of therapy can result in the persistence of relatively resistant strains of microorganisms that

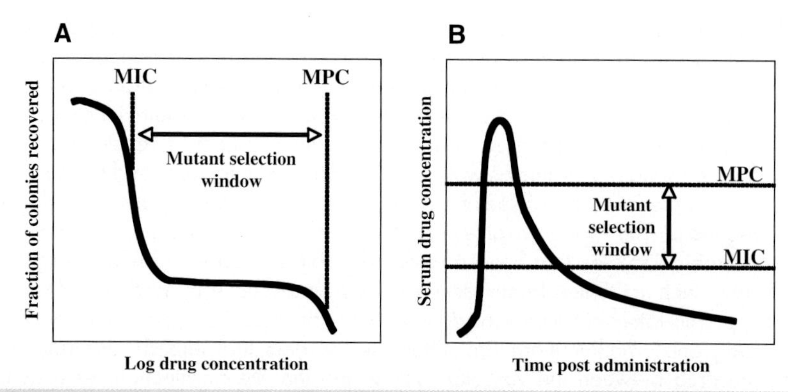

Fig. 3. Mutant selection window (MPC – MIC), expressed in terms of the fraction of microbial colonies that survive exposure to a particular drug concentration (*A*) and the time after drug administration (*B*). (*Adapted from* Zhao X, Drlica K. Restricting the selection of antibiotic-resistant mutants: a general strategy derived from fluoroquinolone studies. Clin Infect Dis 2001;33:S149, S151; with permission.)

require longer exposure periods for successful treatment. The resolution of clinical signs often is not a reliable indicator of elimination of the infection. A meta-analysis of 3-day versus longer antibacterial therapy of cystitis in women confirmed that there was no difference in symptomatic cure rates between the two durations of therapy but that the prolonged treatment was more successful in achieving bacteriologic cure and reducing recurrence of the infection [46]. Collection of clinical samples for culture and sensitivity testing at the conclusion of treatment may be used to determine whether therapy needs to be prolonged or if an alternative drug should be used.

Generally, antimicrobial therapy should be continued for 7 to 10 days or for 4 to 5 days after resolution of fever [38]. Patients that have compromised host defenses, such as those that are leukopenic, should be treated for 10 to 14 days. Chronic infections may require 4 to 6 weeks of treatment.

4. When possible, select narrow-spectrum agents, based on definitive identification of the infectious agent, rather than broad-spectrum drugs. Efficacious antimicrobial therapy is accomplished and emergence of resistance is minimized when the concentration of antibacterial agent achieved at the site of infection is high enough to eliminate susceptible and relatively resistant strains. This objective is most likely to be achieved when attention is focused on the specific relationships between drug dose, tissue concentration of drug, and susceptibility of the target pathogen. Broad-spectrum antimicrobials affect a wide variety of microorganisms (but with varying sensitivity) and may thus select relatively resistant strains of nontarget microorganisms. Even when these collateral effects involve nonpathogenic microorganisms, emergence of resistance is promoted because the propagation of these resistant bystanders increases the reservoir of resistance in the population.
5. Monitor development of resistance by means of well-designed surveillance schemes. Long-term preservation of the effectiveness of antimicrobial agents

relies on the implementation of strategies to monitor emergence of resistance associated with specific practices (eg, use of fluoroquinolones in food animals, treatment of staphylococcal infections using glycopeptides). Although such surveillance usually is performed by governmental regulatory agencies [47], such as the National Antimicrobial Resistance Monitoring System (NARMS) [48], veterinary clinical service facilities also have a responsibility for monitoring antimicrobial agent use and susceptibility profiles of prevailing pathogens. Unfortunately, based on the paucity of reports pertaining to studies in the scientific literature involving small companion animals, little attention is devoted to this responsibility including in veterinary teaching hospitals.

SUMMARY

Development of antimicrobial resistance is an inevitable consequence of exposure of microorganisms to antimicrobial agents. It represents an evolutionary consequence of multiple genetic strategies designed to ensure survival in a hostile and changing environment. Although emergence of resistance cannot be prevented, it can be retarded by minimizing use of antimicrobial agents and avoiding selection of relatively resistant pathogenic and nonpathogenic strains caused by exposure to tissue concentrations that confer a competitive advantage. Most attention in veterinary medicine has focused on the emergence of resistance in food-borne pathogens, with relatively little attention being devoted to small companion animals, despite the frequent use of antimicrobial agents in these animals, evidence that resistance is emerging, and potential for transfer of resistance between companion animals and people. To retard further emergence of resistance in small companion animals, it is imperative that surveillance programs be instituted to monitor development of resistance.

References

[1] Cosgrove S. The relationship between antimicrobial resistance and patient outcomes: mortality, length of hospital stay, and health care costs. Clin Infect Dis 2006;42:S82–9.

[2] McGowan JE. Economic impact of antimicrobial resistance. Emerg Infect Dis 2001;7: 286–92. [Erratum in Emerg Infect Dis 2001;7:765].

[3] Bryson V, Demerec M. Patterns of resistance to antimicrobial agents. Ann NY Acad Sci 1950;53:283–9.

[4] Demerec M. Origin of bacterial resistance to antibiotics. J Bacteriol 1948;56:63–74.

[5] Putman M, Van Veen H, Konings W. Molecular properties of bacterial multidrug transporters. Microbiol Mol Biol Rev 2000;64:672–93.

[6] Mallea M, Chevalier J, Bornet C, et al. Porin alteration and active efflux: two *in vivo* drug resistance strategies used by *Enterobacter aerogenes*. Microbiology 1998;144:3003–9.

[7] Snyder L, Champness W. Conjugation. In: Molecular genetics of bacteria. Washington (DC): ASM Press; 1997. p. 129–46.

[8] Snyder L, Champness W. Transposition and nonhomologous recombination. In: Molecular genetics of bacteria. Washington (DC): ASM Press; 1997. p. 195–213.

[9] Randall L, Woodward M. The multiple antibiotic resistance (*mar*) locus and its significance. Res Vet Sci 2002;72:87–93.

[10] Webber MA, Piddock LJV. Absence of mutations in *marRAB* or *soxRS* in *acrB*-overexpressing fluoroquinolone-resistant clinical and veterinary isolates of *Escherichia coli*. Antimicrob Agents Chemother 2001;45:1550–2.

[11] Giraud E, Cloeckaert A, Kerboeuf D, et al. Evidence for active efflux as the primary mechanism of resistance to ciprofloxacin in *Salmonella enterica* serovar Typhimurium. Antimicrob Agents Chemother 2000;244:1223–8.
[12] Oethinger M, Podglajen I, Kern W, et al. Overexpression of the *marA* or *soxS* regulatory gene in clinical topoisomerase mutants of *Escherichia coli*. Antimicrob Agents Chemother 1998;42:2089–94.
[13] Rich M, Deighton L, Roberts L. Clindamycin-resistance in methicillin-resistant *Staphylococcus aureus* isolated from animals. Vet Microbiol 2005;111:237–40.
[14] Prescott JF, Hanna WJB, Reid-Smith R, et al. Antimicrobial drug use and resistance in dogs. Can Vet J 2002;43:107.
[15] Cohn L, Gary A, Fales W, et al. Trends in fluoroquinolone resistance of bacteria isolated from canine urinary tracts. J Vet Diagn Invest 2003;15:338–43.
[16] Normand E, Gibson N, Taylor D, et al. Trends of antimicrobial resistance in bacterial isolates from a small animal referral hospital. Vet Rec 2000;146:151–5.
[17] Normand E, Gibson N, Reid S, et al. Antimicrobial-resistance trends in bacterial isolates from companion-animal community practice in the UK. Prev Vet Med 2000;46:267–78.
[18] Meunier D, Acar J, Martel J, et al. A seven-year survey of susceptibility to marbofloxacin of pathogenic strains isolated from pets. Int J Antimicrob Agents 2004;24:592–8.
[19] Ganiere J, Medaille C, Mangion C. Antimicrobial drug susceptibility of *Staphylococcus intermedius* clinical isolates from canine pyoderma. J Vet Med B Infect Dis Vet Public Health 2005;52:25–31.
[20] Werckenthin C, Cardoso M, Martel J-L, et al. Antimicrobial resistance in staphylococci from animals with particular reference to bovine *Staphylococcus aureus*, porcine *Staphylococcus hyicus*, and canine *Staphylococcus intermedius*. Vet Res 2001;32:341–62.
[21] Middleton J, Fales W, Luby C, et al. Surveillance of *Staphylococcus aureus* in veterinary teaching hospitals. J Clin Microbiol 2005;43:2916–9.
[22] O'Mahony R, Abbott Y, Leonard F, et al. Methicillin-resistant *Staphylococcus aureus* (MRSA) isolated from animals and veterinary personnel in Ireland. Vet Microbiol 2005;109:285–96.
[23] Rich M, Roberts L, Kearns A. Methicillin-resistant staphylococci isolated from animals. Vet Microbiol 2005;105:313–4.
[24] Hagman R, Greko C. Antimicrobial resistance in *Escherichia coli* isolated from bitches with pyometra and from urine samples from other dogs. Vet Rec 2005;157:193–7.
[25] Rantala M, Lahti E, Kuhalampil J, et al. Antimicrobial resistance in *Staphylococcus* spp., *Escherichia coli* and *Enterococcus* spp. in dogs given antibiotics for chronic dermatological disorders, compared with non-treated control dogs. Acta Vet Scand 2004;45:37–45.
[26] Carattoli A, Lovari S, Franco A, et al. Extended-spectrum β-lactamases in *Escherichia coli* isolated from dogs and cats in Rome, Italy, from 2001 to 2003. Antimicrob Agents Chemother 2005;49:833–5.
[27] Seepersadsingh N, Adesiyun AA, Seebaransingh R. Prevalence and antimicrobial resistance of *Salmonella* spp. in non-diarrhoeic dogs in Trinidad. J Vet Med B Infect Dis Vet Public Health 2004;51:337–42.
[28] Butzler J. Campylobacter, from obscurity to celebrity. Clin Microbiol Infect 2004;10:868–76.
[29] Endtz H, Ruijs G, van Klingeren B, et al. Quinolone resistance in campylobacter isolated from man and poultry following the introduction of fluoroquinolones in veterinary medicine. J Antimicrob Chemother 1991;27:199–208.
[30] Guardabassi L, Schwarz S, Lloyd DH. Pet animals as reservoirs of antimicrobial-resistant bacteria. J Antimicrob Chemother 2004;54:321–32.
[31] Rankin S, Roberts S, O'Shea K, et al. Panton valentine leukocidin (PVL) toxin positive MRSA strains isolated from companion animals. Vet Microbiol 2005;108:145–8.
[32] Sannes M, Kuskowski M, Johnson J. Antimicrobial resistance of *Escherichia coli* strains isolated from urine of women with cystitis or pyelonephritis and feces of dogs and healthy humans. J Am Vet Med Assoc 2004;225:368–73.

[33] Enoch D, Karas J, Slater J, et al. MRSA carriage in a pet therapy dog. J Hosp Infect 2005;60: 186–8.
[34] Malik S, Peng H, Barton M. Antibiotic resistance in staphylococci associated with cats and dogs. J Appl Microbiol 2005;99:1283–93.
[35] Spellberg B, Powers J, Brass E, et al. Trends in antimicrobial drug development: implications for the future. Clin Infect Dis 2004;38:1279–86.
[36] Wise R. The development of new antimicrobial agents. BMJ 1998;317:643–4.
[37] American Veterinary Medical Association. American Veterinary Medical Association judicious therapeutic use of antimicrobials. AVMA Scientific Activities Division, Food Safety Advisory Committee. Available at: www.avma.org/scienact/jtua/jtua98.asp. Accessed January 2006.
[38] American Animal Hospital Association. AAHA guidelines on the judicious use of antimicrobials in dogs. AVMA Scientific Activities Division, Food Safety Advisory Committee. Available at: www.avma.org/scienact/jtua/canine/jtuacanine.asp. 2001. Accessed January 2006.
[39] American Association of Feline Practitioners. American Association of Feline Practitioners basic guidelines of judicious therapeutic use of antimicrobials in cats. AVMA Scientific Activities Division, Food Safety Advisory Committee. Available at: www.avma.org/scienact/jtua/feline/jtuafeline.asp. 2004. Accessed January 2006.
[40] Gonzales R, Bartlett JG, Besser RE, et al. Principles of appropriate antibiotic use for treatment of nonspecific upper respiratory tract infections in adults: background. Ann Intern Med 2001;134:490–4.
[41] Bissett L. Controlling the risk of MRSA infection: screening and isolating patients. Br J Nurs 2005;14:386–90.
[42] Eveillard M, Eb F, Tramier B, et al. Evaluation of the contribution of isolation precautions in prevention and control of multi-resistant bacteria in a teaching hospital. J Hosp Infect 2001;47:116–24.
[43] Drlica K. The mutant selection window and antimicrobial resistance. J Antimicrob Chemother 2003;52:11–7.
[44] Zhao X, Drlica K. Restricting the selection of antibiotic-resistant mutants: a general strategy derived from fluoroquinolone studies. Clin Infect Dis 2001;33(Suppl):S147–56.
[45] Smith HJ, Nichol KA, Hoban DJ, et al. Stretching the mutant prevention concentration (MPC) beyond its limits. J Antimicrob Chemother 2003;51:1323–5.
[46] Katchman E, Milo G, Paul M, et al. Three-day vs longer duration of antibiotic treatment for cystitis in women: systematic review and meta-analysis. Am J Med 2005;118:1196–207.
[47] Centers for Disease Control. Food and Drug Administration, National Institutes of Health. A public health plan to combat antimicrobial resistance. Part 1: domestic issues. Interagency Task Force on Antimicrobial Resistance. Available at: www.cdc.gov/drugresistance/actionplan/. 2001. Accessed January 2006.
[48] Centers for Disease Control. Food and Drug Administration, US Department of Agriculture. National antimicrobial resistance monitoring system (NARMS): enteric bacteria. National Center for Infectious Diseases. Available at: www.cdc.gov/narms/. 1996. Accessed January 2006.

ELSEVIER
SAUNDERS
Vet Clin Small Anim 36 (2006) 1003–1047
VETERINARY CLINICS
SMALL ANIMAL PRACTICE

Principles of Antimicrobial Therapy

Dawn Merton Boothe, DVM, PhD

Department of Anatomy, Physiology, and Pharmacology, 109 Greene Hall,
College of Veterinary Medicine, Auburn University, AL 36849, USA

JUDICIOUS ANTIMICROBIAL USE

"Even experienced practitioners may not realize that giving a patient antibiotics affects not just that patient, but also their environment, and all the other people that come into contact with that environment." With that statement, Dancer [1] summarizes the importance of judicious antimicrobial therapy in veterinary (and human) medicine. Clearly, the most compelling reason for practicing judicious antimicrobial use is to facilitate therapeutic success. The definition of therapeutic success is changing to include both eradication of infection and avoidance of resistance. The two goals do not necessarily go hand in hand. However, if sufficient concentrations of antimicrobials are achieved at the site of infection such that all infecting isolates are killed, then both goals will be met. The mantra "dead bugs don't mutate" should be the driving force behind antimicrobial use.

Judicious antimicrobial use should also be pursued because of public health considerations. Veterinary use of antimicrobials has been intensely scrutinized in the past decades. The focus has largely been oriented toward use of antimicrobials as growth promotants in food animals and subsequent resistant infections in human beings. The focus is shifting toward the household pet, however. This reflects a dramatic increase in the number of household animals as well as a closer relationship between pets and pet owners. Further, many antimicrobials used in small animals are approved for use in people. Additionally, a number of organisms have been transmitted between small animals and their owners. For example, resistant strains of *Staphylococcus intermedius*, *Campylobacter* spp, *Salmonella* spp, and *Escherichia coli* have been cited as possible zoonotic concerns [2,3]. Methicillin-resistant *Staphylococcus aureus* (MRSA) has been isolated in family members and pets in the same household. In dogs, *E coli* strains are phylogenetically similar to pathogenic strains causing infection in human beings; more than 15% of canine fecal deposits in the environment contain *E coli* strains related to virulent human strains [4].

In human medicine, antibiotic stewardship (ie, judicious antimicrobial use) has become the focus for reducing resistance [5]. The veterinary profession would be

E-mail address: boothdm@auburn.edu

0195-5616/06/$ – see front matter
doi:10.1016/j.cvsm.2006.07.002

vetsmall.theclinics.com

prudent to pursue the same path. We have further to go. The age of using antimicrobials for lack of a better therapeutic option, with the belief that the drugs are innocuous, or the design of a dosing regimen based on cost and convenience rather than on pharmacodynamics and pharmacokinetics needs to end. Antimicrobial use must have a minimal impact on the patient, hospital, and community; however, it must do so in a manner that does not forfeit the likelihood of therapeutic success. Not surprisingly, therapeutic decisions concerning antimicrobial therapy for the infected patient are among the most challenging to be made. Unlike most other drug therapies, antimicrobial therapy must take into account microbe, drug, and patient factors (ie, the chemotherapeutic triangle), many of which confound successful therapy to the point of causing failure. Antimicrobial therapy is most likely to be successful when the infecting microbe is killed. This, in turn, is facilitated by identification of the target selection of a drug with a narrow (not broad) spectrum and design of a dosing regimen based on microbial pharmacodynamics and host pharmacokinetics, with adjustments made to accommodate host and microbial factors (Fig. 1).

IDENTIFYING THE NEED FOR ANTIMICROBIAL THERAPY

The first and potentially most important decision to be made regarding antimicrobial therapy is confirming the need. With some exceptions, as a class of drugs, antimicrobials are considered safe. Yet, the pernicious advent of resistance over the previous decades of antimicrobial use has taught the medical professions that antimicrobials are not innocuous drugs. The lack of discreet adverse patient reactions to the antimicrobial should not be mistaken for the lack of adverse events. Unfortunately, the first decision regarding antimicrobial therapy is probably the most difficult. Verifying the presence of infection and its site of location simply may not be possible with current diagnostic aids. Infection often cannot be discriminated from other causes of inflammation. With time, newer detection methods based on molecular diagnostic techniques, such as polymerase chain reaction (PCR), may ultimately prove to be the most important tools in the diagnosis of infectious diseases. Although culture and susceptibility (C&S) testing can be a powerful tool in the guidance of therapy, it may not discriminate between infection, defined as reproducing pathogenic organisms, and colonization, defined as the presence of normal microflora. Indeed, currently, one of the few means by which infection can be confirmed is cytologic revelation of phagocytized organisms.

Indiscriminant use of antimicrobials is discouraged for many reasons; among these are the risk of superinfection, development of resistant organisms, cost, inconvenience, and increased host toxicity. Selection pressure leading to resistant organisms and superinfection go hand in hand. A number of body systems are characterized by normal microflora. Included are external surfaces (skin and conjunctiva of the eye) and internal surfaces (linings of the respiratory, digestive, and urogenital systems). Mutalistic organisms help to maintain microbial balance through host-microbe interactions, providing beneficial effects (eg, lowered environmental pH) and blocking colonization

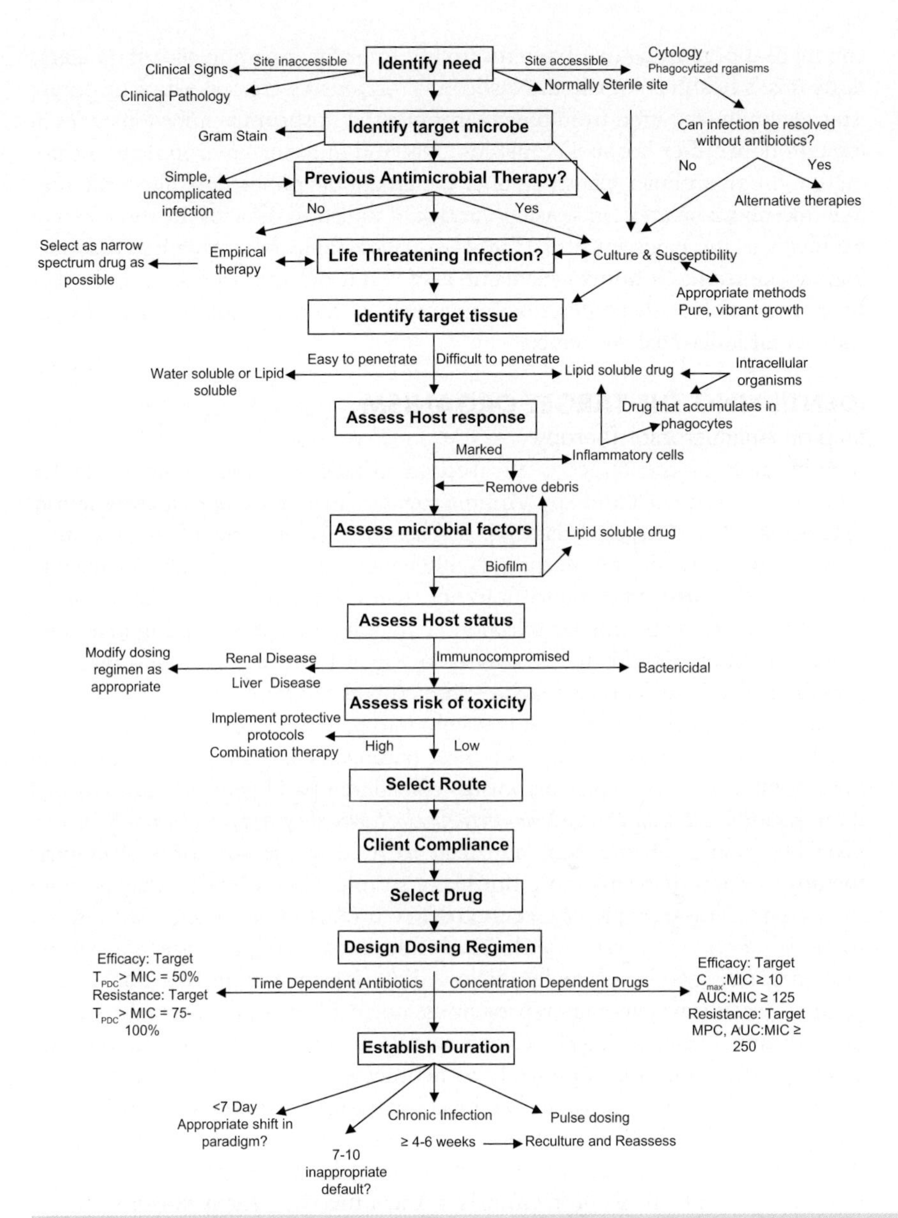

Fig. 1. Decision-making tree for selection of an antimicrobial. AUC, area under the curve; C_{max}, maximum drug concentration; MIC, maximum inhibitory concentration; MPC, mutant prevention concentration; T_{PDC}, time to peak drug concentration.

by more dangerous microbes. Antibiotics secreted by these organisms maintain the composition of aerobic and anaerobic commensal bacteria most appropriate for the health of the host. Most normal florae are commensals in that they neither harm nor help the host. In contrast, opportunistic organisms are commensal organisms that have the ability to become pathogenic, particularly if the host's health is impaired. Nosocomial organisms are opportunistic organisms generally acquired from the environment; a nosocomial infection arises at least 48 hours after hospital admission. Disruption of the environment, including the use of antimicrobials that alter the anaerobic population, alters the normal microflora balance, increasing the risk of infection. One of the more recent examples is the emergence of *Clostridium difficile* infections reaching epidemiologic proportions in human medicine as a result of antimicrobial use; similar circumstances have been described in veterinary medicine [6]. See later discussion on antimicrobial resistance.

IDENTIFYING THE TARGET ORGANISM

Empiric Antimicrobial Therapy

Identification of the target is the second critical decision to be made for judicious antimicrobial therapy. Antimicrobial selection therapy can be empiric, that is, based on historical data [7], or based on isolates identified by culture collected from the site of infection. Neither method guarantees proper identification, particularly if the site of infection is not known, but the risk of being wrong is greater with empiric selection. The utility of Gram staining in antimicrobial selection should not be overlooked as a tool for identifying infection and the isolate, and narrowing the antimicrobial spectrum.

Although historical data provide insight into pathogens (defined as a microbe capable of causing host damage [8]), these pathogens may simply reflect normal flora of infected sites. Many organisms considered pathogenic are also normal flora, including *E coli*, *Pseudomonas aeruginosa*, *Klebsiella pneumoniae*, and *S intermedius*. The source of infection may help to narrow the spectrum of empiric therapy; some organisms are more likely to infect some body systems more than others. For example, the genitourinary tract is often infected with gram-negative aerobes, whereas abdominal infections generally are caused by gram-negative aerobes initially, followed by anaerobes [9,10]. For critical patients, organisms generally represent the normal flora of the alimentary canal or nosocomial organisms [11]. Granulocytopenic or otherwise immunoincompetent patients also are more likely to be infected with aerobic gram-negative organisms. Although, historically "broad-spectrum antibiotics" were considered predictably effective for empiric treatment in these situations, increasingly they are not, and use of a broad spectrum drug increases the development of resistance, even if the drug is effective toward the infecting pathogen.

Unfortunately, the flexibility afforded with empiric antimicrobial selection is decreasing. As early as 1992, Hardie documented that empirical selection often is wrong. In her study of critical care patients treated empirically, initial antimicrobial therapy changed after receipt of C&S data in close to 45% of patients [12]. In a retrospective study, empiric antimicrobial drug therapy was proven wrong by susceptibility data in close to 40% of dogs with pyothorax [13]. More recently, in a teaching hospital setting, *E coli* was the most frequently cultured organism in the urine of dogs, only 50% of the time. More disconcertingly, close to 50% of the organisms were resistant to drugs commonly selected for empiric treatment of bacteria: cephalothin, amoxicillin–clavulanic acid, potentiated sulfonamides, and fluoroquinolones. Fluorquinolones are among the drugs to which *E coli* is considered predictably susceptible, yet 40% of isolates were resistant to veterinary fluoroquinolones in one study [13]. Increasingly, as the need for targeted antimicrobial therapy is realized, the appropriateness of empiric therapy should decrease and the role of culture should accordingly increase. Even culture data, particularly susceptibility data, can be misleading, however, and lead to therapeutic failure if not used appropriately.

Culture and Susceptibility Testing: Putting Sense to the Numbers

C&S data (pharmacodynamic data) increasingly are becoming an important tool in the selection of an antimicrobial. Culture might identify the target organisms, help to confirm the need for therapy, and confirm the susceptibility of the isolate to drugs of interest. Further, testing might allow comparison of the level of susceptibility of the isolate to several potentially effective drugs [14]. Finally, a dosing regimen can be designed. Sequestial cultures can be used to identify developing resistance in patients receiving antimicrobial therapy. C&S testing is particularly important in patients treated with antimicrobials within the past several months [13] and for nosocomial organisms that are generally characterized by complex resistant patterns [15]. Even if antimicrobial therapy must begin immediately (thus empirically) for potentially critical patients, culture of blood, urine, respiratory secretions (collected by bronchoscopy), and other pertinent body fluids (pleural, peritoneal, or cerebrospinal fluid [CSF]) should be carefully sampled before antimicrobial therapy is begun.

It is beyond the scope of this discussion to address the proper techniques of culture collecting, but culture data are only as good as the sampling method used for their collection. The importance of proper culture collection cannot be overemphasized. The risk of improper anaerobic collection is greater than that for aerobic collection; the absence of anaerobes may simply reflect improper techniques. Many aerobes are also facultative anaerobes (eg, coliforms, *Staphylococcus* spp); if cultured aerobically from an anaerobic environment, successful therapy may be impaired by the anaerobic environment (eg, aminoglycosides). Even a properly collected culture may not confirm infection or identify the infecting microbe unless the culture is from an otherwise sterile environment. In nonsterile environments, a culture cannot discriminate colonization by normal flora from infection by pathogenic organisms. The behavior of the culture may give some basis for discrimination, however. Contaminants might be recognized by a characteristic pattern. In general, a complex pattern of resistance is more indicative of infection compared with colonization, although the converse is not true (ie, a pattern of susceptibility is not necessarily indicative of commensal rather than infecting organisms). Nonhemolytic *Staphylococcus* spp or coryneforms cultured from wounds or other sites are rarely pathogenic. Culture of an obligate anaerobe from urine also should be suspect. Multiple organisms may reflect floral colonization rather than a polymicrobial infection [9]. Culture of three or more organisms might cause collection techniques to be suspect. Pure growth is more indicative of infection and the need for therapy, however, if greater than 10^5 colony-forming units (CFUs) are present per milliliter of sample for urinary tract infections or greater than 10^3 CFUs are present per milliliter of sample for respiratory cultures. Unfortunately, colony counts are not feasible for most tissues. Cultures yielding successful growth only after incubation in enriched nutrient broth might be indicative of colonization rather than infection. Treatment of isolates characterized by light growth might be de-emphasized in favor of targeting those isolates with significant growth; indeed, controlling the latter might facilitate control of the former.

Interpreting Culture and Susceptibility Tests

Susceptibility data varies with the method of culture. The two most common methods are agar gel diffusion and tube dilution. Both methods, but especially tube dilution, require rapid growth of organisms. As such, tube dilution data may not be available for some organisms. As an in vitro test, C&S data must eventually be applied to in vivo conditions. As such, many aspects of the procedure are subject to incorrect interpretation or inappropriate applicability to the patient. The Clinical Laboratory Standards Institute (CLSI; formerly the National Committee for Clinical Laboratory Standards) validates interpretive standards as well as provides guidelines for methods and procedures of C&S testing. Only those laboratories that can ensure adherence to these standards and guidelines should be used for C&S testing. Further, because of the inherent risks of inaccuracy associated with C&S testing, results yielded from procedures that are not based on CLSI standards and guidelines should be interpreted with caution. This includes "preliminary data," quick "snap" tests, or other methods intended to generate rapid results.

Tube dilution techniques

Various dilution techniques have been described, ranging from tubes to micro-well plates, with the latter modified for automated devices. For each drug of interest, multiple tubes or wells containing liquid media are modified to contain concentrations of the drug of interest. The dilutions that increase twofold as designated by CLSI guidelines (eg, 0.0312, 0.0625, 0.125, 0.25, 0.5, 1, 2, 4, 8, 16, 32, 64, 128, and 256 μg/mL to 512 μg/mL). Although the concentrations tested are the same for each drug (exceptions include drugs tested as combinations, such as amoxicillin–clavulanic acid and sulfonamide-trimethoprim), the ranges tested for each drug differ. Ultimately, drug concentrations in the well must correlate with plasma drug concentrations (PDC). As such, the range of concentrations tested for each drug (particularly for each drug class) differs. The higher end of the range for each drug approximates the maximum drug concentration (C_{max}) of plasma achieved at the recommended dose of the drug of interest. The lower limit tested for each drug varies with the laboratory; however, it is generally is two to four tube dilutions below the maximum. In the author's opinion, the lower end of the range often is too high, because it does not allow assessment of how susceptible an isolate is.

For testing procedures, each well (drug concentration) is inoculated with a standard number of the infecting isolate. After bacterial growth for the specified time, the tube with the lowest concentration of drug that exhibits no detectable growth is identified as that containing the minimum inhibitory concentration (MIC; in micrograms per milliliter), or the minimum amount of the antimicrobial necessary to inhibit the growth of the isolate cultured from the patient [16,17]. The MIC, which is a measure of antimicrobial potency, represents "what is needed" to inhibit the (in vitro) growth of the cultured organisms (ie, pharmacodynamic data). As such, it represents the target or therapeutic concentration on which antimicrobial therapy dosing regimens can be based. For example, in Fig. 2, the MIC for *E coli* and amoxicillin–clavulanic acid is 8 μg/mL, indicating that the minimum amount of drug that inhibits the isolate in the testing environment is 8 μg/mL. By itself, however, the target of 8 μg/mL offers little direction regarding the potential efficacy of a given drug. Thus, its inclusion on C&S reports is accompanied by a susceptible, intermediate, resistant (SIR) designation. For *E coli* and amoxicillin–clavulanic acid in Fig. 2, the isolate is considered susceptible to the drug.

The CLSI interpretation (SIR) that accompanies the MIC for each drug is based on the "breakpoint MIC" (MIC_{BP}), or the upper limit of susceptibility for each drug (Table 1) [18]. If the MIC of the cultured isolate is sufficiently close or equal to the MIC_{BP} of the drug, the isolate is considered resistant; if the MIC is sufficiently below the MIC_{BP}, the isolate is considered susceptible. For some drugs, as the MIC approaches the MIC_{BP}, the isolate is considered intermediate. For example, for amikacin, an isolate with an MIC of 16 μg/mL or less would be designated as susceptible, an isolate with an MIC of 64 μg/mL or greater would be designated as resistant, and an isolate with an MIC of 32 μg/mL would be considered intermediate. For enrofloxacin, isolates characterized by an MIC of 4 μg/mL or greater (the approximate plasma peak drug concentration [PDC] achieved at 20 mg/kg) are designated as resistant, those with an MIC of 0.5 μg/mL (surpassed at the lowest labeled dose in normal dogs) are considered as susceptible, and those with an MIC of 1 or 2 μg/mL are designated as intermediate. Concentrations between 0.5 and 4 mcg/ml might be considered intermediate (indicated as "F" for flexible by some laboratories), but the close proximity of these MIC to the breakpoint is indicative of first-step resistance and the need to use a dose not less than 20 mg/kg [13,24]. Indeed, any intermediate designation should cause selection of the drug to be made with care. As the organism approaches MIC, the risk of therapeutic failure increases and use of the drug might be limited to combination antimicrobial therapy or to treatment at sites where drug accumulation well above that achieved in plasma might be expected (eg, urine, white blood cells for some drugs). Thus, the prudent clinician should consider an intermediate designation as resistant.

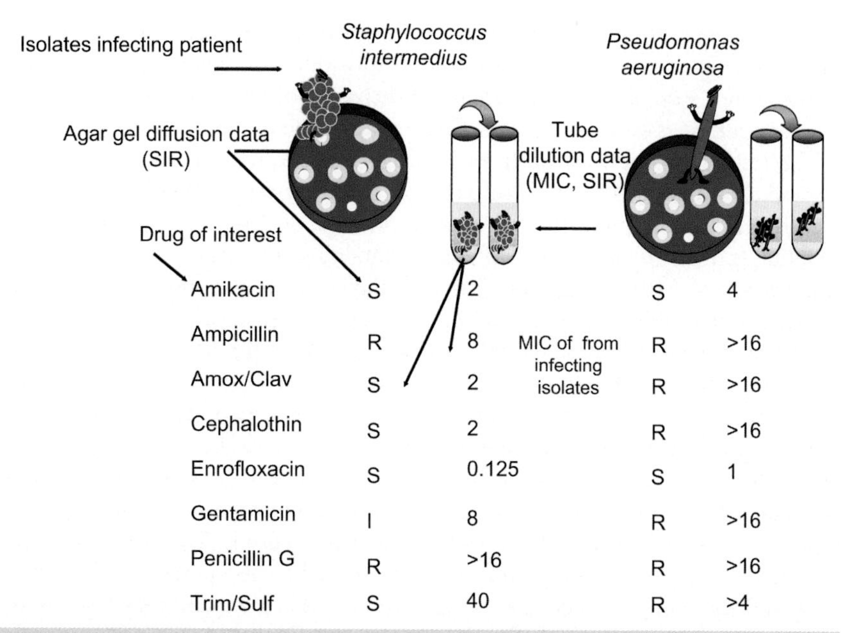

Fig. 2. Susceptibility report generated from dilution procedures for two organisms isolated from the external ear canal of a dog. In this example, four different concentrations were tested toward each isolate (see text for interpretation of the diagram of figures). Amox/Clav, amoxicillin–clavulanic acid; I, intermediate; R, restrictive; S, selective; Sulf/Trim, sulfamethoxazole-trimethoprim.

The MIC_{BP}, as promulgated by the CLSI, incorporates pharmacodynamic and pharmacokinetic considerations. Three criteria are used to determine an MIC_{BP} for each drug [17]. The first is pharmacologic. The upper limit of the MIC_{BP} must be lower than the concentration of drug that can be achieved in blood or at the site of infection. The primary pharmacokinetic parameter currently considered by the CLSI is the C_{max}, or peak PDC achieved when the drug is administered at the recommended route and (labeled) dose. However, CLSI increasingly is considering other pharmacokinetic data [18]. Generally, the highest dose is considered as a basis for C_{max} if flexible doses are approved. The second criterion is epidemiologic. The MIC_{BP} must fit within clusters of organisms having comparable susceptibilities. The third criterion is clinical. The MIC_{BP} must be clinically relevant; the isolates defined as susceptible should respond clinically to the drug at the dose studied, and in vitro data must correlate adequately with in vivo findings [19].

Because pharmacokinetic data in the target species are considered the same regardless of the infecting organism, the MIC_{BP} on which susceptibility to a drug is based is generally the same for any organism tested toward the drug. Exceptions do exist, however, and are likely to continue to emerge as population pharmacodynamic patterns change in response to antimicrobial use. The best examples are organisms capable of β-lactamase production. Acquisition of genes necessary for the synthesis of these enzymes can result in sufficient destruction of selected β-lactam drugs such that the concentration at the site of infection is reduced, necessitating a proportional reduction in the MIC_{BP}. Accordingly, the CLSI has provided lower interpretive standards for such organisms (generally *Staphylococcus* spp). For example, whereas the susceptible MIC_{BP} for ampicillin is 0.25 μg/mL for *Staphylococcus* spp, for other organisms less capable of β-lactamase production, an MIC_{BP} of 32 μg/mL has been determined (Fig. 2; see Table 1). *Pseudomonas* spp are more susceptible to extended-spectrum penicillins compared with other isolates; accordingly (see Table 1), these organisms are associated with a higher MIC_{BP}.

Across time, the population pharmacodynamics of a microbe toward a drug, particularly a drug in high use, are likely to increase as drug exposure continues. Thus, the criteria on which the MIC_{BP} is based also should change. Intermittently, the CLSI validates new interpretive criteria. The information is provided in two publications, one each describing human (CLSI M100-S16E, 2006) or animal (CLSI M31-A2E, 2002) interpretive criteria. These publications are not generally available to the public, however, and the MIC_{BP} must be obtained through alternative sources. Because interpretive standards are based on sample population data, the MIC_{BP} of a drug should be the same for any laboratory in the United States. As such, the diagnostic laboratory performing C&S testing can be contacted for these standards. Initial interpretive standards are generally also delineated on package inserts (including sources like the *Physician's Desk Reference* for human drugs), although the cited standards may not be corrected to reflect new CSLI standards once the drug label has been approved.

Although automated C&S techniques increase the accuracy and ease of C&S testing, automation also has limitations. Only a limited number of drugs and dilutions can be tested. Ideally, concentrations tested by tube dilutions should include a range that allows the clinician to detect not only a resistant isolate [17] but also, it should allow detection of an isolate that is very susceptible to the drug of interest (ie, the MIC is several magnitudes lower than the MIC_{BP}). Armed with such information, the clinician may then select a drug based on susceptibility rather than simply resistance. A drug for which the MIC is several magnitudes lower than the MIC_{BP} might be preferable to one for which the MIC is approaching the breakpoint. Although both isolates might be designated as susceptible, the latter has likely undergone a first step toward resistance and is not only more difficult to eradicate but is more likely to progress to multistep resistance. Unfortunately, in general, automated systems used by most diagnostic laboratories test over a limited range of concentrations close to the MIC_{BP}.

The limited range of C&S testing is also indicated in the presence of a greater than or equal to ($\geq$) or less than or equal to ($\leq$) designation, along with the MIC and the S (less than or equal to) or R (greater than or equal to) designation. For S, the $\leq$ indicates that the isolate was inhibited at the lowest

Table 1
Interpretive standards for disk diffusion and equivalent minimum inhibitory concentration breakpoints for selected antimicrobials

Drug	Breakpoint[a] (μg/mL) susceptible	Breakpoint MIC[a] (μg/mL) resistant
Amikacin*	≤16	≥64
Amoxicillin with clavulanic acid*	≤4/2[b]	≥8/4
	≤16/2[c]	≥32/16
Ampicillin*,[d]	≤0.25[b]	≥0.5
	≤8[c]	≥32
	≤0.25[i]	≥8
	≤8[e]	≥16
Azithromycin	≤4	≥8
Carbenicillin	≤16	≥64
Cefazolin*	≤8	≥32
Cefotaxime	≤8	≥64
Cefoxitin	≤8	≥32
Cefpodoxime	≤2	≥8
Ceftazidime	≤8	≥32
Ceftiofur*,[i]	≤2	≥8
Ceftizoxime	≤8	≥32
Ceftriaxone	≤8	≥64
Cefuroxime	≤4	≥32
Cephalexin	≤8	≥32
Cephalothin*,[g]	≤8	≥32
Chloramphenicol*	≤8	≥32
	≤8[i]	≥16
Ciprofloxacin[p] (see also enrofloxacin)	≤1	≥4
Clarithromycin	≤1	≥8
	≤8	≥32
Clindamycin*,[h]	≤0.5	≥4
Difloxacin*	≤0.5	≥4
Doxycycline	≤4	≥16
Enrofloxacin*	≤0.5	≥4
Erythromycin	≤0.5	≥8
	≤0.25[i]	≥1
Florfenicol[i]	≤2	≥8
Gentamicin*	≤4	≥16
Imipenem/cilastin*	≤4	≥16
Kanamycin*	≤16	≥64
Lincomycin	≤0.5	≥4
Marbofloxacin	≤1	≥4
Meropenem	≤4	≥16
Metronidazole	≤8	≥32
Nitrofurantoin	≤32	≥128
Orbifloxacin*	≤1	≥8
Oxacillin*,[f]	≤2	≥4
Penicillin G	≤8[c]	≥16
	≤0.12[b]	≥0.25

(*continued on next page*)

Table 1
(continued)

Drug	Breakpoint[a] (μg/mL) susceptible	Breakpoint MIC[a] (μg/mL) resistant
Piperacillin	≤16[b]	≥128
	≤64[e]	≥128
Rifampin*	≤1	≥4
Sulfadiazine	≤2	≥4
Tetracycline*,[n]	≤4	≥16
Ticarcillin*	≤64[e]	≥128
	≤16[d]	≥128
Ticarcillin with clavulanic acid*	64/2[e]	≥128/2
	16/2[c]	≥128/2
Trimethoprim/ sulfamethoxazole*,[k]	≤2/38[l]	≥4/76
	≤0.5/9.5[m]	
Vancomycin*	≤4[o]	≥32
	≤1[i]	≥32
	≤4	

Abbreviation: MIC, minimum inhibitory concentration.

[a]Clinical Laboratory Standards Institute. Interpretive standards that are based on animal pathogens are designated by an asterisk.

[b]When testing staphylococcal organisms.

[c]When testing gram-negative enteric organisms.

[d]Ampicillin is used to test amoxicillin.

[e]When testing *Pseudomonas* spp.

[f]Ofloxacin is used to treat methicillin, cloxacillin.

[g]Cephalothin is used to test all first-generation cephalsoprins. It does not represent cefazolin, which should be tested separately if a gram-negative organism.

[h]Clindamycin is used to test lincomycin, which is less susceptible to *Staphylococcus* spp.

[i]When testing *Streptococcus* spp.

[j]When testing pathogens associated with food animal respiratory disease.

[k]Trimethoprim-sulfamethoxazole is used to test trimethoprim-sulfadiazine and ormetoprim-sulfadimethoxine.

[l]For urinary tract infections.

[m]For soft tissue infections.

[n]Used to test chlortetracycline, oxytetracycline, minocyclines, doxycycline.

[o]When testing enterococci.

[p]A human criterion, not adjusted to reduced oral bioavailability (mean of 40%) in dogs and negligible (0%–20%) in cats.

concentration tested. The actual MIC is not known but is at most the concentration indicated (if $\leq$) or half of the concentration indicated (if $<$). For example, if the MIC of amikacin for *E coli* is 2 μg/mL or less, no growth was evident in the test tube or well containing 4 μg/mL, which was the lowest concentration tested. Thus, for the isolate tested, the MIC for amikacin is 2 μg/mL or less. This might also have been reported as < 4 μg/mL. An MIC may also be accompanied by a greater than ($>$) designation, which is indicated as resistance (see Fig. 2). In this case, growth was not inhibited at the highest concentration tested, which generally is one tube dilution below the MIC_{BP}. For example, the resistant MIC_{BP} for amikacin is 64 μg/mL or greater. The highest concentration that would be tested would be 32 μg/mL. Growth in that tube would be reported as greater than 32 μg/mL or ≥64 μg/mL.

One other method of C&S testing bears mentioning. For selected situations, the preferred method of the author is the "E-test" (epsilon test), a method that combines the advantages of agar gel diffusion with those of tube dilutions. The E-test is composed of a strip that contains concentrations of the drug of interest (one drug per strip) that increase more often than twofold. Although E-tests are tedious, and thus expensive, an advantage is the wide range of drug concentrations tested. Not only can the impact of increasing the dose be considered (concentrations tested exceed the C_{max} achieved at recommended doses), but in the author's opinion, the low range of concentrations tested allows assessment of how susceptible the isolate is, which is a critical consideration when trying to avoid resistance. The use of E-testing is increasingly being used in human medicine to identify selected isolates that have undergone first-step mutations leading to resistance. Some veterinary diagnostic laboratories currently offer E-testing for selected drugs.

Population pharmacodynamic indices

The MIC on C&S reports (see Fig. 2) reflects the MIC of each isolate collected from the patient. In contrast, population pharmacodynamic data reflect the MIC determined from multiple isolates of the same organism collected from a sample population (ideally, at least 100 patients). Population pharmacodynamic information might be found in package inserts of antimicrobials, drug information texts (eg, *Physician's Desk Reference*), and scientific literature, including journal articles. Pertinent pharmacodynamic (MIC) population statistics include the range (the lowest and highest MICs recorded for the organism), mode (the most frequently reported MIC), median (the 50th percentile MIC [MIC_{50}]), and 90th percentile MIC (MIC_{90}; 90% of the tested isolates are inhibited [in vitro] at or below this drug concentration) (Fig. 3). Pharmacodynamic data generated for package inserts or scientific reports may incorporate dilutions other than the serial twofold dilutions directed by the CLSI. Because MIC data are not continuous, statistical representation may include log transformations (eg, if mean is reported) rather than range and median.

Understanding the behavior of an organism toward a class of antimicrobial drugs can be facilitated by examining population pharmacodynamic data. For example, comparison of the MIC_{90} among different organisms reveals the relative susceptibility of various organisms to the same drug. Using fluoroquinolones as an example, *P aeruginosa* tends to be resistant to many drug classes, and when susceptible, the MIC_{90} tends to be high, often approaching or surpassing the MIC_{BP}. *Pasteurella multocida* is often characterized by a lower level of susceptibility to many drugs. Nevertheless, particularly in the face of antimicrobial use, population MICs tend to increase as resistance develops. *E coli* collected from dogs and cats offers an example of bimodal

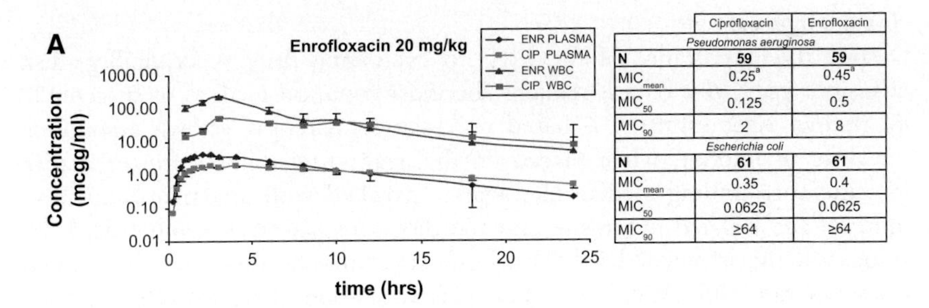

	Ciprofloxacin	Enrofloxacin
Pseudomonas aeruginosa		
N	**59**	**59**
MIC_{mean}	0.25[a]	0.45[a]
MIC_{50}	0.125	0.5
MIC_{90}	2	8
Escherichia coli		
N	**61**	**61**
MIC_{mean}	0.35	0.4
MIC_{50}	0.0625	0.0625
MIC_{90}	≥64	≥64

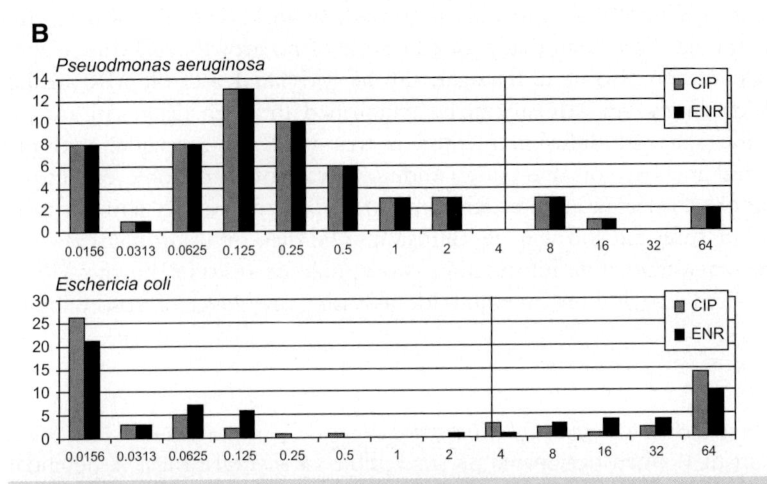

Fig. 3. Design of a dosing regimen based on pharmacokinetic/pharmacodynamic (PK/PD) statistics. (*A*) PK statistics. Enrofloxacin at a dose of 20 mg/kg generated a plasma C_{max} of 4 μg/mL. Formation of ciprofloxacin increases the C_{max} to 6 μg/mL. Because enrofloxacin is a concentration-dependent drug, despite an MIC_{BP} of 4 μg/mL (indicated by vertical line), to target the suggested C_{max}/MIC of 10, only isolates with an MIC of 0.5 μg/mL or less should be treated at 20 mg/kg. At 5 mg/kg, the combined C_{max} is approximately 1.2 mg/mL, limiting treatment to isolates with an MIC of less than 0.125 μg/mL. Accumulation of either drug in white blood cells yields concentrations much higher than in plasma, which may help to treat infections associated with inflammatory debris. ENR, enrofloxacin; CIP, ciprofloxacin; WBC, white blood cell. (*B*) PD statistics. *Pseudomonas aeruginosa* is characterized by a normal distribution, but for *Escherichia coli*, development of resistance in a large proportion of the population results in a bimodal distribution. Thus, although the MIC_{50} for *P aeruginosa* is higher than that for *E coli* (table inset), the MIC_{90} for *E coli* is indicative of a high level of resistance. These data suggest that empiric use of enrofloxacin for either isolate may result in a fair proportion of failures, even at the highest dose. The data also suggest that if an *E coli* isolate is known to be susceptible, chances are that the MIC is quite low and a dose lower than 20 mg/kg might be considered. For *P aeruginosa*, however, many of the susceptible isolates probably have undergone the first step toward resistance and the highest dose is more prudent. (*Data from* Refs. [13,24,97].)

distribution: although its mode and MIC_{50} toward fluorinated quinolones are low (0.06 μg/mL), its MIC_{90} is much higher than the MIC_{BP}. As such, *E coli* isolates tend to be quite susceptible or quite resistant toward the fluoroquinolones [12].

Agar gel diffusion

Despite the importance of the MIC to evaluating drug susceptibility, disk diffusion (eg, Kirby Bauer) remains the most common method of susceptibility testing. Agar diffusion is based on disks containing a known amount of the drug of interest; when placed on the agar, drug diffuses from the disk into the surrounding media. The agar is streaked with a standardized inoculum of the isolated organism, and the disks are placed in standardized positions on the inoculated gel. Drug diffuses from the disk into the agar at a known rate [20]. After a standard period, a zone of no microbial growth (measured in millimeters) is measured around the disk. The rate of drug diffusion is standardized such that a specific zone of no growth, reflecting a specific concentration of drug in the agar, can be correlated with the MIC of the drug. Accordingly, an MIC_{BP} can be established for each drug. An advantage of the agar gel diffusion method is that it allows testing of multiple drugs simultaneously on one plate. Additionally, growth of some organisms (eg, anaerobes, selected gram-positive and gram-negative) is too slow for tube dilution but sufficient for agar gel diffusion. The disk diffusion method only provides semiquantitative information (susceptible or resistant but no MIC), however, and provides no method for assessing the level of susceptibility [17].

Evaluation of the relative efficacy of antimicrobials

An organism is often designated as susceptible to several drugs. A potential advantage of C&S methods that provide MIC data is the ability to rank the drugs according to relative susceptibility if concentrations tested extend sufficiently below the MIC_{BP}. Relative susceptibility cannot be compared among drugs based on the MIC alone, however. For example, if the MICs for cephalexin and ticarcillin, respectively, toward *Staphylococcus* spp are 4 and 16 μg/mL, cephalexin is more potent than ticarcillin toward inhibition of *Staphylococcus* spp growth. It may not be more effective, however. To compare the potential efficacy of the drugs for an isolate, the MIC must be compared among drugs taking into account the pharmacokinetics, that is, what is achieved at the site in the target patient. Ideally, the parameter used to determine what is achieved is the tissue concentration at the site of infection, which is information that is generally not available. A reasonable surrogate might be the CLSI MIC_{BP}, however, which takes into account pharmacokinetic indicators of what is achieved in the target species at the recommended dose. Although the resistant MIC_{BP} of each drug might be used to standardize the MIC, a more conservative approach would be the susceptible MIC_{BP}. For cephalexin and *Staphylococcus* spp, the MIC of 4 μg/mL is compared with the susceptible MIC_{BP} of 8 μg/mL. Because this is a time dependent drug, only one half-life can elapse between doses before dosing should be reconsidered (see discussion on time-dependent drugs). For ticarcillin, 16 μg/mL is compared with 128 μg/mL, yielding an eightfold difference, which allows at least 3 drug half-lives between dosing intervals for ticarcillin. As such, ticarcillin has the greater potential for efficacy based on C&S data alone.

Although the susceptibility of one isolate toward different drugs cannot be compared directly using the MIC, the susceptibility of two isolates toward the same drug can be directly compared based on the MIC. This might be demonstrated in isolates cultured from a patient or by comparing the MIC_{90} of the two organisms. For example, if *S intermedius* and *P aeruginosa* were cultured from the ear of a dog and C&S testing revealed an MIC for amikacin of 2 and 8 μg/mL, respectively, for each isolate, *S intermedius* is more susceptible to amikacin than is *P aeruginosa*. From a clinical standpoint, this comparison may not be particularly useful, but the same approach might be used when considering population data as a basis for drug selection. For example, the original package insert accompanying difloxacin indicates MIC_{90}s of 0.11 and 1.8 μg/mL, respectively, for *E coli* and *Proteus* spp. As such, *E coli* might be considered more susceptible to difloxacin than *Proteus* spp. If the MIC_{90} of each organism is compared with the C_{max} on the same package insert (1.8 μg/mL at 5 mg/kg), the prudent clinician would reconsider the use of difloxacin for the treatment of *Proteus* spp.

The pharmacokinetic/pharmacodynamic (PK/PD) relation between the MIC of the infecting organism ("what is needed") and the MIC_{BP} ("what is achieved") can also guide the design of a dosing regimen (see Fig. 3) [21–23]. The approach depends on whether the drug is a time-dependent or concentration-dependent drug. Simplistically, the closer the MIC (or for population statistics, the MIC_{90}) is to the MIC_{BP} (or if not available, the C_{max}), the higher the dose (concentration-dependant) or the more frequent the dosing (time dependant) of the antimicrobial should be to facilitate adequate drug concentrations at the infection site. The MIC can also be used to calculate a specific dose for a drug as long as the volume of distribution (Vd) of the drug is known ($\text{Dose} = \text{MIC} \cdot \text{Vd}$).

MIC data collected from the same organism in the same patient as a result of sequential cultures can indicate an increasing pattern of resistance. Development of multiple drug resistance may be indicated if the MIC has increased for several or more drugs. The clinical relevancy of the increase is less clear if the increase is only one tube dilution in magnitude and only for one to two drugs, however. In the presence of increasing resistance, antimicrobial therapy must be modified by increasing the dose or shortening the interval, changing to a more effective drug, or adding another drug.

Pitfalls of culture and susceptibility testing

Despite the usefulness of C&S testing, the information nonetheless reflects an in vitro testing system [17,20] that must be applied to in vivo situations. Results can be misleading, even with ideal culture technique and conditions; the controlled system of the culture simply cannot accurately represent the dynamic infection in the patient. As such, C&S results must be interpreted in the context of potential host and microbial factors that can alter concentrations of active drug at the tissue site. Further caveats that may limit the applicability of the data to some patients include the following:

1. Time, space, and other limitations preclude testing of all drugs. For some drug classes, one drug serves as a model for other members in the class. In some instances, cross-susceptibility and resistance justify this approach (eg, fluorinated quinolones might represent all veterinary fluorinated quinolones [12], ampicillin accurately predicts amoxicillin but not amoxicillin–clavulanic acid, sulfamethoxazole-trimethoprim predicts other "potentiated" sulfonamides). Exceptions to the relevance of model drugs to other members in the class do occur, however. For example, cephalothin (which is no longer available) represents first-generation cephalosporins; yet, cefazolin generally is less susceptible to *S aureus* and more susceptible to *E coli* than is cephalothin. The spectrum of third- and fourth-generation cephalosporins is markedly disparate; thus, the class is not well represented by a model drug. Among the aminoglycosides, gentamicin is more effective than amikacin toward *Staphylococcus* spp and tobramycin is more effective against *Serratia* spp, whereas tobramycin and amikacin are more effective than gentamicin against *P aeruginosa*. Model drugs also may not represent levels of susceptibility well. Whereas resistance to one veterinary fluoroquinolone generally reflects cross-resistance to others, among susceptible isolates, difloxacin and orbifloxacin are more often characterized by MICs that are closer to the breakpoint compared with ciprofloxacin, enrofloxacin, or marbofloxacin [12].
2. Many laboratories include model drugs approved for use in human beings but not other animals. Because the MIC_{BP} is based, in part, on kinetic parameters (particularly the C_{max}), species differences in the disposition of the drug might yield a different MIC_{BP}. Nevertheless, these differences may not be reflected in the interpretive criteria. Exceptions have been made for some human drugs for which the CLSI has generated interpretive standards for animals, based on published data. For other drugs, human standards are used and the testing laboratory should indicate this fact. Amikacin offers an example of a drug for which interpretive standards might be similar. The C_{max} for amikacin in dogs (65 μg/mL) after an intravenous dose of 20 mg/kg. The human resistant MIC_{BP} of 64 μg/mL is a reasonable approximation for dogs. In contrast, criteria for ciprofloxacin are not as applicable to dogs and should not be used for cats. The oral bioavailability of ciprofloxacin in dogs is approximately 40% (and 20% or less in cats) versus close to 80% in human beings. Accordingly, the MIC_{BP} in dogs might be expected to be approximately half that of human beings. This may explain, in part, why some isolates are susceptible to ciprofloxacin yet resistant to enrofloxacin. For other isolates (eg, *Pseudomonas*), ciprofloxacin is more potent than enrofloxacin.
3. For any C&S method, active metabolites may not be included in the interpretive standards; however, the metabolite may contribute markedly to activity. For ceftiofur, interpretive standards are based on the parent and active metabolites. Enrofloxacin is de-ethylated by most animals to ciprofloxacin, however, and the two compounds act in an additive fashion. Up to 40% of the area under the curve (AUC) of the plasma drug concentration may be

represented by ciprofloxacin in dogs, with the magnitude somewhat dependent on dose (greater proportion at the higher dose) [12,24]. Mean ciprofloxacin concentrations in a dog receiving enrofloxacin at a dose of 20 mg/kg approximate 2 μg/mL, yielding a total antimicrobial activity of 6 μg/mL (rather than 4 μg/mL for enrofloxacin alone). Yet, current interpretive standards do not take into account ciprofloxacin formed from enrofloxacin; as such, the efficacy of enrofloxacin may be underestimated by C&S methods.

4. The C&S testing may fail to represent in vivo behavior of bacterial organisms. A selected example is provided by extended-spectrum β-lactamases that destroy selected third- and fourth-generation cephalosporins (eg, oxyiminocephalosporins), including ceftazidime, cefotaxime, and cefpodoxime. These enzymes, produced particularly well by fecal coliforms, are transmitted by plasmids. They cannot generally be detected using standard susceptibility procedures but require special (expensive) methods of detection that many laboratories have yet to incorporate in testing procedures [25]. Isolates are not capable of destroying clavulanic acid, and thus should retain susceptibility to combinations with this drug.
5. Finally, the kinetics contributing to interpretative criteria of C&S testing are largely based on total plasma drug concentrations. As such, testing does not take into account binding of drug to proteins (which will overestimate efficacy of protein-bound drugs) or the fact that infections are in the tissue rather than in the plasma. These considerations are discussed more in depth in the section on drug factors affecting efficacy.

CULTURE AND SUSCEPTIBILITY TESTING: FROM LABORATORY TO LABRADOR

Relationships Between Minimum Inhibitory Concentration, Plasma Drug Concentration, and Drug Efficacy

The chemotherapeutic triangle indicates that the efficacy of an antimicrobial is dependent on many interactive host, drug, and microbial factors. Among the relationships that affect efficacy is the PK/PD relationship. The pharmacodynamic component is the MIC of the infecting isolate (or a population statistic such as MIC_{90}). The pharmacokinetic component varies, but most often is the C_{max} or AUC [26–28]. This relationship, and thus therapeutic response, is influenced by many host and microbial factors. Although the MIC of a (presumed) infecting isolate offers a target concentration for antimicrobial therapy, simply achieving the MIC in plasma is rarely sufficient to ensure efficacy.

The relation between the MIC of the infecting organisms and drug concentrations achieved at the site of infection (magnitude and duration) is complex and difficult to predict. Ultimately, mathematic models that integrate the major determinants of efficacy (bactericidal activity, relation between PDC and MIC, duration of postantibiotic effect [PAE], and susceptibility versus resistance) may prove most predictive [29].

Bactericidal Versus Bacteriostatic Antimicrobials

Antimicrobials are classified in vitro according to their ability to kill (bactericidal) versus simply inhibit (bacteriostatic) microbial growth. For example, using the tube dilution method, if media from tubes yielding no visible growth are inoculated on agar plates, the test tube that contains the lowest concentration of drug and does not yield growth contains the minimum bactericidal concentration (MBC). For bacteriostatic drugs, the MBC is several tube dilutions higher than the MIC, indicating that the organisms are still alive but that growth has been suppressed. For such organisms, the concentration necessary to kill the organisms is much higher than the concentration necessary to inhibit their growth [16,17]. The MBC of these drugs may not be achievable in the patient unless the dose of the drug is much higher than that recommended, which may increase the risk of adverse events. In contrast, a drug is considered to be bactericidal if the MBC is equal or close to (within one tube dilution) the MIC. The bactericidal designation of the drug is also based on killing curves, which detect log changes in the number of surviving isolates. For organisms noted to be susceptible to bactericidal drugs, achieving sufficient drug to kill rather than simply inhibit the microbe is more achievable than for bacteriostatic drugs. The categorization of bacteriostatic versus bacteriocidal activity of a drug often is associated with its mechanism of action. In general, drugs that target cell walls (eg, β-lactams, glycopeptides), cell membranes (polymyxin B, colistin), or DNA (fluorinated quinolones) tend to act bactericidal in vitro. In contrast, drugs that target ribosomes (eg, tetracyclines, macrolides, lincosamides) or metabolic pathways (sulfonamides) tend to act bacteriostatic in vitro. Exceptions exist: aminoglycosides target ribosomes so effectively that they are classified as bactericidal, and the combination of a sulfonamide with a "potentiating" dipyrimidine results in a two-point inhibition of folic acid production. Whereas each drug alone would act in a bacteristatic fashion, combined, the drugs act in a bactericidal fashion.

Host defenses must be effective to kill those organisms whose growth is merely inhibited. Bactericidal concentrations are paramount to therapeutic success in immunocompromised hosts (eg, viral infections, granulopoietic patients, use of immunohibitory drugs) or immunocompromised sites (eg, septicemia, meningitis, valvular endocarditis, osteomyelitis) [11,16].

The bacteriocidal versus bacteriostatic designation of a drug can be misleading, however. A drug cannot act in a bactericidal manner if insufficient drug concentrations are achieved at the site of the infection. Likewise, concentrations of static drug may be sufficient to kill, particularly if the drug is accumulated in the active form at the site of infection. Drug combinations may facilitate bactericidal actions of drugs, although the converse is also true if drugs that antagonize one another are used in combination [12].

Time-Dependent Versus Concentration-Dependent Drugs

An important PK/PD characteristic of drug efficacy that has emerged in the past decade is the relation between the MIC and the magnitude and time course of PDC. Two categories have been described: concentration dependent (sometimes referred to as dose dependent) and time dependent. As with the bactericidal versus bacteriostatic categorization, much of the data supporting concentration dependency versus time dependency reflects in vitro studies. These studies are supported by in vivo studies, including human clinical response or animal models of infection. Studies have attempted to identify the pharmacokinetic parameter most likely to predict drug efficacy [28]. Efficacy of concentration-dependent drugs, which are best represented by the fluoroquinolones and aminoglycosides, is best predicted by the magnitude of the PDC (C_{max}) compared with the MIC of the infecting organism (C_{max}/MIC, sometimes referred to as the inhibitory quotient [IQ]) [30–37]. For such drugs, the magnitude of the C_{max}/MIC should be a minimum of 8 to 10, and it should be higher for more difficult infections (eg, *P aeruginosa* or infections caused by multiple organisms) [28]. For concentration-dependent drugs, a dose that is too low is particularly detrimental. In a mouse model of *E coli* peritonitis, the antibacterial efficacy of ciprofloxacin but not imipenem (a time-dependent drug) was improved by doubling the dose. Concentration-dependent drugs generally can be administered at longer intervals (ie, once a day) [38–40]. The duration that the PDC is above the MIC does not seem to be as important as the magnitude of the PDC for concentration-dependent drugs; in fact, efficacy may be enhanced by a drug-free period (ie, a long interval between doses) (Fig. 4) [30,31,41–44]. This may reflect, in part, the phenomenon of adaptive resistance [45], which is a period of refractoriness to bactericidal effects. The phenomenon has been well documented for the aminoglycosides toward gram-negative organisms but seems to occur for the quinolones as well. Adaptive resistance occurs rapidly (within 1–2 hours) of antimicrobial therapy. In human beings, adaptive resistance to aminoglycosides may last for up to 16 hours after a single dose of an aminoglycoside, with a partial return of bacterial susceptibility at 24 hours and complete recovery at approximately 40 hours [45]. The mechanism may reflect reversible downregulation of aminoglycoside active transport.

In contrast to concentration-dependent drugs, time-dependent drugs (eg, β-lactams) are characterized by efficacy that is enhanced if the PDC remains above the MIC for most (at least 50%) of the dosing interval. Efficacy is best predicted by percentage of time that the PDC is above the MIC ($T > MIC$) [27,28,31,37,41,46,47]. Although increasing the dose also may be beneficial for time-dependent drugs, shortening the dose interval is more cost-effective [28]. This may be particularly true for drugs with a short half-life. Because drug concentrations decrease by 50% every drug half-life, doubling the dose adds only one drug elimination half-life to the dosing interval. Because drug elimination is first order, to extend the dosing interval two half-lives requires quadrupling the dosing interval; the addition of a third half-life requires an eightfold increase, and so on. Amoxicillin, with a half-life of less than 2 hours, offers a good example of inappropriate dosing regimens. Peak plasma amoxicillin concentrations following oral administration of 10 mg/kg approximate 6 μg/mL in the dog. At 50% of a 12 hour dosing regimen (6 h or 3 half-lives), concentrations will have declined to approximately 0.75 μg/mL. Accordingly, any isolate with an MIC $\geq$ 1 μg/mL should not be treated at 12 hour intervals. Yet, isolates with an MIC $\leq$ 16 μg/mL are considered susceptible (Table 1).

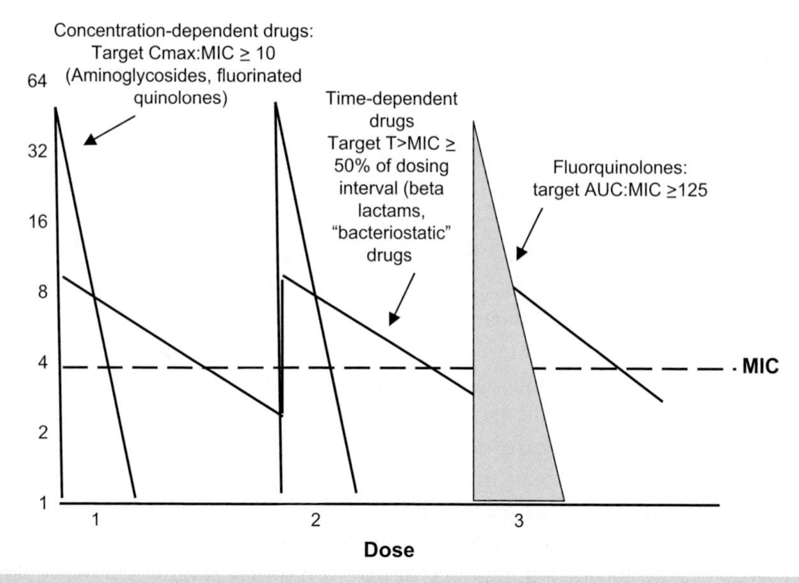

Fig. 4. Two categories of drugs have been described based on the relation between tissue concentration and MIC that is most predictive of efficacy. For concentration-dependent drugs, efficacy is best predicted by a peak tissue (plasma) concentration or C_{max} that is at least 10-fold higher than the microbe MIC (C_{max}/MIC $\geq$ 10). For time-dependent drugs, efficacy is best predicted by tissue (plasma) drug concentrations that exceed the MIC (T > MIC) for at least 50% of the dosing interval and, to prevent resistance, 100% of the dosing interval. For fluoroquinolones, a more consistent predictor of efficacy is the ratio of the drug concentration AUC (in µg · min/mL over a 24-hour period) to the MIC (AUC/MIC). For efficacy, a target of 125 or greater is recommended, particularly for gram-negative isolates. To avoid resistance, however, a target of 250 or greater is recommended.

Cefpodoxime offers an example of a β-lactam whose half-life is probably sufficiently long (5 to 6 hours) to allow once-daily administration for isolates whose MIC is $\leq$ 4 µg/mL. This is based on its package insert data, which indicates that in a sample population of dogs at 24 hours, concentrations 12 hours after a dose of 10 mg/kg approximated 4 µg/mL. For any isolate with an MIC $\geq$ 4.0 µg/mL, once-daily dosing may be insufficient for efficacy. Note, however, if the goal is to avoid resistance for time dependent drugs, the T > MIC should be 80–100% of the dosing interval. For cefpodoxime, drug concentrations fall to 0.5 µg/mL at 24 hours. Thus, only isolates with an MIC of 0.5 µg/mL or less might be treated prudently once daily. For time-dependent drugs with a short half-life, administration by constant rate infusion [48] or slow release products [49] should be considered. A higher dose for time-dependent drugs may be necessary, in addition to a shorter interval, to ensure that the targeted PDC concentration is reached in tissues that are difficult to penetrate. Conversely, efficacy should be enhanced for those time-dependent drugs that accumulate and subsequently persist in tissue, such as macrolides [50], or for drugs that accumulate in phagocytes.

The relation between the PDC and MIC and time versus concentration dependency might be explained, in part, by the mechanism of antimicrobial action. Efficacy of the aminoglycosides or fluorinated quinolones depends on drug binding to the target (ribosome and topoisomerase or DNA-gyrase, respectively); once sufficient binding occurs, protein synthesis or DNA activity, respectively, is prevented and does not reinitiate. β-Lactams substitute as a substrate for cell wall synthesis, however, and as long as the organism is growing, it is synthesizing cell wall. The glycopeptides (eg, vancomycin), which also target the cell wall, are also time dependent.

As with all aspects of antimicrobial therapy, the optimal relation between the PDC and MIC that determines the efficacy of a drug is not so simple and varies with organisms and drugs. The optimal relation between the PDC and MIC and the parameter that best predicts antimicrobial efficacy (eg, C_{max}/MIC, T > MIC) have not been established definitively for all antimicrobials [23,38,39,41]. Increasingly, a third PK/PD index is becoming the preferred predictor of efficacy for fluorinated quinolones: AUC/MIC [51,52]. An AUC/MIC of 60 or greater for gram-negative isolates is generally associated with bacteriostatic actions, whereas bactericidal actions occur at an AUC/MIC of 125 or greater, which is the recommended target for fluoroquinolones (particularly for gram-negative organisms). A lower AUC/MIC, such as 60, has been suggested for selected gram-positive organisms, although this target remains controversial. At an AUC/MIC of 125 or greater, the risk of resistance is decreased, despite relatively slow bacterial killing; a ratio of 250 or greater is associated with rapid bacterial killing [28]. Boothe and colleagues [53] demonstrated that an AUC/MIC of 125 or greater (or C_{max}/MIC $\geq$ 10) generally was reached by fluorinated quinolones only at the high dose for susceptible isolates of *Proteus mirabilis*, *E coli*, and *S intermedius* and only for ciprofloxacin, enrofloxacin, or marbofloxacin. Although the predictors described for efficacy are oriented toward successful eradication of infection, successful targeting of the predictors does not necessarily avoid resistance. In general, higher or longer microbe exposure to drug is required to minimize the advent of resistance. For the AUC/MIC ratio, a target of 250 or greater is recommended, and for the equation T > MIC, a target of 80% to 100% of the dosing interval is recommended to avoid resistance. For concentration-dependent drugs, a second dose, and for time-dependent drugs with a short half-life, constant rate infusion should be considered to avoid resistance, respectively.

Postantibiotic effect

The PAE exhibited by a drug is defined in vitro as the time that must lapse after a culture has been treated with an antibiotic before the number of CFUs in the culture increases from baseline (or untreated controls) by 10-fold. Clinically, it indicates the ability of a drug to inhibit bacterial growth after the drug is no longer present [54–57]. The impact of the PAE on antimicrobial efficacy can be profound, particularly for concentration-dependent drugs. It is the PAE that allows some of these drugs to be administered at long intervals

[17,21,23,41,56,58]. The PAE may be absent for some organisms or some patients (eg, some immunocompromised patients) [54]. In general, concentration-dependent drugs seem to exhibit a longer PAE; further, the duration of the PAE may vary with the magnitude of the plasma PDC (ie, longer with a higher PDC [59]) and is enhanced by combination antimicrobial therapy [60–62]. In addition, PAEs vary with each drug and each organism [63]. Against *P aeruginosa*, gentamicin exhibits a PAE of 4 to 5 hours [64], but it has a PAE of 5 to 10 hours for *Staphylococcus* spp [65].

Presumably, the dosing interval of an antimicrobial should equal the time for which the PDC is above the MIC plus the duration of the PAE [22]. Although the PAE is based on in vitro observations, the clinical relevancy of many of the studies focusing on the relation between drug concentrations, MIC, and efficacy is not clear [66].

Mutant Prevention Concentration

Presumably, the MIC reported with C&S testing represents most but not all of the isolates in the patient. Should the MIC be determined for each bacterium (CFU) causing infection, however, the pattern is likely to be described by a normal distribution whose mean is represented by the MIC of the cultured isolate. Once a population of isolates reaches 10^7 CFUs (depending on the drug), chance mutation yields at least a single CFU that is resistant to any antimicrobial drug [22]. Thus, a proportion of the population is characterized by an MIC higher than most of the isolates. These isolates have probably undergone a first-step mutation, indicating low-level resistance. Should the dosing regimen of the drug be designed to target the MIC of the cultured isolate, most of the isolates are inhibited. Although the infection might be eradicated, surviving (resistant) isolates face less competition and can proliferate unimpeded [67,68]. In healthy patients in whom infection has been controlled, emergence of these first-step mutants may not be an issue. In patients at risk (eg, immunosuppression, unhealed injuries, etc.), however, mutants emerge as a new population characterized by a higher MIC. The mutant prevention concentration (MPC) is the concentration of the drug necessary to prevent (or inhibit) the emergence of the first-step mutants. An alternative definition of the MPC is the highest MIC of the isolates in the patient. The mutant selection window consists of a lower boundary reflecting the cultured MIC (generally representing the wild-type or natural isolates) and a higher boundary (the MPC) reflecting the drug concentration necessary to inhibit the most resistant of the single-step mutants (Fig. 5). Achieving drug concentrations in this window facilitates stepwise or multistep mutations that eventually confer a high level (higher drug concentrations) of resistance [69]. Although MIC-based strategies of antimicrobial therapy may result in eradication of infection, they also readily select for resistant mutants. If the MPC rather than the MIC is targeted as the in vitro measure of an antibiotic, two concurrent resistance mutation steps (ie, 10^{14} CFUs) must occur. Conversely, failure to achieve the MIC at the site of infection minimizes selection pressure and may reduce the risk of resistance, although therapeutic failure is more likely. Increasingly, reference to the MPC

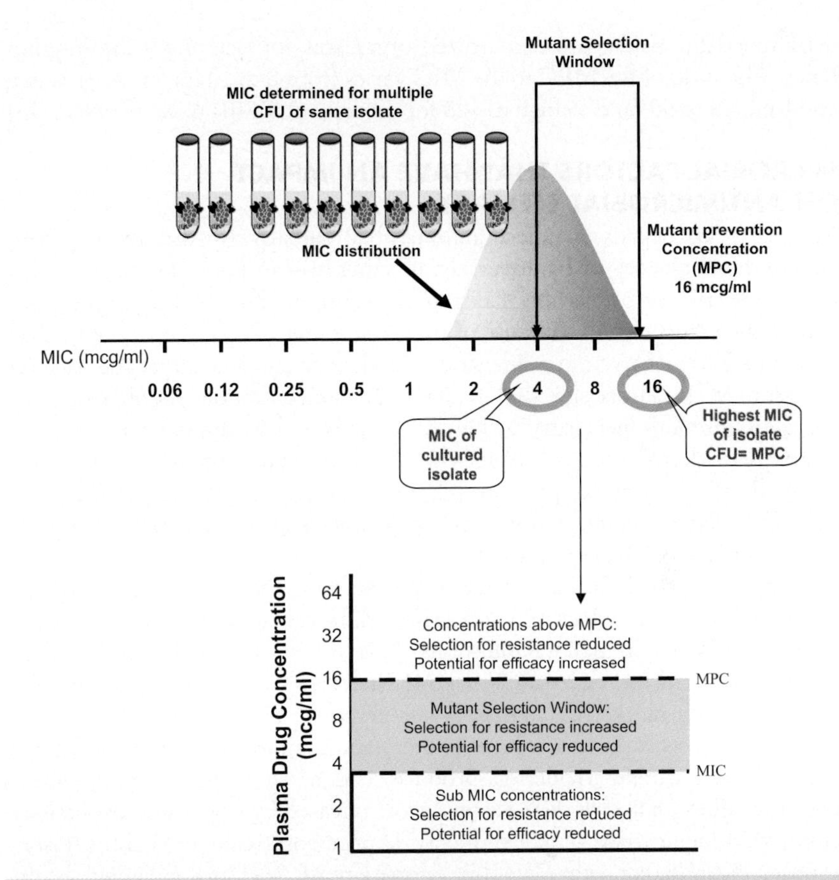

Fig. 5. The mutant selection window describes a range of plasma or tissue drug concentrations, which, if achieved in the patient, is likely to promote the emergence of resistant isolates. The lower threshold of the window is represented by the MIC of the cultured infecting isolate. The upper threshold is represented by the MPC. The MPC is the highest MIC of the infecting isolate present in the patient, or the concentration of drug that is necessary to inhibit the growth of all CFUs of the infecting isolate. If the dosing regimen is designed to target the cultured MIC, even if successful, isolates with a higher MIC survive. In normal patients, proliferation may be prevented by host defenses. If proliferation does occur, however, the emergent population is characterized by a higher MIC indicative of stepwise resistance. Repetition of the process is likely to yield multistep resistance isolates characterized by a MIC that cannot be achieved in the patient.

rather than the MIC can be expected when predicting antimicrobial efficacy [70] as long as the mechanism of resistance measured by the MPC is clinically relevant [71].

Unfortunately, determining the MPC is costly, requiring multiple testing steps and large numbers (10^{10}) of cells. As such, current culture techniques cannot be applied for its determination. Additionally, the MPC of an isolate for a drug cannot be predicted by the MIC [69]. For example, the MPC has been determined for wild-type standardized organisms for veterinary fluoroquinolones. The ratio of the MPC to the MIC varies from 6 to 10 for the *E coli* isolate and from 23 to 50 (and as high as 125 for difloxacin) for the *S aureus* isolate [72].

MICROBIAL FACTORS THAT HAVE AN IMPACT ON ANTIMICROBIAL EFFICACY

Microbes can negatively affect antimicrobial therapy by directly impairing antimicrobial efficacy or by adversely affecting host response to infection. Materials released from microbes facilitate invasion, impair cellular phagocytosis, and damage host tissues. Because of these and other effects, the size of the bacterial inoculum clearly can influence antibiotic efficacy. The larger the bacterial inoculum at the target site, the greater is the concentration (number of molecules) of antibiotic necessary to kill the organisms and the greater is the risk of antibiotic destruction by enzymes produced by microorganisms. The "inoculum effect" of extended-spectrum β-lactamase resistance describes the increasing MIC of the organisms toward cephalosporins at a larger (10^7) compared with a smaller (10^5) inoculum [73].

Many other factors facilitate infection or protect microbes. Infection in epithelial tissues is facilitated by bacterial adherence. Pathogen attachment to host cells is a crucial early step in mucosal infections. This step is accomplished through bacterial virulence factors called adhesins [74]. Materials secreted by organisms often contribute to the marked inflammatory host response, which not only leads to clinical signs of infection but contributes to therapeutic failure. Most staphylococci associated with canine pyoderma produce "slime," a material that facilitates bacterial adhesion to cells. Soluble mediators released by organisms (eg, hemolysin, epidermolytic toxin, leukocidin) may damage host tissues or alter the host response. *Nocardia* spp stimulate the formation of calcium-containing "sulfur granules" that impair drug penetration to the organisms.

Biofilm formation is among the more recently recognized protective mechanisms enacted by microbes. *Pseudomonas* spp and other gram-negative organisms are particularly adept at producing biofilm. Biofilms are microcolonies of pathogenic and host microbes embedded in a polysaccharide matrix (slime or glycocalyx) produced by the bacteria [74]. Dental plaque is the prototypic example of the impact that biofilm might have on antimicrobial therapy [74]. Normal microflora of the skin or mucous membranes in the biofilm are lost with shedding of the skin surface or by the excretion of mucus; new cells and mucus are rapidly colonized by biofilm, forming bacteria. Microbes released from the surface may colonize new surfaces and subsequently produce new biofilms. The surrounding glycocalyx protects microbes against hostile environmental factors, including antimicrobials. Translocation of the normal microflora to otherwise sterile tissues (which can be facilitated by the presence of foreign bodies) may lead to acute infections (again, associated with biofilm) and an accompanying inflammatory response. Persistent chronic bacterial infections may reflect biofilm-producing bacteria; persistent inflammation associated with immune complexes contributes to clinical signs. Unfortunately, bacteria growing in biofilms more easily resist antimicrobial killing and immune defenses of the host. The nature of microbial biofilm behavior is difficult to predict because it often is not present in liquid (planktonic) culture, where organisms exist as individuals rather than as a consortium [74]. Biofilm can facilitate organism growth in foreign bodies in the host, including catheters. The nidus of bacteria may ultimately cause infection, as was demonstrated in dogs undergoing experimental catheterization of the portal vein. Organism growth in catheters, presumably associated with biofilm, ultimately led to bacteremia and septicemia in some dogs [75]. However, organism growth in catheters does not necessarily lead to infection, and organisms isolated from urinary catheter tips are not necessarily organisms causing urinary tract infection.

Antimicrobial Resistance

Mechanisms of transmission

The role of resistance in therapeutic failure of antimicrobials is well established [16,76]. Antimicrobial resistance might be inherent to the microorganisms or acquired through chromosomal mutations or transfer of genetic information. Inherent resistance is exemplified by the lack of efficacy of aminoglycosides against anaerobic organisms, because the drugs must be actively transported into the cell (oxygen dependent), or by the resistance of gram-positive organisms, which lack an outer cell membrane, to polymyxin B, which targets the same. Generally, spectrums of antimicrobials (listed on package inserts) reflect inherent resistance patterns. Acquired resistance, conversely, generally renders a previously susceptible organism resistant. As such, it is not necessarily predictable and can occur during the course of therapy (leading to changes in a C&S pattern).

Development of antimicrobial resistance is facilitated by several factors [77]; among the most important is exposure to antibiotics. The normal flora of the gastrointestinal tract is extremely diverse, with anaerobes predominating. Among the aerobes, *E coli* are the major gram-negative organisms and *Enterococcus* spp are the major gram-positive organisms [78]. Environmental microbes maintain an ecologic niche through suppression of the competition by section of antibiotics. As such, commensal organisms are constantly being exposed to antibiotics. The microbe producing the antibiotic as well as surrounding normal flora is resistant to the antibiotic, however. Thus, genes for resistance develop along with genes directing antibiotic production, and organisms are "primed" to develop resistance [78]. The use of synthetic antimicrobials is less likely to induce resistance, perhaps because there is less risk of previous exposure of the flora to these drugs.

Rapid microbial turnover in the gastrointestinal tract supports the development of resistance by ensuring active DNA, and thus mutation potential (see previous discussion). Chromosomal (DNA) mutations (10^{-14}–10^{-10} per cell division) are DNA mistakes that have been missed by bacterial repair mechanisms. These mistakes occur spontaneously and randomly, whether or not the antibiotic is present. Every time an antibiotic is administered, the normal flora is exposed to varying concentrations of the drug. If the mutation that confers resistance occurs in the presence of the antibiotic, the surviving mutant can progress to a single-step mutation, conferring a low level of resistance (see discussion on MPC). The MIC of the organism is likely to increase. Further microbial turnover can lead to multistep mutations and rapid emergence of high-level resistance (eg, unlimited regulation of β-lactamase production) characterized by increasingly higher MICs. Stepwise mutations can lead to more specific resistance, such as clinical resistance to fluorinated quinolones, which reflects stepwise mutation in DNA-gyrase. Information for nonspecific mechanisms that is shared among organisms can result in multiple organisms developing multiple drug resistance. Microflora of the gastrointestinal tract can serve as a reservoir of resistance genes; a single drug (via integrins, plasmids, and transposons) facilitates the rapid transfer of multiple drug resistance among organisms.

Shared resistance among bacteria reflects the ability of bacteria to incorporate extrachromosomal DNA carrying the information for resistance from other (including non-self) organisms. Extrachromosomal DNA (including plasmids and bacteriophages) encodes for resistance to multiple drugs and can be transmitted vertically (to progeny) or horizontally across species and genera. Transposons are individual or clusters of resistance genes bound by integrins or repeated DNA sequences (two conserved DNA segments on either side of a resistant gene) [78]. Transposons move resistance genes back and forth between chromosomes to plasmids. As such, bacterial resistance is extremely mobile and can spread rapidly [78]. Among the mechanisms by which genetic resistance information is shared is (sexual) conjugation. Conjugation occurs particularly in gram-negative organisms and is often accompanied by genetic material that confers bacterial pathogenicity as well as altered metabolic functions. *Enterococcus* spp and selected other gram-positive bacteria transfer resistance to glycopeptides through conjugative transposons [78]. Transduction, which requires a specific receptor, involves transfer of information by a bacterial virus (bacteriophage) and is especially implemented in *Staphylococcus* spp. Resistance, including methicillin, can be transferred between coagulase-negative and -positive *Staphylococcus* spp [1]. Transformation involves transfer of naked DNA from one lysed bacterium; this mechanism of transfer tends to be limited to (in human beings) pneumococci and meningococci.

Although present for eons, acquired antimicrobial resistance is increasingly becoming problematic, although not uniformly so among organisms. The ability of organisms to develop resistance to an antimicrobial varies with the species and strain. Many organisms remain predictably susceptible to selected drugs (eg, *Brucella* spp, *Chlamydia* spp), whereas others are becoming problematic (*P multocida*). Others have proven be a therapeutic challenge because of resistance that rapidly impairs the efficacy of even new antimicrobials (eg, *E coli*, *Klebsiella pneumoniae*, *Salmonella* spp, *S aureus*, *Streptococcus pneumoniae*). In general, these organisms have developed MDR. MDR is now considered the normal response to antibiotics for gram-positive cocci, including pneumococci, enterococci, and staphylococci [79]. Among these, *Staphylococcus* spp are considered to be the most problematic; they are intrinsically virulent, able to adapt to many different environmental conditions, and tend to be associated with life-threatening infections [79].

In people, mortality associated with *S aureus* bacteremia is 20% to 40%; it is now the leading cause of nosocomial infections in human medicine. Unfortunately, MRSA is now a community-acquired infection in human beings, and its recent acquisition of virulence factors has increased the risk of morbidity and mortality. The term *methicillin-resistant Staphylococcus aureus* refers to those staphylococci organisms that are resistant to semisynthetic β-lactams, including methicillin. The term was coined in the early 1960s when these penicillinase-resistant drugs were relatively new [79]. *Staphylococcus* spp resistance to penicillin appeared as early as 1942; by the late 1960s, more than 80% of medically relevant isolates were resistant to penicillin. Today, more than 90% of isolates (human) produce penicillinase [79]. Although low-level resistance can be overcome by administration of a "protector," such as clavulanic acid, high-level resistance also involves production of a penicillin-binding protein that has a low affinity for the β-lactam ring, which cannot be overcome by protection [79]. The gene conferring methicillin resistance has been detected in MRSA organisms infecting dogs [80,81].

Antibiotics are associated with the induction, selection, and propagation of MRSA. The wide use of cephalosporins, in particular, may have contributed significantly to the advent of MRSA [1]; indeed, the increase in MRSA in human patients receiving cephalosporins indicates that it is no longer simply a hospital-acquired infection [1]. Detection of MRSA on C&S testing generally is based on resistance to oxacillin, which is more stable in disks used for testing. Variability in testing methods can profoundly alter results, however; as such, cefoxitin might be a more appropriate indicator of MDR in these organisms [81]. Alternative procedures, such as PCR or latex agglutination, have been used to detect the gene responsible for MRSA.

Over the 30 to 40 years since the methicillin-resistant classification was coined, the infections associated with the organisms have led to increasing mortality and morbidity. Susceptibility to a number of alternative antimicrobials, including fluorinated quinolones, aminoglycosides, and glycopeptides (vancomycin), is now decreasing.

E coli is another organism that seems to develop resistance rapidly when exposed to selected antibiotics. Most resistance often leads to MDR. More disconcerting, resistance developed by *E coli* seems to be easily conferred to and from more pathogenic organisms, such as *Salmonella* spp. *E coli* is among the organisms that has developed resistance to the fluorinated quinolones. Even a single dose of a fluorinated quinolone has been associated with changes in the resistant pattern of commensal coliforms [82,83]. Fluorinated quinolone–resistant *E coli* has been documented in the urinary tract and other tissues of dogs [12,84]. Previous work by the author found approximately 30% of *E coli* (n = 300, with most cultured from the urinary tract) resistant to all veterinary fluorinated quinolones; the MIC_{90} of most of these organisms was greater than 64 μg/mL, suggesting a high level of multistep resistance [12]. Further, resistance in *E coli* cultured from the urine of dogs admitted to a veterinary teaching hospital was characterized by more than 40% resistance to drugs most commonly selected empirically (unpublished data, D.M. Boothe, DVM, PhD,

2005). As with MRSA, the advent of resistance by *E coli* as well as other gram-negative organisms has been associated with increased cephalosporin use [1].

Avoiding antimicrobial resistance

Action should be taken to avoid antimicrobial resistance not only for the patient but for the medical community. Clearly, some patients are at risk for resistant infections (unpublished data, D.M. Boothe, DVM, PhD, 2005); previous antimicrobial therapy is one of the most important factors associated with resistance. Although the risk of resistance can be associated with the dose of drug (see discussion on mutant selection window and MPC), it likely can be correlated with duration as well.

Pharmaceutical companies have been able to manipulate antimicrobial drugs in a variety of ways such that resistance is minimized, and these options can be selected in an attempt to minimize resistance. For example, bacterial resistance has been decreased by synthesizing smaller molecules that can penetrate smaller porins (eg, the extended-spectrum penicillins ticarcillin and piperacillin), "protecting" the antibiotic (eg, with clavulanic acid, which "draws" the attention of the β-lactamase away from the penicillin), modifying the compound so that it is more difficult to destroy (eg, amikacin, which is a larger and more difficult to reach molecule than gentamicin), and developing lipid-soluble compounds that are more able to achieve effective concentrations at the site of infection (eg, doxycycline compared with other tetracyclines). With each innovative approach to reducing resistance, however, microbes are able to circumvent the drug in a disconcertingly short time. The use of probiotics or prebiotics to minimize emergence of resistance in the gastrointestinal tract is controversial and requires additional scientific evidence [85].

Once the decision to treat is made, the single most important action that can be taken to reduce the incidence of resistance is to ensure that adequate drug concentrations are reached at the site of infection. Adequate implies bacterial killing and not simply inhibition. Intravenous administration should be considered in selected situations, such as life-threatening conditions or prophylactic therapy. For tissues that are difficult to penetrate, doses should be maximized and based on the MIC. Therapeutic drug monitoring might be used in selected situations to assure an adequate C_{max} has been achieved. The proper dosing interval should be used for time-dependent antibiotics. Topical therapy might support systemic therapy in selected situations. Host factors should be considered in the design of the dosing regimen. Drugs inherently more resistant to bacterial inactivation should be selected (eg, amikacin rather than gentamicin). Combination antimicrobial therapy (eg, β-lactamase–protected antimicrobial combinations, combination of β-lactams with aminoglycosides) also reduces the incidence of resistance; for example, the use of a fluoroquinolone reduced the advent of resistance to cephalosporins in one study [15].

Probably the single most effective means by which antimicrobial resistance might be reduced is by de-escalation. The increasing presence of drug-resistant bacterial infections among hospitalized patients has resulted in greater numbers of patients receiving inappropriate antimicrobial treatment [86]. In some human intensive care units, some isolates are characterized by a resistance prevalence of 86%, a finding mirrored in our veterinary hospital for ampicillin. In people, this resistance results in increased morbidity and mortality as well as increased costs [87].

Risk factors for resistance include but are not limited to increased antibiotic use, host factors (including severity of illness and length of hospital stay), and lack of adherence to infection control practices [88]. To reduce antimicrobial resistance in the intensive care unit, hospitals are developing strategies that involve a multitiered approach, including the following:

1. Improving infection control (eg, selective decontamination procedures; prevention of horizontal transmission via handwashing, glove and gown use, alternatives to soap, improving the workload and facilities for health care workers)
2. Improving appropriate antimicrobial use (eg, adhering to prescribed formularies, requiring prior approval for using certain antibiotics, setting limits on the duration of antimicrobial therapy, narrowing the spectrum of empiric antibiotics, rotating the use of antimicrobial drugs on a regular schedule) [87,88]
3. Primary prevention via a decrease in the length of hospital stay, decreased use of invasive devices, and newer approaches [87], such as selective digestive decontamination and vaccine development

Improved information systems technology also plays a role. Each proposed or implemented strategy has theoretic benefits and limitations, but good data on their efficacy in controlling antimicrobial resistance are limited [87,88]. Nevertheless, clearly, decreased antimicrobial use is associated with a decrease in the advent of resistance.

Among the more rational paradigms is antibacterial de-escalation, an approach to empiric antibacterial use in the hospital setting for patients with serious bacterial infections [86]. Antibacterial de-escalation attempts to balance the need to provide appropriate initial antibacterial treatment while limiting the emergence of antibacterial resistance. The goal of de-escalation is to prescribe an initial antibacterial regimen that covers the most likely bacterial pathogens associated with infection while minimizing the risk of emerging antibacterial resistance [86]. The three-pronged approach includes narrowing the antibacterial regimen through culture, assessing the susceptibility of bacterial pathogens for dose determination, and choosing the shortest course of therapy clinically acceptable. De-escalation does not include denial of the use of antimicrobials for patients in need; rather, reduction is used based on establishment of need. Judicious antimicrobial use combined with a reduction in the use of selected antimicrobials in a human hospital setting has been demonstrated to reduce the percentage of resistance [89].

Host Factors That Have an Impact on Antimicrobial Efficacy

Careful consideration must be given to host factors that can reduce concentrations of active drug at the site of infection [16,32,90]. The impact of host factors on antimicrobial efficacy is often underestimated. The effects can be profound and should be anticipated as dosing regimens are individualized for the patient [90]. Changes in the health of the host can lead to changes in drug disposition, which can result in lower than anticipated PDCs [21]. The volume at which a drug is distributed can be affected by the fluid compartments, which vary with age, species, and hydration status. Distribution to target organs can be affected profoundly by cardiovascular responses, particularly in the shock patient. Elimination of the drug must be considered when selecting antimicrobials for the critical patient. Changes in glomerular filtration cause parallel changes in renal excretion of drugs. Serum creatinine concentrations should be used to modify doses or intervals of potentially toxic drugs that are excreted renally [91]. Likewise, severe changes in hepatic function may indicate selection of an antimicrobial drug not dependent on hepatic function for activation or excretion.

More problematic is the host inflammatory response, which can profoundly alter drug efficacy [16,90]. Although acute inflammation may increase drug delivery and drug concentration to the site of infection because of increased blood flow, increased capillary permeability, and increased protein release at the site (the latter effect increases the concentration of total but not necessarily active drug), chronic inflammation may do the opposite. Purulent exudate presents an acidic, hyperosmolar, and hypoxic environment that impairs the efficacy of many antimicrobials. Hemoglobin and degradative products of inflammation can bind antimicrobials [92]. Selected drugs, including aminoglycosides (and probably highly protein-bound drugs) are bound to, and thus inactivated by, the proteinaceous debris that accumulates with inflammation. Some antimicrobials can inhibit neutrophil function. Accumulation of cellular debris associated with the inflammatory process can present a barrier to passive antibiotic distribution. The deposition of fibrous tissue at the infected site further impairs drug penetrance and distribution.

Local pH becomes more acidic as degradative products, such as lysosomes, nucleic acids, and other intracellular constituents from white blood cells, accumulate. The efficacy of many antibiotics can subsequently be impaired. In human beings, a pH ranging from 5.5 to 6.8 can adversely affect host defenses and antimicrobial activity. White blood cell oxidative bursts and phagocytosis are diminished in the presence of a low pH. Some antibiotics are inactive at a low pH. Erythromycin loses all its activity at a pH less than 7. Similar effects have been reported for β-lactam antibiotics. Although β-lactam antibiotics are weak acids, and therefore less ionized in an acidic environment, they are destroyed at pH 6.0 or less. The activities of cefoxitin, piperacillin, and imipenem are significantly less at pH 6.0 than at pH 6.5; of these drugs, piperacillin is least affected. The activity of clindamycin is similarly decreased. In addition, the accumulation of some drugs in white blood cells is impaired in an acidic environment. Changes in pH also lead to changes in the concentration of unionized, and thus active, drug. Weak bases, such as aminoglycosides and fluorinated quinolones, are predominantly ionized in an acidic environment and are less effective than in a less acidic environment, partially because of impaired diffusibility.

Low tissue oxygen tension, which can accompany pus, reduces white blood cell phagocytic and killing activity; slows the growth of organisms, making them less susceptible to many drugs; and specifically prevents the efficacy of aminoglycosides, which depend on active transport into bacterial organisms. The aerobic component (ie, facultative aerobes) of a mixed infection may also be resistant to aminoglycoside therapy, because the oxidative transport systems of such organisms (eg, *E coli*) may shut down in an anaerobic environment. β-Lactams are less effective in a hyperosmolar environment, which might occur as inflammatory debris accumulates and osmotic destruction of organisms is reduced.

The host response to infection and its impact on antimicrobial therapy may vary with the organ system infected. For example, in respiratory tract infections, mucus produced by the host can directly interfere with antimicrobial therapy. Aminoglycoside efficacy may be decreased by chelation with magnesium and calcium in the mucus (hence the rationale for using chelating agents such as tris-EDTA in combination). Antibiotics may bind to glycoproteins, and mucus may present a barrier to passive diffusion. In addition, some antibiotics may alter the function of the mucociliary apparatus by increasing mucous viscosity or by decreasing ciliary activity (eg, tetracyclines).

In general, in the presence of inflammation, selection of a lipid-soluble drug may facilitate movement of drug through inflammatory debris. Further, drugs that accumulate in phagocytic cells should be considered such that drug released at the site might increase concentrations.

Host factors that facilitate drug efficacy

Not all host factors have a negative impact on antimicrobial efficacy. The accumulation of drug in urine was previously discussed (see the article on treatment of urinary tract infections elsewhere in this issue). Another site of drug concentration is the phagocytic leukocyte in the peripheral circulation and at the site of inflammation. Active concentrates of some antimicrobials (eg, macrolides, lincosamides, fluorinated quinolones) may increase concentrations up to 20 to 100 or more times the PDC [16,24,93–99]. Thus, drugs that achieve only bacteriostatic concentrations in plasma may become bactericidal inside the cell, particularly against organisms that locate and survive inside cells. Accumulation of drug has been assumed as a reason for azithromycin efficacy in pulmonary infections despite low plasma drug concentrations [50].

DRUG FACTORS THAT HAVE AN IMPACT ON ANTIMICROBIAL EFFICACY

Mechanisms of Drug Action

Knowledge of the mechanism of action target of a particular antimicrobial is important for several reasons:

1. The mechanism of action of a drug determines whether or not the antimicrobial can act in a bactericidal or bacteriostatic manner (assuming proper

concentrations are achieved at the tissue site). See previous section on bactericidal versus bacteriostatic antimicrobials.

2. The therapeutic efficacy of some antimicrobials can be impaired by host factors that alter the mechanism of action of the drug. Knowledge of the mechanism of action facilitates anticipation of therapeutic failure. For example, β-lactams are less effective in a hypertonic environment such as might occur in the renal medullary interstitium or in the presence of inflammatory debris.
3. The mechanism of antimicrobial resistance often reflects the mechanism of resistance. Identifying mechanisms by which resistance might be avoided or minimized requires an appreciation of these mechanisms.
4. Understanding or anticipating host toxicity occassionally can be improved by understanding the mechanism of action of some antimicrobials.
5. A final need for understanding antimicrobial mechanisms of action is to provide a basis for the selection of antimicrobials to be used in combination. Such drugs should be selected based on mechanisms of action that complement rather than antagonize one another.

The cell wall is an important target for several antimicrobials (eg, β-lactams, glycopeptides), protecting the hypertonic intracellular environment of the organism from the hypotonic environment [16]. A variety of proteins located in the cell wall (penicillin-bound proteins) are important in the formation of the cell wall during division of growth of the organisms. These proteins are the target of several antimicrobial agents. Destruction of the peptidoglycan layer, which provides support to the cell wall, increases the permeability of the cell wall to the hypotonic environment, resulting in osmotic lysis of the cell. Intracellular structures are also major targets for various antimicrobial agents. Binding of ribosomes (eg, tetracyclines, phenicols, aminoglycosides, macrolides, lincosamides), the site of protein synthesis in the cell, can inhibit protein formation or result in the formation of faulty proteins that eventually prove detrimental to the organism. The nuclear material of microbes is another target; interference with cellular DNA (eg, fluorinated quinolones, metronidazole) or RNA (rifampin) inhibits cellular division as well as initial cellular functions. Generally, impaired DNA synthesis results in cell death. Other intracellular targets include selected metabolic pathways, such as folic acid synthesis (sulfonamides), which, when interfered with, prevents formation of materials vital to the microorganism.

Drug Disposition

Absorption

Care must be taken when selecting the antibiotic that the disposition of the drug meets the needs of the patient (see previous discussion of host factors). The availability of drug preparations determines drug selection in many instances, because not all drugs are available for administration by all routes. To maximize plasma, and thus tissue, drug concentrations, intravenous administration is the preferred route for critically ill patients or for tissues that are difficult to penetrate; intramuscular and subcutaneous administration are the second and third choices, respectively. Oral absorption of antimicrobials, however, is preferred as the long-term route of administration, for nonhospitalized patients, and when drug therapy is targeting the gastrointestinal tract.

Note that although a drug may be 100% bioavailable after oral administration (ie, the drug is completely absorbed), the rate of absorption may be sufficiently slow that the peak effect is minimized (although the duration of the drug in circulation may be prolonged). Efficacy may be impaired, particularly for organisms with a high MIC or for concentration-dependent drugs. Slow-release preparations, orally or parenterally administered, should be used cautiously, because prolonged absorption (controlled rate of release) may be so slow that therapeutic concentrations are not achieved. The risk of resistance is increased in such situations. Topical administration is the sole route for drugs that are too toxic to the host to administer systemically. Care must be taken, however, with drugs applied to skin whose surface has been damaged. Sufficient drug absorption may occur to render the patient at risk of developing toxicity. Drugs applied to the ear canal may be ototoxic, particularly in the presence of a perforated eardrum.

Distribution

Once in circulation, the antimicrobial must distribute well to target tissues (ie, the site of infection). Anatomically, capillaries can be categorized to one of three types, with each representing an increasing barrier to drug penetration [100]. Sinusoidal capillaries, found primarily in the adrenal cortex, pituitary gland, liver, and spleen, present essentially no barrier to drug movement. Fenestrated capillaries, such as those located in the kidneys and endocrine glands, contain pores (50–80 nm in size) that facilitate movement between the plasma and interstitium. Because the ratio of capillary surface area to interstitial fluid volume is so large, unbound drug movement from plasma into the interstitium occurs rapidly in these tissues [100,101]. Continuous capillaries, such as those found in the brain, CSF, testes, and prostate, present a barrier of endothelial cells with a tight junction [100]. For such tissues, this presents an additional barrier that is difficult to penetrate for drugs that are not lipid soluble. Muscle and adipose tissue also contain continuous capillaries. Studies examining the relation between plasma drug concentrations and tissue, and specifically interstitial tissue concentrations, are handicapped by differences in methodology. Many are based on tissue homogenates, which is an inappropriate model because it includes at least three compartments: vascular, interstitial, and intracellular. More recent studies that use microprobes for collection of interstitial fluid are preferred. In general, preliminary data in the author's laboratory indicate interstitial concentrations of drugs equal to or exceeding plasma drug concentrations in tissues characterized by fenestrated capillaries. For infections in tissues with nonfenestrated capillaries, drug doses generally should be higher, especially for water-soluble drugs (eg, β-lactams and aminoglycosides, selected sulfonamides, selected tetracyclines). Comparison of MIC data with tissue (non-homgenate) drug concentrations may be useful when designing dosing regimens for such tissues.

Examples of different distribution patterns might be predicted somewhat based on the Vd. Although the Vd of a drug does not indicate to which tissues drug is distributed, it can be used to approximate the likelihood of tissue penetration. For example, water-soluble drugs tend to be distributed only to extracellular fluid, and thus often have a Vd that approximates that of extracellular fluid (ie, 0.2–0.3 L/kg). In contrast, a lipid-soluble drug can penetrate all membranes more easily and is thus more likely to be distributed to total body water; the Vd often approximates or exceeds 0.6 L/kg. Drugs with a Vd greater than 0.6 L/kg may be accumulated in tissues. Care must be taken even with tissue characterized by excellent blood flow. For example, distribution of β-lactams, aminoglycosides, and selected sulfonamides into bronchial secretions is generally less than 30% of that in plasma [92,102,103].

Lipid-soluble antimicrobials should be used for infections that are more difficult to treat, including those associated with a tissue reaction or caused by intracellular organisms, and when the site of infection presents a distribution barrier. The tissue distribution of aminoglycosides and most β-lactam antimicrobials is limited to extracellular fluid; in contrast, many other antibiotics (eg, fluorinated quinolones, macrolides, trimethoprim-sulfonamide combinations) are distributed well to all body tissues, including the prostate gland and eye [53]. Care must be taken even with tissues normally characterized by excellent blood flow. For example, despite excellent blood flood flow to alveoli, distribution of β-lactams, aminoglycosides, and selected sulfonamides into bronchial secretions is generally less than 30% of that in plasma [92,102,103]. Successful antimicrobial therapy may initially be facilitated by inflammation in sites presenting a blood-tissue barrier; once inflammation resolves, however, drug distribution may again decrease. The blood-brain or CSF barrier represents a particularly challenging site because it not only prevents movement of antimicrobials into the CNS but actively transports or destroys some antimicrobials (eg, penicillins, selected cephalosporins). Imipenem, trimethoprim-sulfonamide, and fluorinated quinolones can achieve bactericidal concentrations for some infections in the CNS (particularly in organisms with a low MIC), and chloramphenicol can achieve bacteriostatic concentrations [104]. On the other hand, some tissues may facilitate treatment of infection by accumulating drugs. For tissues that concentrate the drug, C&S testing may underestimate susceptibility. Examples include drugs that undergo renal or biliary excretion, and thus may exceed the PDC from 30-fold to several hundred fold. Urine is easily targeted with drugs renally excreted. However, care must be taken not to assume that high concentrations in the urine equate to higher concentrations in other tissues of the urinary system. Other components of the urinary tract, such as the kidney and particularly the prostate, will be more difficult to penetrate, however. Phagocytic accumulation of selected drugs (eg, fluorinated quinolones, macrolides, selected lincosamides) up to several hundred fold higher than in plasma may facilitate treatment of intracellular infections (eg, *Brucella* spp, cell-wall deficient organisms, intracellular parasites, facultative intracellular organisms like *Staphylococcus* spp) [34,93–95]. Note, however, that drug accumulation does not necessarily enhance efficacy toward intracellular organisms. The accumulated drug is sequestered into subcellular organelles, where it cannot reach the organism. Yet, accumulated drug released by dying phagocytes at the site of infection might still increase concentrations to which the infecting microbe is exposed. Boeckh and colleagues [98] demonstrated that phagocytic white blood cell accumulation of enrofloxacin resulted in drug delivery to inflamed tissues in dogs, supporting that accumulation may facilitate therapeutic success. Drugs that do not accumulate in white blood cells (ie, achieve a less than onefold up to approximately fivefold concentration compared with plasma) include the β-lactams, aminoglycosides, and metronidazole. Drugs that are moderately accumulated in white blood cells include chloramphenicol (one-to-fivefold) and selected sulfonamides (three-to-fivefold) [99]. Finally, C&S testing also underestimates the efficacy of drugs that can be applied topically at the site of infection. In such situations, several thousand fold concentrations of the MIC may be reached. The rationale for collecting C&S data for such infections might be controversial, but identification of the organism and some indication of susceptibility are prudent, particularly if initial therapy fails. Certainly, susceptibility testing will support systemic therapy, which generally should accompany topical therapy.

Protein-binding of a drug to plasma proteins may affect antimicrobial efficacy directly and indirectly. Directly, only unbound drug is pharmacologically active. Bound drug is retained in the vasculature; within interstitial fluids or inside the cell, rebinding of unbound drug again renders the drug ineffective. The indirect impact of protein binding on drug efficacy reflects C&S interpretation. C&S testing is based on the MIC determined in the absence of protein. Pharmacokinetics on which the MIC_{BP} are based (with the C_{max} being a major consideration) are generally based on total drug rather than on the fraction unbound. For a drug insignificantly protein bound, this disconnect is generally not significant. As the fraction increases, however, C&S testing may markedly overestimate efficacy: a drug that is 50% protein bound actually yields only 50% of the C_{max} in active drug. Thus, the breakpoint MIC of such drugs should be lowered by the fraction bound. However, CLSI has not yet taken protein binding into consideration when determining interpretive criteria. Antimicrobials that are highly protein bound (eg, doxycycline) also may be less rapidly effective because distribution of unbound drug into the target tissue may take longer [92,105]. Further, once the unbound drug distributes into tissue, it may become bound once again to inflammatory or other proteins. Reports on pharmacokinetic studies in general are also based on total rather than unbound drug. Yet, the Vd and clearance (thus, elimination half-life) may be affected by protein binding [105]. Attempts should be made to base therapeutic decisions on unbound drug.

Drug movement into bacteria must also be considered. Gram-negative organisms offer a challenge different than that of gram-positive organisms. The efficacy of all antimicrobials depends on the drug reaching and penetrating the cell wall of the target organism. Although the cell wall of gram-positive organisms is often relatively accessible to chemotherapeutic agents, that of gram-negative organisms is protected beneath several layers of cell wall–associated structures. Proteins imbedded in the outermost membrane, known as porins or outer membrane proteins, form pores through which small molecules (including drugs) can penetrate. Although lipid-soluble drugs may be able to diffuse passively (to some degree) through this outer covering as well as through porins, for water-soluble drugs (eg, β-lactams, aminoglycosides), the porins are the predominant method by which drugs are able to access the cell wall, and thus subsequent movement into the organism [16]. The size of porins varies between organisms, contributing to the differences in drug resistance that often characterize these microorganisms. For example, *Pseudomonas* spp have extremely small porins, which exclude the penetration of many drugs. The efficacy of the extended penicillins (ie, ticarcillin, piperacillin) results, in part, because of their smaller molecular weight, and thus ease of penetration. Other proteins in the outside layer of gram-negative organisms act as active transport mechanisms, which may transport small molecules, including drugs, into the cell. Organisms can change the lipid or cationic component of the lipopolysaccharide (LPS), thus impeding drug penetrability.

The roles of drug pK_a and the environmental pH of a target tissue on drug efficacy have already been addressed. Ionization may impair drug movement through the LPS for drugs that passively move through this layer.

Drug elimination

The route through which the drug is eliminated is an important consideration for several reasons. First, if the target tissue is also a route of elimination for that drug, higher drug concentrations can be expected at the site. Second, if the drug is toxic to an organ of elimination, use of the drug should be avoided if the organ is already diseased. Finally, if the drug is toxic to any tissue, the drug should be used cautiously in the presence of disease in the organ of elimination or dosing regimens should be appropriately modified.

Adverse Drug Events

Actions that minimize host toxicity enhance therapeutic success. Host cells are eukaryotic, whereas the bacteria are prokaryotic. As such, targets of antibacterial therapy are sufficiently different from mammalian cells so that, as a class, antibacterials (but not antifungals) tend to be safe. For example, β-lactam antibiotics are among the safest antimicrobials because they target cell walls–a structure not present in mammalian cells. Often, even if cellular structures are present in the microbe and host, differences in the structure result in different antimicrobial binding properties. For example, sulfonamides and fluorinated quinolones tend to be safe because the antibiotics have a much greater affinity for the bacterial target enzymes than the mammalian enzymes. As with other drugs, the incidence of predictable (type A) drug reactions to most antimicrobial therapy correlates with maximum drug concentration or PDC. Aminoglycoside-induced nephrotoxicity and ototoxicity are an exception, however; toxicity tends to be related to duration of exposure and is more likely if minimum or trough PDCs are above a maximum [106–108]. Occasionally, toxicity of antimicrobials does reflect their mechanism of action if the microbial target occurs in mammalian cells and is structurally similar. For example, colistin and polymyxin target microbial and bacterial cell membranes. Administration of either drug is associated with a high incidence of nephrotoxicity (probably because the drug is concentrated in renal tubular cells); subsequently, their use is generally limited to the topical route of administration. Drugs that inhibit protein synthesis by binding to ribosomes (eg, tetracyclines, chloramphenicol) may cause (limited) antianabolic effects in the host at sufficiently high doses. For most antimicrobial drugs, host toxicity may occur through mechanisms unrelated to its mechanism of action.

Aminoglycosides cause nephro- and ototoxicity, not because of their ribosomal inhibition (their antibacterial mechanism of action) but because they actively accumulate in renal tubular (or otic hair) cells (as they do in bacterial organisms) and lysosomes to concentrations that cause lysosomal disruption. Topical application is more likely to cause ototoxicity with aminoglycoside and other drugs. Fluorinated quinolones cause retinal degeneration in cats through mechanisms yet to be defined. Tilmicosin causes (potentially lethal) β-adrenergic stimulation; the caustic nature of doxycycline can cause esophageal erosion in cats.

Many antimicrobials cause diarrhea due to the effect on smooth muscles (eg, erythromycin) or bacterial microflora. Allergies are a less common adverse reaction caused by antimicrobials. Some drugs cause anaphylactoid reactions because of direct mast cell degranulation. True allergic reactions should be differentiated from anaphylactoid reactions (more common with intravenous administration [eg, fluorinated quinolones]). The latter may occur with the first dose and may be dose dependent. Anaphylactoid reactions can be minimized by administration of a small first dose before therapy. In contrast, drug-induced allergies generally require previous administration or duration of therapy sufficient to allow antibody formation to the drug, which acts as a hapten (generally 10–14 days, although as few as 5 days for sulfonamides). Few drug allergies have been documented in animals. Among the most notorious are reactions to the potentiated sulfonamides.

Adverse reactions to antimicrobials may reflect their antimicrobial success. Many orally administered drugs cause disruption of normal gastrointestinal microflora (see previous discussions). For example, *Streptococcus* spp are generally associated with opportunistic infections. Infections caused by members of this genus (*Streptococcus pyogenes* in human beings and *Streptococcus canis* in other animals) are associated with streptococcal toxic shock syndrome (STSS) and necrotizing fasciitis (NF) [109]. These syndromes seem to reflect the presence of lysogenic bacteriophage-encoded superantigen genes encoded in the bacterial organisms [109]. The superantigen genes are powerful inducers of T-cell proliferation; the presence of the superantigens then causes release of host cytokines in quantities that may be sufficient to cause lethal effects. In one study, a bacteriophage-encoded streptococcal superantigen gene was identified in most *S canis* isolates. Induction of these genes can lead to bacterial lyses and subsequent release of proinflammatory and other destructive cytokines. Indeed, use of the fluorinated quinolones has been associated with STSS and NF in dogs [110].

Release of endotoxins is another example of therapeutic success potentially leading to therapeutic failure. Release of endotoxins is a side effect of antimicrobials that occurs with therapeutic success and may influence antimicrobial selection for the patient infected with a large number of gram-negative organisms [38]. Endotoxins cause further release of cytokines and other mediators of septic shock. Most of these effects are mediated by the inner lipid A component of the LPS molecule, which becomes exposed after antimicrobial therapy. In human patients experiencing endotoxic shock, the outcome of antimicrobial therapy has been related to plasma endotoxin levels. A number of antibiotics cause release of endotoxin from gram-negative organisms. Attempts have been made to correlate the amount of endotoxin released to the class of antimicrobial, and specifically to its mechanism of action.

Continued bacterial growth or rapid cell lysis and death have been suggested to be important criteria for endotoxin release after antimicrobial therapy. In contrast, the rates of bacterial killing and antimicrobial efficacy do not seem to be related to the rate and amount of endotoxin release. The amount of endotoxin release varies among the antimicrobial classes, and even within the classes. Release can be related to the mechanism of action. Among the drugs traditionally used to treat septicemia, aminoglycosides have been associated with the least and β-lactams with the greatest endotoxin release (with imipenem or meropenem, which causes the least amount of endotoxin release among the β-lactams [111]). The different amounts of endotoxin released by β-lactams may reflect different affinities of the drugs for different penicillin-binding proteins. The release of endotoxin by quinolones is variable, depending on the study. In a study of mouse *E coli* peritonitis, however, imipenem and ciprofloxacin caused less endotoxin release than did cefotaxime [38]. Selected third-generation cephalosporins also seem to be associated with less endotoxin release. In a study of septicemic patients with acute pyelonephritis, the amount of endotoxin released did not differ among cefuroxime, ciprofloxacin, and netilmicin, and each was deemed safe in the septicemic patient [112].

The release of endotoxin may also be dose (concentration) dependent. For example, endotoxin release is greater at half the recommended dose of ciprofloxacin (3 mg/kg versus 7 mg/kg) according to the previously described model [38]. Actions that might minimize the sequelae of endotoxin release after antimicrobial therapy have not been established. Presumably, administering a dose more slowly may decrease the rate of endotoxin release. Binding and subsequent inactivation of endotoxin by antimicrobials have been documented, particularly for cationic antimicrobials, such as the quinolones, aminoglycosides, and polymyxin [38,113]. The clinical relevance of endotoxin binding by antimicrobials has yet to be established.

ENHANCING ANTIMICROBIAL EFFICACY

Selecting the Route

Drugs may be selected based on their route of administration. Not all drugs are available for parenteral or oral administration. Parenteral and particularly intravenous administration is indicated for life-threatening infections or whenever tissue concentrations need to be maximized. Parenteral drugs are also indicated for the vomiting animal. Oral drugs are indicated for long-term use, outpatient therapy, and treatment of gastrointestinal tract illness. Topical therapy may be selected to enhance drug delivery while minimizing toxicity. Topical therapy with lipid-soluble drugs might best be limited to situations in which systemic therapy of the same drug is implemented, however, thus avoiding the development of subtherapeutic drug concentrations in tissues other than the site of topical application, as might occur if topical administration alone is implemented. The use of transdermal gels to systemicaly deliver drugs is strongly discouraged. Studies thus far have failed to demonstrate effective antimicrobial drug delivery (see Veterinary Compounding in Small Animals in this same issue).

Designing the Dosing Regimen

The dosing regimen should be designed not only to ensure antimicrobial efficacy but to minimize the advent of resistance. The best approach is to ensure that sufficient drug reaches the site of infection to kill the infecting microbe.

Antimicrobial therapy must be implemented in a timely fashion. An effective dose of antimicrobials administered at the first appearance of a clinical infection has much greater therapeutic effect than therapy initiated a week later. Although labeled dosing recommendations generally should be followed, exceptions increasingly must be made as more is learned regarding the optimization of antimicrobial therapy. In general, to maximize efficacy, doses should be increased, particularly for serious or chronic infections, tissues that are difficult to penetrate, or infections associated with detrimental changes at the site of infection. Product labels may not reflect new findings regarding antimicrobial efficacy, because pharmaceutical companies may choose not to endure the costs associated with gaining approval for a new label that reflects the new dosing regimen. Dose modification beyond that on the label should be based on C&S data, current literature, and clinical signs of the patient. Therapy should be designed not only to ensure efficacy but to minimize the advance of resistance.

Design of a dosing regimen increasingly must be based on a combination of pharmacokinetics and pharmacodynamics. The closer the MIC is to the drug concentrations achieved at the site of infection, the higher is the dose (concentration-dependent drugs) or the shorter is the interval (time-dependent drugs). If infection is in tissue that is difficult to penetrate, the dose should be increased further. In human medicine, doses of β-lactams are increased up to 10-fold when treating CNS infections. A marked host inflammatory response should cause an additional adjustment; use of a drug accumulated in phagocytes might be preferred. The duration of antimicrobial therapy is controversial. Febrile patients should be treated until they have been afebrile for 4 to 5 days [9,11]. Chronic infections may require 6 to 8 weeks or more of therapy. The longer that therapy is implemented, the greater is the risk of resistance developing. In human medicine, the focus on killing the infecting microbe increasingly is leading to a shorter duration of higher doses [114,115]. Exceptions are made for infections characterized by slow growth, slow healing or chronic inflammation. Duration of antimicrobial therapy may also vary with the severity of illness; 10 to 14 days is generally recommended for granulocytopenic, septicemic, and seriously ill patients, whereas less than 7 to 10 days of therapy may be sufficient for patients with less severe infections. If the mantra of "dead bugs don't mutate" is to be believed, higher doses for a shorter period of time may be the approach in the near future.

References

[1] Dancer SJ. The problem with cephalosporins. J Antimicrob Chemother 2001;48:463–78.
[2] Guardabassi L, Schwarz S, Lloyd DH. Pet animals as reservoirs of antimicrobial-resistant bacterial. J Antimicrob Chemother 2004;54:321–32.
[3] Damborg P, Olsen KE, Moller Nielsen E, et al. Occurrence of Campylobacter jejuni in pets living with human patients infected with C. jejuni. J Clin Microbiol 2004;42(3): 1363–4.
[4] Phillips I, Casewell M, Cox T, et al. Does the use of antibiotics in food animals pose a risk to human health? A critical review of published data. J Antimicrob Chemother 2004;53: 28–52.
[5] Owens RC, Fraser GL, Stogsdill P. Antimicrobial stewardship programs as a means to optimize antimicrobial use. Pharmacotherapy 2004;24(7):896–908.
[6] Safdar N, Maki DG. The commonality of risk factors for nosocomial colonization and infection with antimicrobial-resistant *Staphylococcus aureus*, enterococcus, gram-negative bacilli, *Clostridium difficile*, and *Candida*. Ann Intern Med 2002;136:834–44.
[7] Yoshikawa TT. Empiric antimicrobial therapy. In: Ristuccia AM, Cunha BA, editors. Antimicrobial therapy. New York: Raven Press; 1984. p. 125–35.
[8] Casadevall A, Pirofski L. What is a pathogen? Ann Med 2002;34:2–4.
[9] Kapusnik J, Miller RT, Sande MA. Antibacterial therapy in critical care. In: Schoemaker WC, Ayers S, Grenvik A, et al, editors. Textbook of critical care. 2nd edition. Philadelphia: WB Saunders; 1989. p. 780–801.
[10] Greene CE. Infectious diseases of the dog and cat. Philadelphia: WB Saunders; 1990.
[11] Schimpff SC, Johngh CA, Caplan ES. Infections in the critical care patient. In: Schoemaker WC, Ayers S, Grenvik A, et al, editors. Textbook of critical care. 2nd edition. Philadelphia: WB Saunders; 1989. p. 767–80.
[12] Hardie EM. Sepsis versus septic shock. In: Murtaugh RJ, Kaplan PM, editors. Veterinary emergency and critical care medicine. St. Louis (MO): Mosby-Yearbook; 1992. p. 176–93.
[13] Boothe DM, Boeckh A, Simpson B, et al. Comparison of pharmacodynamic and pharmacokinetic indices of efficacy for five fluoroquinolones toward pathogens of dogs and dats. J Vet Int Med, in press.
[14] Washington JA. In vitro testing of antimicrobial agents. Infect Dis Clin North Am 1989;3: 375–88.
[15] Schwaber M, Cosgrove SE, Gold H. Fluoroquinolones protective against cephalosporin resistance in gram negative nosocomial pathogens. Emerg Infect Dis 2004;10(1): 94–9.

[16] Neu HC. Principles of antimicrobial use. In: Brody TM, Larner J, Minneman KP, et al, editors. Human pharmacology: molecular to clinical. St. Louis (MO): Mosby; 1994. p. 616–701.
[17] Amsterdam D. Susceptibility testing of antimicrobials in liquid media. In: Lorian V, editor. Antibiotics in laboratory medicine. Baltimore (MD): Williams & Wilkins; 1996. p. 52–112.
[18] Mouton JW. Breakpoints: current practice and future perspectives. Int J Antimicrob Agents 2003;19:323–31.
[19] Wiedemann B, Atkinson BA. Susceptibility to antibiotics: species incidence and trends. In: Lorian V, editor. Antibiotics in laboratory medicine. Baltimore: Williams & Wilkins; 1996. p. 900–1168.
[20] Acar JR, Goldstein FW. Disk susceptibility testing. In: Lorian V, editor. Antibiotics in laboratory medicine. Baltimore (MD): Williams & Wilkins; 1996. p. 1–51.
[21] Thompson WL. Optimization of drug doses in critically ill patients. In: Schoemaker WC, Ayers S, Grenvik A, et al, editors. Textbook of critical care. 2nd edition. Philadelphia: WB Saunders; 1989. p. 1181–210.
[22] Brown SA. Minimum inhibitory concentrations and postantimicrobial effects as factors in dosage of antimicrobial drugs. J Am Vet Med Assoc 1987;191:871–2.
[23] Schentag JJ, Nix DE, Adelman MH. Mathematical examination of dual individualization principles (I): relationships between AUC above MIC and area under the inhibitory curve for cefmenoxime, ciprofloxacin and tobramycin. Ann Pharmacother 1991;25: 1050–7.
[24] Boeckh A, Boothe DM, Wilkie S, et al. Time course of enrofloxacin and its active metabolite in peripheral leukocytes of dogs. Vet Ther 2001;2:334–44.
[25] Bradford PA. Extended spectrum β lactamases in the 21st century: characterization, epidemiology and detection of this important resistant threat. Clin Microbiol Rev 2001;14: 933–51.
[26] Corvaisier S, Mairie PH, Bouvierd MY, et al. Comparisons between antimicrobial pharmacodynamic indices and bacterial killing as described by using the Zhi model. Antimicrob Agents Chemother 1998;42:1731–3.
[27] Nicolau DP. Predicting antibacterial response from pharmacodynamic and pharmacokinetic profiles. Infection 2001;29(Suppl 2):11–5.
[28] McKinnon PS, Davis SL. Pharmacokinetic and pharmacodynamic issues in the treatment of bacterial infectious diseases. Eur J Clin Microbiol Infect Dis 2004;23:271–88.
[29] Li RC, Zhu ZY. The integration of four major determinants of antibiotic action: bactericidal activity, postantibiotic effect, susceptibility, and pharmacokinetics. J Chemother 2002; 14(6):579–83.
[30] John JF. What price success? The continuing saga of the toxic:therapeutic ratio in the use of aminoglycoside antibiotics. J Infect Dis 1988;158:1–6.
[31] Carbon C. Single-dose antibiotic therapy: what has the past taught us? J Clin Pharmacol 1992;32:686–91.
[32] Korzeniowski OM. Effects of antibiotics on the mammalian immune system. Infect Dis Clin North Am 1989;3:469–77.
[33] Mallera R, Ahrneb H, Holmenc C, et al. Once- versus twice-daily amikacin regimen: efficacy and safety in systemic gram-negative infections. J Antimicrob Chemother 1993;31: 939–48.
[34] Nördstrom L, Ringberg H, Cronberg S, et al. Does administration of an aminoglycoside in a single daily dose affect its efficacy and toxicity? J Antimicrob Chemother 1990;25: 159–73.
[35] Powell SH, Thompson WL, Luthe MA, et al. Once-daily vs. continuous aminoglycoside dosing: efficacy and toxicity in animal and clinical studies of gentamicin, netilmicin, and tobramycin. J Infect Dis 1983;147:918–32.

[36] Blaser J. Efficacy of once- and thrice-daily dosing of aminoglycosides in in-vitro models of infection. J Antimicrob Chemother 1991;27(Suppl C):21–8.
[37] Mouton JW, Dudley NM, Cars O, et al. Standardization of pharmacokinetic/pharmacodynamic (PK/PD) terminology for anti-infective drugs: an update. J Antimicrob Chemother 2005;55:601–7.
[38] Nitsche D, Schulze C, Oesser S, et al. Impact of effects of different types of antimicrobial agents on plasma endotoxin activity in gram-negative bacterial infections. Arch Surg 1996;131(2):192–9.
[39] Wetzstein HG. The in vitro postantibiotic effect of enrofloxacin. In: Proceeding of the 18th World Bariatrics Congress. Bologna; 1994. p. 615–8.
[40] Marchbanks CR, McKiel JR, Gilbert DH, et al. Dose ranging and fractionation of intravenous ciprofloxacin against *Pseudomonas aeruginosa* and *Staphylococcus aureus* in an in vitro model of infection. Antimicrob Agents Chemother 1993;37:1756–63.
[41] Schentag JJ. Correlation of pharmacokinetic parameters to efficacy of antibiotics: relationships between serum concentrations, MIC values, and bacterial eradication in patients with gram-negative pneumonia. Scand J Infect Dis 1991;(Suppl 74):218–34.
[42] Vanhaeverbeek M, Siska G, Douchamps J, et al. Comparison of the efficacy and safety of amikacin once or twice-a-day in the treatment of severe gram-negative infections in the elderly. Int J Clin Pharmacol Ther 1993;31:153–6.
[43] Moore RD, Lietman PS, Smith CR. Clinical response to aminoglycoside therapy: importance of the ratio of peak concentration to minimal inhibitory concentration. J Infect Dis 1987;155:93–9.
[44] Karlowsky JA, Zhanel GG, Davidson RJ. Postantibiotic effect in Pseudomonas aeruginosa following single and multiple aminoglycoside exposures in vitro. J Antimicrob Chemother 1994;33(5):937–47.
[45] Barclay ML, Begg EJ. Aminoglycoside adaptive resistance: importance for effective dosage regimens. Drugs 2001;61(6):713–21.
[46] Slavik RS, Jewesson PJ. Selecting antibacterials for outpatient parenteral antimicrobial therapy: pharmacokinetic-pharmacodynamic considerations. Clin Pharmacokinet 2003; 42(9):793–817.
[47] Preston SL. The importance of appropriate antimicrobial dosing: pharmacokinetic and pharmacodynamic considerations. Ann Pharmacother 2004;38(Suppl 9):S14–8.
[48] MacGowan AP, Bowker KE. Continuous infusion of beta-lactam antibiotics. Clin Pharmacokinet 1998;35(5):391–402.
[49] Hoffman A, Danenberg HD, Katzhendler I, et al. Pharmacodynamic and pharmacokinetic rationales for the development of an oral controlled-release amoxicillin dosage form. J Control Release 1998;54(1):29–37.
[50] Bishai W. Comparative effectiveness of different macrolides: clarithromycin, azithromycin, and erythromycin. In: Johns Hopkins Division of Infectious Diseases Antibiotic Guide F. 2003.
[51] Schentag JJ, Meagher AK, Forrest A. Fluoroquinolone AUC/MIC break points and the link to bacterial killing rates. Part 2: human trials. Ann Pharmacother 2003;37: 1518–21.
[52] Schentag JJ, Meagher AK, Forrest A. Fluoroquinolone AUC/MIC break points and the link to bacterial killing rates. Part 1: in vitro and animal models. Ann Pharmacother 2003;37: 1287–98.
[53] Boothe DM, Boeckh A, Boothe HW, et al. Tissue concentrations of enrofloxacin and ciprofloxacin in anesthetized dogs following single intravenous administration. Vet Ther 2001;2:120–8.
[54] Levison ME, Bush LM. Pharmacodynamics of antimicrobial agents. Bactericidal and postantibiotic effects. Infect Dis Clin North Am 1989;3:415–22.
[55] Craig WA, Gudmundsson S. Postantibiotic effect. In: Lorian V, editor. Antibiotics in laboratory medicine. Baltimore (MD): Williams & Wilkins; 1996. p. 296–330.

[56] Spivey JM. Clinical frontiers: the postantibiotic effect. Clin Pharm 1992;11:865–75.
[57] Vogelman B, Gudmundsson S, Leggett J, et al. Correlation of antimicrobial pharmacokinetic parameters with therapeutic efficacy in an animal model. J Infect Dis 1988;158: 831–47.
[58] Hostacka A. Serum sensitivity and cell surface hydrophobicity of Klebsiella pneumoniae treated with gentamicin, tobramycin and amikacin. J Basic Microbiol 1998;38(5–6): 383–8.
[59] Mayer I, Nagy E. Post-antibiotic and synergic effects of fluoroquinolones and ceftazidime in combination against Pseudomonas strains. Acta Biol Hung 2001;52(2–3):241–8.
[60] Sood P, Mandal A, Mishra B. Postantibiotic effect of a combination of antimicrobial agents on *Pseudomonas aeruginosa*. Chemotherapy 2000;46(3):173–6.
[61] Majtan V, Majtanova L. Postantibiotic effect of some antibiotics on the metabolism of *Pseudomonas aeruginosa*. J Basic Microbiol 1998;38(3):221–7.
[62] Athamna A, Athamna M, Medlej B, et al. In vitro post-antibiotic effect of fluoroquinolones, macrolides, beta-lactams, tetracyclines, vancomycin, clindamycin, linezolid, chloramphenicol, quinupristin/dalfopristin and rifampicin on Bacillus anthracis. J Antimicrob Chemother 2004;53(4):609–15.
[63] Wang MG, Zhang YY, Zhu DM, et al. Postantibiotic effects of eleven antimicrobials on five bacteria. Acta Pharmacol Sin 2001;22(9):804–8.
[64] Isaksson B, Maller R, Nilsson LE, et al. Postantibiotic effect of aminoglycosides on staphylococci. J Antimicrob Chemother 1993;32(2):215–22.
[65] Levin S, Karakusis PH. Clinical significance of antibiotic blood levels. In: Ristuccia AM, Cuhna BA, editors. Antimicrobial therapy. New York: Raven Press; 1984. p. 113–24.
[66] Blondeau JM, Hansen G, Metzler K, et al. The role of PK/PD (pharmacokinetic/pharmacodynamic) parameters to avoid selection and increase of resistance: mutant prevention concentration. J Chemother 2004;16:1–19.
[67] Gould IM, MacKenzie FM. Antibiotic exposure as a risk factor for emergence of resistance: the influence of concentration. Soc Appl Microbiol 2002;31(Suppl):78S–84S.
[68] Drlica K. The mutant selection window and antimicrobial resistance. J Antimicrob Chem 2003;52:11–7.
[69] Olofsson SK, Marcusson LL, Lingren PK, et al. Selection of ciprofloxacin resistance in Escherichia coli in an in vitro kinetic model: relation between drug exposure and mutant prevention concentration. J Antimicrob Chemother 2006;57:1116–21.
[70] Smith JH, Nicholl KA, Hoban DJ, et al. Stretching the mutant prevention concentration (MPC) beyond its limits. J Antimicrob Chemother 2003;51:1323–5.
[71] Wetzstein HG. Comparative mutant prevention concentrations of pradofloxacin and other veterinary fluoroquinolones. Presented at the American Society of Microbiology, 103rd General Meeting. Washington (DC), May 7–11, 2003. p. Z-010.
[72] Helfand MS, Bonomo RA. β-Lactamases: a survey of protein diversity. Curr Drug Targets Infect Disord 2003;3:9–23.
[73] Coutee L, Alonso S, Reveneau N, et al. Role of adhesin release for mucosal colonization by a bacterial pathogen. J Exp Med 2003;197(6):735–42.
[74] Marsh PD. Dental plaque as a microbial biofilm. Caries Research 2004;38: 204–11.
[75] Howe LM, Boothe DM, Boothe HW. Detection of portal and systemic bacteremia in dogs with severe hepatic disease and multiple portosystemic shunts. Am J Vet Res 1999;60(2): 181–5.
[76] Tomasz A. Multiple antibiotic resistant pathogenic bacteria. N Engl J Med 1994;330: 1247–51.
[77] Lederberg J, Shope RE, Oaks SC, editors. Emerging infections: microbial threats to health in the United States. Washington (DC): National Academy Press; 1992.
[78] Fluit AC, Schmitz FJ. Resistance integrins and super integrins. Clin Microbial Infect 2004;10:272–88.

[79] Kariuki S, Hart CA. Global aspects of antimicrobial-resistant enteric bacteria. Curr Opin Infect Dis 2001;14:479–586.
[80] Lowy FD. Antimicrobial resistance: the example of *Staphylococcus aureus*. J Clin Invest 2003;111:1265–73.
[81] Gortel K, Campbell KL, Kakoma I, et al. Methicillin resistance among staphylococci isolated from dogs. Am J Vet Res 1999;60(12):1526–30.
[82] Kania SA, Williamson NL, Frank LA. Methicillin resistance of staphylococci isolated from the skin of dogs with pyoderma. J Am Vet Med Assoc 2004;65:1285–8.
[83] Hooton T. Fluoroquinolones and resistance in the treatment of uncomplicated urinary tract infection. Int J Antimicrob Agents 2003;22(Suppl):S65–72.
[84] Wagenlehner F, Stöwer-Hoffmann J, Schneider-Brachert W, et al. Influence of a prophylactic single dose of ciprofloxacin on the level of resistance of *Escherichia coli* to fluoroquinolones in urology. Int J Antimicrob Agents 2000;15:207–11.
[85] Cooke CL, Singer RS, Jang SS, et al. Enrofloxacin resistance in *Escherichia coli* isolated from dogs with urinary tract infections. J Am Vet Med Assoc 2002;220:190–2.
[86] Conly J. Alpha and omega of microbes, antibiotics and probiotics: judicious use is the key. [editorial]. Canadian Family Physician 2004;50:525–7.
[87] Kollef M. Appropriate empirical antibacterial therapy for nosocomial infections: getting it right the first time. Current Opinion Drugs 2003;63(20):2157–68.
[88] Hall CS, Ost DE. Effectiveness of programs to decrease antimicrobial resistance in the intensive care unit. Semin Respir Infect 2003;18(2):112–21.
[89] Rice LB. Controlling antibiotic resistance in the ICU: different bacteria, different strategies. Cleve Clin J Med 2003;70(9):793–800.
[90] Regal RE, DePestel DD, VandenBussche HL. The effect of an antimicrobial restriction program on *Pseudomonas aeruginosa* resistance to beta-lactams in a large teaching hospital. Pharmacotherapy 2003;23(5):618–24.
[91] Brumbaugh G. Antimicrobial susceptibility and therapy: concepts and controversies. Parts I and II. Proc Am Coll Vet Intern Med 1990;8:525–32.
[92] Lesar TS, Zaske DE. Modifying dosage regimens in renal and hepatic failure. In: Ristuccia AM, Cuhna BA, editors. Antimicrobial therapy. New York: Raven Press; 1984. p. 95–111.
[93] Bergan T. Pharmacokinetics of tissue penetration of antibiotics. Rev Infect Dis 1981;3: 45–66.
[94] Easmon CSF, Crane JP. Uptake of ciprofloxacin by macrophages. J Clin Pathol 1985;38: 442–4.
[95] Tulkens PM. Accumulation and subcellular distribution of antibiotics in macrophages in relation to activity against intracellular bacteria. In: Fass RJ, editor. Ciprofloxacin in pulmonology. San Francisco (CA): W Zuckschwerdt Verlag; 1990. p. 12–20.
[96] Hawkins EH, Boothe DEM, Aucoin D, et al. Accumulation of enrofloxacin and its metabolite, ciprofloxacin, in alveolar macrophages and extracellular lung fluid of dogs. J Vet Pharmacol Ther 1998;21:18–23.
[97] Boeckh A, Boothe D, Boothe H, et al. Effect of Wbc accumulation of enrofloxacin on its concentration at a site of inflammation [abstract]. Proceedings of the American College of Veterinary internal Medicine Annual Forum, 2002. Dallas, TX.
[98] Boothe HW, Jones SA, Wilkie WS, et al. Evaluation of the concentration of marbofloxacin in alveolar macrophages and pulmonary epithelial lining fluid after administration in dogs. Am J Vet Res 2005;66(10):1770–4.
[99] Labro MT. Interference of antibacterial agents with phagocyte functions: immunomodulation or "Immuno-Fairy Tales"? Clin Microbiol Rev 2000;13(40):625–50.
[100] Ryan DM. Pharmacokinetics of antibiotics in natural and experimental superficial compartments in animals and humans. J Antimicrob Chemother 1993;31(Suppl D):1–16.
[101] Barza M. Tissue directed antibiotic therapy: antibiotic dynamics in cells and tissues. Clin Infect Dis 1994;19:910–5.

[102] Braga PC. Antibiotic penetrability into bronchial mucus: pharmacokinetic and clinical considerations. Curr Ther Res 1989;49(2):300–27.
[103] Bergogne-Bérézin E. Pharmacokinetics of antibiotics in respiratory secretions. In: Pennington JE, editor. Respiratory infections: diagnosis and management. 2nd edition. New York: Raven Press; 1988. p. 608–31.
[104] LeFrock JL, Prince RA, Richards ML. Penetration of antimicrobials into the cerebrospinal fluid and brain. In: Ristuccia AM, Cuhna BA, editors. Antimicrobial therapy. New York: Raven Press; 1984. p. 397–413.
[105] Craig WA, Ebert SC. Protein binding and its significance in antibacterial therapy. Infect Dis Clin North Am 1989;3:407–14.
[106] Bennett WM, Plamp CE, Gilbert DN, et al. The influence of dosage regimen on experimental gentamicin nephrotoxicity: dissociation of peak serum levels from renal failure. J Infect Dis 1979;140:576–80.
[107] Maller R, Ahrne H, Eilard T, et al. Efficacy and safety in systemic infections when given as a single daily dose or in two divided doses. J Antimicrob Chemother 1991;27(Suppl C): 121–8.
[108] Reiner NE, Bloxham DD, Thompson WL. Nephrotoxicity of gentamicin and tobramycin given once daily or continuously in dogs. J Antimicrob Chemother 1978;4(Suppl A):85–101.
[109] Ingrey KT, Ren J, Prescot JF. A fluoroquinolone induces a novel mitogen-encoding bacteriophage. Infect Immun 2003;71(6):3028–33.
[110] Miller CW, Prescott JF, Mathews KA, et al. Streptococcal toxic shock syndrome in dogs. J Am Vet Med Assoc 1996;209:1421–6.
[111] Trautmann M, Zick R, Rukavina T, et al. Antibiotic-induced release of endotoxin: in-vitro comparison of meropenem and other antibiotics. J Antimicrob Chemother 1998;41(2): 163–9.
[112] Giamarellos-Bourboulis EJ, Perdios J, Gargalianos P, et al. Antimicrobial-induced endotoxaemia in patients with sepsis in the field of acute pyelonephritis. J Postgrad Med 2003;49(2):118–22.
[113] Aoki H, Kodama M, Tani T, et al. Treatment of sepsis by extracorporal elimination of endotoxin using polymyxin B-immobilized fiber. Am J Surg 1994;167:412–7.
[114] File TM. A new dosing paradigm: high-dose, short-course fluoroquinolone therapy for community-acquired pneumonia. Clinical Cornerstone 2003;(Suppl 3):S21–8.
[115] Guay DP. Short-course antimicrobial therapy of respiratory tract infections. Drugs 2003;63(20):2169–84.

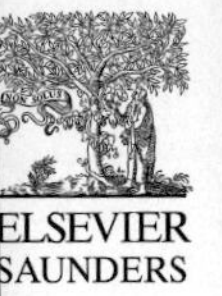

ELSEVIER
SAUNDERS

Vet Clin Small Anim 36 (2006) 1049–1060

VETERINARY CLINICS
SMALL ANIMAL PRACTICE

Antimicrobial Use in the Surgical Patient

Lisa M. Howe, DVM, PhD[a,*], Harry W. Boothe, Jr, DVM, MS[b]

[a]Surgical Sciences Section, Department of Small Animal Clinical Sciences, College of Veterinary Medicine and Biomedical Sciences, Texas A&M University, College Station, TX 77843-4474, USA
[b]Small Animal Surgery, Department of Clinical Sciences, College of Veterinary Medicine, Auburn University, Auburn, AL 36849-5540, USA

Preventing infection in the veterinary surgical patient without established infection at the time of surgery is essential for a good outcome. Risk of infection in the surgical patient is based on the susceptibility of the surgical wound to microbial contamination [1]. Surgical site infections (SSIs) are a complication that results in increased expense in the veterinary patient [2,3]. Adhering to strict surgical asepsis and the appropriate use of antimicrobial prophylaxis are important in preventing SSIs [2–4]. Antimicrobial prophylaxis is the use of antimicrobial agents in surgical patients without established infection [4–8]. Although a reduced incidence of SSIs occurs with prophylactic antimicrobial use, inappropriate use results in unnecessary costs, increased antimicrobial resistance, and superinfection [7–10]. Prophylactic antimicrobials are relatively commonly used inappropriately in human and veterinary surgery [7–10]. Likewise, the appropriate selection and use of therapeutic antimicrobials in patients that develop postoperative infection or have infection at surgery are also important. Therapeutic antimicrobials are used to treat established localized or systemic infections [2]. Selection of antimicrobial agents for prophylactic and therapeutic use should be based on knowledge of expected flora, ability of the antimicrobial to reach the target tissue at appropriate concentrations, bacterial resistance patterns, drug pharmacokinetics, pharmacodynamics, and culture and susceptibility testing results (therapeutic use) [4,11,12]. Consideration of these factors can reduce antimicrobial therapy failure, associated morbidity, mortality, and expenses.

ANTIMICROBIAL PROPHYLAXIS

Antimicrobial prophylaxis refers to the use of antimicrobial agents in surgical patients without established infection at the time of surgery [13–19]. The intent of prophylactic antimicrobials is to decrease the number of microorganisms to a level that the host defense mechanisms can effectively eradicate [20]. Factors

*Corresponding author. *E-mail address:* lhowe@cvm.tamu.edu (L.M. Howe).

0195-5616/06/$ – see front matter

doi:10.1016/j.cvsm.2006.05.001
vetsmall.theclinics.com

influencing indications for antimicrobial prophylaxis include incision location, category and length of the surgery, placement of implants, overall health of the patient, and level of contamination [14–19].

Surgical wounds are classified into one of four categories: clean (class I in the human literature), clean-contaminated (class II), contaminated (class III), and dirty (class IV) [4,21,22]. Clean wounds are noncontaminated, and surgery is performed using aseptic technique. These are surgical wounds in which the gastrointestinal, genitourinary, oropharyngeal, or respiratory tract is not entered [23,24]. Clean-contaminated wounds are those in which contaminated areas of the body (eg, gastrointestinal system, genitourinary system) are entered under controlled conditions without unusual contamination. Clean surgical wounds in which a drain is placed are also classified as clean-contaminated wounds, as are procedures in which minor breaks in surgical asepsis have occurred [2,22]. Contaminated surgical wounds have visibly inflamed tissue, are associated with trauma or a major breach of surgical asepsis, or include procedures in which gastrointestinal contents or infected urine is spilled [2,22]. These wounds have the potential to become infected. Dirty wounds are heavily laden with foreign material, necrotic tissue, or pus. Dirty wounds also include procedures in which fecal contamination occurs or a viscus is perforated before surgery [2,22].

Clean wounds typically have an infection rate less than 5%, so antimicrobial prophylaxis is generally not necessary [25–27]. Prophylactic antimicrobials may be indicated in a clean procedure lasting 90 minutes or longer, however, and in selective orthopedic procedures, particularly those in which a prosthesis or osteosynthetic material (eg, wire, screw, plate) is used [28]. The risk of postoperative infection in small animals undergoing a 90-minute clean surgical procedure is double that of animals undergoing a 60-minute procedure [25]. Whittem and colleagues [11] demonstrated in a randomized, controlled, blind clinical trial that the use of prophylactic antimicrobials significantly reduced the incidence of postoperative infection in dogs undergoing clean orthopedic procedures. Additionally, clean procedures in which nonmetallic prostheses are implanted, such as pacemakers, mesh, and bone cement, are indications for prophylactic antimicrobial use [2,29]. Veterinary patients with prostheses that undergo a surgical procedure (including dental prophylaxis) may also require antimicrobial prophylaxis regardless of the classification of the wound [2].

Antimicrobial prophylaxis is indicated in some clean-contaminated wounds, depending on such factors as location of the incision, length of the procedure, and immunocompetency and overall health of the patient [2,28]. Infection rates reported for clean-contaminated wounds range from approximately 4.5% to 10%, with fractures of the pelvis and long bones becoming infected most frequently [25,30,31].

The reported infection rate for contaminated wounds in veterinary patients ranges from approximately 6% to 29% [2,25–27]. Early aggressive wound therapy, including debridement, lavage, and drainage, can potentially alter the fate of contaminated wounds. Antimicrobial prophylaxis is indicated in contaminated procedures and should be based on anticipated bacterial contaminants, with the choice of therapeutic antimicrobials based on culture and susceptibility testing results. Perioperative antimicrobial use is appropriate in the management of dirty infected wounds. Therapeutic antimicrobial selection should be based on culture and susceptibility testing results [2].

Host factors that may influence the need for antimicrobial prophylaxis include general considerations (eg, age, immunocompetence), concurrent debilitating disorders (eg, diabetes mellitus, hyperadrenocorticism, protein-losing enteropathy), and nutritional status [2,22,25,32]. Other risk factors for the development of SSIs include length of anesthesia (independent of length of surgery), use of propofol as an anesthetic agent, and overuse or inappropriate use of antimicrobials [25,28,33,34]. Lack of surgical asepsis and traumatic tissue handling also contribute to SSIs. Antimicrobial prophylaxis should never be used as a substitute for appropriate surgical asepsis and atraumatic tissue handling.

To be effective, prophylactic antimicrobials must be present in appropriate levels at the surgical site during the time of contamination [5,9,35]. Time of contamination is during the surgical procedure. In small animal surgical patients, pathogens most commonly responsible for SSIs are *Staphylococcus aureus*, other *Staphylococcus* spp, *Escherichia coli*, and *Pasteurella* spp (particularly in cats) [27,36]. Cefazolin, a first-generation cephalosporin, is frequently used during surgery in the veterinary patient [36]. When administered intravenously (20–22 mg/kg), cefazolin achieves appropriate concentrations in most tissues to prevent bacterial growth of common wound contaminants [36]. Cephalothin is also effective against a similar range of organisms but is less effective against gram-negative bacteria [4]. With surgery of the large intestine or other areas containing anaerobic organisms, prophylactic antimicrobials with anaerobic and enteric gram-negative coverage, such as cefoxitin, should be considered [2,36]. For the critically ill patient, combination antimicrobial therapy may be necessary prophylactically. Newer broad-spectrum antimicrobial agents that are used therapeutically should be avoided in surgical prophylaxis so as to reduce emergence of resistant bacterial strains [10,37]. Most third- and fourth-generation cephalosporins are less effective than cefazolin against organisms likely to cause SSIs (eg, *Staphylococcus* spp) [37].

Margin of safety is an additional consideration when selecting antimicrobial agents for prophylaxis. Avoid drugs that are likely to result in toxicity, organ damage, other adverse reactions, or interactions with other medications. For example, Pasco and coworkers [38] reported acute postoperative azotemia in seven dogs given nafcillin for surgical prophylaxis. One dog was euthanatized because of lack of response to therapy, two dogs had persistent isosthenuria, and four dogs recovered. On cessation of nafcillin as a prophylactic antimicrobial, no further cases of acute postoperative azotemia were recorded in dogs over the next 15 months.

Timing of Prophylactic Antimicrobials

Timing and duration of administration of prophylactic antimicrobials are critical and often misunderstood principles. Because the initial dose of a prophylactic antimicrobial is administered intravenously around 30 to 60 minutes before skin incision creation, the term *perioperative* antimicrobial use is also appropriate [39]. Burke [40] determined that the greatest reduction in infection rates occurred when an antimicrobial was given immediately before or at the time of contamination. Additionally, systemic antimicrobials had no benefit when given 3 hours after contamination. Hence, administration of prophylactic antimicrobials after completion of surgery is not likely to be beneficial in preventing infection. In longer surgical procedures (>90 minutes), prophylactic antimicrobial administration should be repeated every 1 to 3 hours (typically every 2 hours with cefazolin). In a surgical series of 131 human patients undergoing colorectal surgery, Morita and colleagues [41] demonstrated that with prolonged surgery (>4 hours), the incidence of infection was decreased with frequent repeated intraoperative dosing of the prophylactic antimicrobial cefmetazole, a second-generation cephalosporin. Operations exceeding 4 hours after the initial antimicrobial dose had surgical wound infection rates of 8.5% in patients receiving repeat dosing compared with 26.5% in those patients not receiving repeat dosing [41]. Richardson and coworkers [42] demonstrated that when cefazolin was administered every 60 minutes during canine total hip replacement surgery (starting when the patient was positioned on the table), a mean of 15 times the minimum inhibitory concentration needed to kill 90% of the contaminants (MIC_{90}) was achieved at the surgical site. Timing of the second dose of prophylactic antimicrobial is influenced by many factors, including the targeted bacteria, dose administered, and half-life and pharmacokinetics of the antimicrobial used [41,42]. For general surgical prophylaxis, the authors typically administer cefazolin intravenously 30 to 60 minutes before the start of surgery and repeat it every 2 hours during surgery.

Although it is relatively common for veterinary surgeons to continue antimicrobial prophylaxis as long as 24 to 48 hours after closure of the surgical wound, prophylactic antimicrobials should be discontinued at the conclusion of the exposure period (ie, surgery) [10]. Further treatment has minimal effect on the incidence of postoperative infection [4,35,43,44]. Continued use of prophylactic antimicrobials beyond the conclusion of the exposure period contributes to the development of resistant bacteria, superinfections, and nosocomial infections [9,45–47]. As mentioned previously, contaminated and dirty and/or infected wounds are typically treated therapeutically after surgery with an appropriate antimicrobial for the length of time deemed necessary to resolve the infection (typically 2 to 3 days after resolution of clinical signs) [36].

THERAPEUTIC ANTIMICROBIALS

The veterinary surgeon often encounters a patient with contaminated or dirty wounds that needs postoperative therapeutic antimicrobial coverage. Veterinarians also occasionally encounter a patient with an SSI that requires treatment. Therapeutic antimicrobials are indicated in these patients, and appropriate antimicrobial selection is based on many of the same factors used to select prophylactic agents, including anticipated flora, bacterial resistance patterns, and ability of the drug to reach the target tissue at appropriate concentrations [36,48]. Ideally, therapeutic antimicrobial selection should be based on culture and susceptibility testing results. Select the antimicrobial agent that is most likely to eliminate microorganisms effectively at the site of infection, least likely to produce adverse effects or toxicity, and least likely to affect the host's immune system negatively [48]. Often, the initial selection of a therapeutic antimicrobial is made empirically while awaiting culture and susceptibility testing results. Empiric selection should be based on clinical judgment, microbe factors, antimicrobial characteristics (including mechanism of action), and infection severity. Antimicrobial selection may need to be altered once culture and susceptibility testing results are available. When choosing between several potentially effective antimicrobials, select the antimicrobial agent that reaches the target tissue, is least toxic, is least expensive, and is easiest to administer [2,36,48]. Length of therapy depends at least on the infection being treated and the toxicity of the antimicrobial selected. For simple infections, therapeutic antimicrobials are typically continued for at least 2 to 3 days beyond complete resolution of clinical signs [36]. With many surgical infections, adjuvant therapy is needed, including foreign body removal, infected nidus removal, debridement of necrotic tissue, drainage of fluid collections, or lavage and other appropriate local wound therapies.

LOCAL ANTIMICROBIAL USE IN THE SURGICAL PATIENT

Antimicrobials may be used locally to treat selected wounds in veterinary surgical patients. Advantages of local antimicrobial use in wounds include selective bacterial toxicity, combined efficacy when used with systemic antibiotics, activity in the presence of organic debris, and achievement of effective levels regardless of tissue perfusion [49,50]. Numerous disadvantages of local antimicrobial use include cost, narrow antimicrobial spectrum, systemic toxicity, bacterial resistance, creation of "superinfections," and increased nosocomial infections [49]. Antimicrobials like ampicillin, penicillin, carbenicillin, tetracycline, kanamycin, and cephalosporins are occasionally added to lavage solutions for local wound administration [49]. Antimicrobial powders should not be used in wounds or body cavities because they act as foreign bodies [49]. Addition of antimicrobials to peritoneal or thoracic lavage fluids is not beneficial and may induce chemical peritonitis, pleuritis, or adhesion formation similar to that seen with antiseptic use in peritoneal or thoracic cavities [51–53]. Avoid direct administration of any antimicrobial or antiseptic agent into the abdominal and thoracic cavities [51–53]. Further, levels of antimicrobials in tissues are less reliably and safely achieved when using local antimicrobials [51–53].

With septic arthritis, joint lavage is essential to help remove deleterious material from the joint. With joint infection, surgical debridement and copious lavage are often indicated [54]. Use of antiseptics or antimicrobials in the lavage solution is controversial and may cause a chemical synovitis [55,56]. In some instances, however, the advantages of joint lavage with antiseptics or antimicrobials may outweigh the risks [54].

TOPICAL ANTISEPTIC AND ANTIMICROBIAL AGENTS IN THE SURGICAL PATIENT

Topical agents may be applied to wounds to help cleanse them or improve healing. Several antiseptic agents are available; however, only a few are appropriate to use in open wounds with exposed tissues. Antiseptic lavage agents appropriate to use in open wounds include dilute chlorhexidine diacetate solution (0.05%) and dilute povidone-iodine solution (0.1%–1%) [57–59]. When using dilute chlorhexidine or dilute povidone-iodine solution to lavage wounds, use appropriate concentrations so that a beneficial bactericidal effect without tissue toxicity is achieved [49,51–59]. Dilute chlorhexidine (0.05%) is the preferred wound lavage agent because of its wide spectrum of antimicrobial activity, sustained residual activity, and activity in the presence of organic debris or blood [49,60]. Povidone-iodine solutions should be used at low concentrations (0.1%–1%) because they are more bactericidal and less toxic to tissues than at higher concentrations [49,57]. Frequent reapplication (every 4 to 6 hours) of povidone-iodine is required because it has reduced residual activity compared with chlorhexidine and is inactivated in the presence of organic matter[60]. Tris-ethylenediaminetetraacetic acid (EDTA) solution (for gram-negative bacteria, including *Pseudomonas* spp) is also occasionally selected as a lavage agent [49]. Other antiseptic lavage solutions, such as hydrogen peroxide (damages tissues and is a poor antiseptic) and Dakin's solution (0.25% dilute bleach solution), should be avoided [60].

Topical antimicrobial agents relatively commonly applied to superficial wounds include triple-antibiotic ointment, silver sulfadiazine, nitrofurazone, and gentamicin sulfate. Triple-antibiotic ointment (bacitracin, neomycin, and polymyxin) is effective against a broad spectrum of bacteria commonly found in superficial skin wounds, but it has poor efficacy against *Pseudomonas* spp [60,61]. Triple-antibiotic ointment can enhance wound re-epithelialization [61]. The agent is poorly absorbed, so systemic toxicity is rare. Triple-antibiotic ointment is more effective in preventing infections than in treating them. Silver sulfadiazine is effective against most gram-positive and gram-negative bacteria and many fungi [60,61]. This agent penetrates necrotic tissues, enhances wound epithelialization, and is considered one of the topical antimicrobials of choice to treat burn wounds [49,60]. Nitrofurazone ointment is commonly used in veterinary patients and has a broad gram-positive spectrum. This agent has hydrophilic properties that enable it to draw body fluid from the wound, which helps in the absorption of tenacious exudates by bandages [60,61]. Nitrofurazone may delay wound epithelialization, however [60]. Nitrofurazone powder should not be used in open wounds. Gentamicin sulfate ointment is especially effective in controlling gram-negative growth and is often used before and after grafting of wounds that have not responded to triple-antibiotic ointment [60,61]. As with parenterally administered antimicrobials, selection of topical antimicrobial agents should be based on efficacy against anticipated organisms and lack of adverse and/or toxic reactions.

ANTIMICROBIAL CONSIDERATIONS FOR SPECIFIC PROCEDURES

Each type of surgical procedure and each body system encountered have their own unique risks and potential pathogens that could result in SSIs. The veterinary surgeon needs to be aware of these considerations to make the most appropriate selection of prophylactic and therapeutic antimicrobials.

Gastrointestinal Surgery

The gastrointestinal tract harbors the largest number and variety of microbial organisms of any body system. Because the stomach has a low pH (an acid "barrier"), there are fewer organisms present compared with other parts of the gastrointestinal tract [2]. Additionally, the rapid transit time of the stomach and proximal small intestine keeps bacterial levels of the enteric contents below 10^3 per gram in fasted patients [2]. Gram-positive cocci and enteric gram-negative bacilli are prevalent in the stomach and upper gastrointestinal tract [2]. Cefazolin is typically an appropriate prophylactic antimicrobial choice for surgery of the esophagus, stomach, and upper gastrointestinal tract. The distal small intestine, however, contains large numbers of aerobic and anaerobic organisms [2]. In the colon, facultative and strict anaerobic organism numbers increase markedly and typically greatly outnumber aerobic organisms [2]. Examples of organisms found in the lower gastrointestinal tract include enteric gram-negative bacilli, enterococci, and anaerobic organisms, such as *Bacteroides* spp [2,48]. Prophylactic antimicrobial selection for patients undergoing surgery of the lower gastrointestinal tract should include agents that have an appropriate spectrum and such drugs as cefoxitin and cefotetan. Large numbers of enteric gram-negative bacilli and anaerobes may also be found in the hepatobiliary system. Surgery of the liver or biliary tract may also warrant selection of a second-generation cephalosporin for prophylactic use [48].

Genitourinary Surgery

Under normal circumstances, the urinary system is free of bacteria, although the genitalia and external openings may be contaminated with enteric or skin organisms [2]. Likewise, the noninfected uterus and prostate typically are free of bacteria. Hence, routine ovariohysterectomy is not an indication for prophylactic antimicrobial use unless other risk factors exist [48]. The infected uterus or prostate, however, is often heavily contaminated with *E coli*, *Streptococcus* spp, and anaerobes [48]. Patients with uterine or prostatic infection typically require appropriate antimicrobial use during surgery and therapeutically [48]. Empiric selection and use of single or multiple antimicrobial agents is often initiated, with culture and susceptibility results guiding further therapy. For routine cystotomy and calculus removal, cefazolin is generally adequate for prophylactic antimicrobial coverage.

Integumentary Surgery

Routine surgery of the integumentary system (eg, tumor resections, skin flaps) does not require antimicrobial prophylaxis unless the skin is already contaminated or infected, surgery is lengthy, or host factors dictate prophylaxis. Free skin grafting or large axial pattern flap procedures may require antimicrobial prophylaxis using cefazolin, particularly because surgery can occasionally be lengthy. Additionally, with free skin grafts, topical antimicrobial therapy (antimicrobial ointment or creams and 0.05% chlorhexidine for cleaning) is often used after surgery [62].

Orthopedic and Neurologic Surgery

Patients undergoing short clean orthopedic or neurologic procedures in which no implants are placed often do not need the administration of prophylactic antimicrobials. Implants are used in many orthopedic and neurologic procedures, however, and prophylactic cefazolin is indicated because *Staphylococcus* spp are most likely to be encountered [11,48]. Additionally, with many neurologic procedures, an SSI would be catastrophic. Hence, the use of prophylactic cefazolin directed toward the common skin contaminants is indicated [11]. In human surgery, antimicrobial prophylaxis usually is not indicated for routine lumbar discectomy; however, it is considered beneficial for patients undergoing prolonged spinal procedures or for those receiving implants or fusions [63].

Thoracic, Cardiac, and Respiratory System Surgery

For patients undergoing a thoracotomy for short procedures, antimicrobial prophylaxis may not be indicated unless other risk factors are identified. With cardiovascular procedures, including pacemaker implantation, the prophylactic use of cefazolin is indicated [48]. *Staphylococcus* spp, *Streptococcus* spp, and, occasionally, gram-negative bacilli may be encountered in the upper respiratory system [2]. The lower respiratory system is not normally a significant source of infection in the healthy animal, although bacterial organisms are often encountered [2]. Prophylactic antimicrobial administration (cefazolin) is indicated in patients undergoing respiratory tract surgery, especially resection of infected lung tissue or tracheal ring prostheses for correction of tracheal collapse.

Head and Neck Surgery

Surgery of the head and neck that does not involve a contaminated or infected area, the eye, or incision through oral or pharyngeal mucosa does not need antimicrobial prophylaxis. Incisions through the oral or pharyngeal mucosa usually necessitate the use of prophylactic antimicrobials directed against common contaminants, including *Staphylococcus* spp, *Streptococcus* spp, facultative bacteria, and anaerobes [48]. Clindamycin or ampicillin is often indicated prophylactically in patients undergoing dental surgery [64–66].

Total ear canal ablation with lateral bulla osteotomy (TECA with LBO), particularly in dogs, is often performed in situations of chronically infected ears that have been treated with a variety of antimicrobials and have a likelihood of resistant bacteria. One study demonstrated that during TECA with LBO, there is substantial contamination of subcutaneous tissues with bacteria from excised tissues from the osseous bulla [67]. Contamination with *E coli* or *Streptococcus canis* occurred in 94% of these surgical procedures. In this study, cefazolin was effective against only 70% of the bacterial isolates. Culture and susceptibility testing of samples from the tympanic cavity is critical for appropriate selection of therapeutic antimicrobials in dogs undergoing TECA with LBO [68].

SUMMARY

Appropriate use of antimicrobials for the veterinary surgical patient is an important part of the practice of veterinary surgery. Prophylactic antimicrobials, when indicated, should be administered following current recommendations, including (1) selection of an appropriate prophylactic antimicrobial agent based on anticipated flora, (2) administration of the selected antimicrobial intravenously 30 to 60 minutes before making the skin incision, 3) repeat dosing of the antimicrobial every 1 to 3 hours during surgery, and 4) discontinuation of antimicrobial use at the conclusion of surgery (the exposure period). By identifying the risk of infection, having knowledge of potential contaminating organisms, being aware of the choices of antimicrobial therapy, and weighing the risks and benefits of each option, veterinary surgeons can devise individualized plans for antimicrobial prophylaxis and, when necessary, appropriate therapeutic intervention after surgery.

References

[1] Bowler PG, Duerden BI, Armstrong DG. Wound microbiology and associated approaches to wound management. Clin Microbiol Rev 2001;14(2):244–69.

[2] Cockshutt J. Principles of surgical asepsis. In: Slatter D, editor. Textbook of small animal surgery. 3rd edition. Philadelphia: Elsevier Science; 2003. p. 149–55.

[3] Glickman LT. Veterinary nosocomial (hospital-acquired) Klebsiella infections. J Am Vet Med Assoc 1981;179(12):1389–92.

[4] Wilcke JR. Use of antimicrobial drugs to prevent infections in veterinary patients. Probl Vet Med 1990;2(2):298–311.

[5] Vasser PB, Paul HA, Enos LR, et al. Infection rates in clean surgical procedures: a comparison of ampicillin prophylaxis vs. a placebo. J Am Vet Med Assoc 1985;187(8):825–7.

[6] Holmberg DL. Prophylactic use of antibiotics in surgery. Vet Clin North Am Small Anim Pract 1978;8(2):219–27.

[7] Holmberg DL. Prophylactic antibiotics, friend or foe. Vet Comp Orthop Traumatol 1990; 1:18–9.

[8] Daude-Lagrave A, Carozzo C, Fayolle P, et al. Infection rates in surgical procedures: a comparison of cefalexin vs. a placebo. Vet Comp Orthop Traumatol 2001;14:146–50.

[9] Classen DC, Evans RS, Pestotnik SL, et al. The timing of prophylactic administration of antibiotics and the risk of surgical-wound infection. N Engl J Med 1992;326(5):281–6.

[10] Bratzler DW, Houck PM. Antimicrobial prophylaxis for surgery: an advisory statement from the National Surgical Infection Prevention Project. Clin Infect Dis 2004;38(12):1706–15.

[11] Whittem TL, Johnson AL, Smith CW, et al. Effect of perioperative prophylactic antimicrobial treatment in dogs undergoing elective orthopedic surgery. J Am Vet Med Assoc 1999;215(2):212–6.

[12] DiPiro JT, Edmiston CE, Bohnen JMA. Pharmacodynamics of antimicrobial therapy in surgery. Am J Surg 1996;171(6):615–22.

[13] Ludwig KA, Carlson MA, Condon RE. Prophylactic antibiotics in surgery. Annu Rev Med 1993;44:385–93.
[14] Cho CY, Lo JS. Dressing the part. Dermatol Clin 1998;16(1):25–47.
[15] Paluzzi RG. Antimicrobial prophylaxis for surgery. Med Clin North Am 1993;77(2): 427–41.
[16] Oishi CS, Carrion WV, Hoaglund FT. Use of parenteral prophylactic antibiotics in clean orthopedic surgery. A review of the literature. Clin Orthop 1993;296:249–55.
[17] Court-Brown CM. Antibiotic prophylaxis in orthopedic surgery. Scand J Infect Dis 1990;70(Suppl):74–9.
[18] Gyssens IC. Preventing postoperative infections: current treatment recommendations. Drugs 1999;57(2):175–85.
[19] Queiroz R, Grinbaum RS, Galvao LL, et al. Antibiotic prophylaxis in orthopedic surgeries: the results of an implemented protocol. Braz J Infect Dis 2005;9(3):283–7.
[20] Page CP, Bohnen JM, Fletcher JR, et al. Antimicrobial prophylaxis for surgical wounds: guidelines for clinical care. Arch Surg 1993;128(1):79–88.
[21] Haas AF, Grekin RC. Antibiotic prophylaxis in dermatologic surgery. J Am Acad Dermatol 1995;32(2 Pt 1):155–76.
[22] Ad Hoc Committee of the Committee on Trauma. Division of Medical Sciences, National Academy of Sciences, National Research Council. Postoperative wound infections: the influence of ultraviolet irradiation of the operating room and various other factors. Ann Surg 1964;160(Suppl):33–81.
[23] Smeak DD, Olmstead ML. Infections in clean wounds: the roles of the surgeon, environment, and host. Compend Contin Educ Pract Vet 1984;6(7):629–34.
[24] Lee JT. Contemporary wound surveillance issues. New Horiz 1998;6(Suppl 2):S20–9.
[25] Brown DC, Conzemius MG, Shofer F, et al. Epidemiologic evaluation of postoperative wound infections in dogs and cats. J Am Vet Med Assoc 1997;210(9):1302–6.
[26] Vasser PB, Levy J, Dowd D, et al. Surgical wound infection rates in dogs and cats: data from a teaching hospital. Vet Surg 1988;17(2):60–4.
[27] Johnson JA, Murtaugh RJ. Preventing and treating nosocomial infection. Part 2. Wound, blood and gastrointestinal infections. Compend Contin Educ Pract Vet 1997;19(6): 693–703.
[28] Eugster S, Schalwalder P, Gaschen F, et al. A prospective study of postoperative surgical site infections in dogs and cats. Vet Surg 2004;33(5):542–50.
[29] Leaper DJ. Prophylactic and therapeutic role of antibiotics in wound care. Am J Surg 1994;167(1A):15S–9S.
[30] Romatowski J. Prevention and control of surgical wound infection. J Am Vet Med Assoc 1989;194(1):107–14.
[31] Nichols RL. Surgical infections: prevention and treatment—1965–1995. Am J Surg 1996;172(1):68–74.
[32] Cruse PJE, Foord R. The epidemiology of wound infection: a 10 year prospective study of 62,939 wounds. Surg Clin North Am 1980;60(1):27–40.
[33] Beal MW, Brown DC, Shofer FS. The effects of perioperative hypothermia and the duration of anesthesia on postoperative wound infection rate in clean wounds: a retrospective study. Vet Surg 2000;29(2):123–7.
[34] Heldmann E, Brown DC, Shofer F. The association of propofol usage with postoperative wound infection rates in clean wounds: a retrospective study. Vet Surg 1999;28(4):256–9.
[35] Polk HC, Lopez-Mayor JF. Postoperative wound infection: a prospective study of determinant factors and prevention. Surgery 1969;66(1):97–103.
[36] Seim HB, Fossum TW. Surgical infections and antibiotic selection. In: Fossum TW, editor. Small animal surgery. 2nd edition. St. Louis (MO): Mosby; 2002. p. 60–8.
[37] Weed HG. Antimicrobial prophylaxis in the surgical patient. Med Clin North Am 2003;87(1):59–75.

[38] Pasco PJ, Ilkiw JE, Kass PH, et al. Case-control study of the association between intraoperative administration of nafcillin and acute postoperative development of azotemia. J Am Vet Med Assoc 1996;208(7):1043–7.
[39] Barie PS, Eachempati SR. Surgical site infections. Surg Clin North Am 2005;85(6):1115–35.
[40] Burke JF. The effective period of preventative antibiotic action in experimental incisions and dermal lesions. Surgery 1961;50:161–8.
[41] Morita S, Nishisho I, Nomua T, et al. The significance of the intraoperative repeated dosing of antimicrobials for preventing surgical wound infection in colorectal surgery. Surg Today 2005;35(9):732–8.
[42] Richardson DC, Aucoin DP, DeYoung DJ, et al. Pharmacokinetic disposition of cefazolin in serum and tissue during canine total hip replacement. Vet Surg 1992;21(1):1–4.
[43] Linton RR. The prophylactic use of the antibiotics in clean surgery. Surg Gynecol Obstet 1961;112(2):218–21.
[44] Ketcham AS, Lieberman JE, West JT. Antibiotic prophylaxis in cancer surgery and its value in staphylococcal carrier patients. Surg Gynecol Obstet 1963;117:1–8.
[45] Nichols RL, Condon RE, Barie PS. Roundtable discussion: antibiotic prophylaxis in surgery—2005 and beyond. Surg Infect 2005;6(3):349–61.
[46] McDonald M, Grabsch E, Marshall C, et al. Single- versus multiple-dose antimicrobial prophylaxis for major surgery: a systematic review. Aust NZ J Surg 1998;68(6):388–96.
[47] Manian FA, Meyer PL, Setzer J, et al. Surgical site infections associated with methicillin-resistant *Staphylococcus aureus*: do postoperative factors play a role? Clin Infect Dis 2003;36(7):863–8
[48] Dunning D. Surgical wound infection and the use of antimicrobials. In: Slatter D, editor. Textbook of small animal surgery. 3rd edition. Philadelphia: Elsevier Science; 2003. p. 113–22.
[49] Hedlund CS. Surgery of the integumentary system. In: Fossum TW, editor. Small animal surgery. 2nd edition. St. Louis (MO): Mosby; 2002. p. 134–48.
[50] Howell-Jones RS, Wilson MJ, Hill KE, et al. A review of the microbiology, antibiotic usage and resistance in chronic skin wounds. J Antimicrob Chemother 2005;55(2):143–9.
[51] Monnet E. Pleura and pleural space. In: Slatter D, editor. Textbook of small animal surgery. 3rd edition. Philadelphia: Elsevier Science; 2003. p. 387–405.
[52] Kirby BM. Peritoneum and peritoneal cavity. In: Slatter D, editor. Textbook of small animal surgery. 3rd edition. Philadelphia: Elsevier Science; 2003. p. 414–45.
[53] Bondar VM, Rago C, Cottone FJ, et al. Chlorhexidine lavage in the treatment of experimental intra-abdominal infection. Arch Surg 2000;135(3):309–14.
[54] Bubenik LJ, Smith MM. Orthopaedic infections. In: Slatter D, editor. Textbook of small animal surgery. 3rd edition. Philadelphia: Elsevier Science; 2003. p. 1862–75.
[55] Bertone A, McIlwraith CW, Powers BE, et al. Effect of four antimicrobial lavage solutions on the tarsocrural joint of horses. Vet Surg 1986;15(4):305–15.
[56] McIlwraith CW. Treatment of infectious arthritis. Vet Clin North Am Large Anim Pract 1983;5(2):363–79.
[57] Amber EI, Henderson RA, Swaim SF, et al. A comparison of antimicrobial efficacy and tissue reaction of four antiseptics on canine wounds. Vet Surg 1983;12(2):63–8.
[58] Sanchez IR, Swaim SF, Nusbaum KE, et al. Effects of chlorhexidine diacetate and povidone-iodine on wound healing in dogs. Vet Surg 1988;17(6):291–5.
[59] Sanchez IR, Nusbaum KE, Swaim SF, et al. Chlorhexidine diacetate and povidone-iodine cytotoxicity to canine embryonic fibroblasts and *Staphylococcus aureus*. Vet Surg 1988;17(4):182–5.
[60] Waldron DR, Zimmerman-Pope N. Superficial skin wounds. In: Slatter D, editor. Textbook of small animal surgery. 3rd edition. Philadelphia: Elsevier Science; 2003. p. 259–73.

[61] Swaim SF, Henderson RA. Wound healing. In: Small animal wound management. Baltimore (MD): Williams & Wilkins; 1997. p. 1–12.
[62] Swaim SF. Skin grafts. In: Slatter D, editor. Textbook of small animal surgery. 3rd edition. Philadelphia: Elsevier Science; 2003. p. 321–8.
[63] Dimmick J, Lipsett P, Kostuik J. Spine update: antimicrobial prophylaxis in spine surgery: basic principles and recent advances. Spine 2000;25(19):2544–8.
[64] Harvey CE, Thornsberry C, Miller BR, et al. Antimicrobial susceptibility of subgingival bacterial flora in cats with gingivitis. J Vet Dent 1995;12(4):157–60.
[65] Harvey CE, Thornsberry C, Miller BR, et al. Antimicrobial susceptibility of subgingival bacterial flora in dogs with gingivitis. J Vet Dent 1995;12(4):151–5.
[66] Johnson JT, Kachman K, Wagner RL, et al. Comparison of ampicillin/sulbactam versus clindamycin in the prevention of infection in patients undergoing head and neck surgery. Head Neck 1997;19(5):367–71.
[67] Vogel PL, Komtebedde J, Hirsh DC, et al. Wound contamination and antimicrobial susceptibility of bacteria cultured during total ear canal ablation and lateral bulla osteotomy in dogs. J Am Vet Med Assoc 1999;214(11):1641–3.
[68] Hettlich BF, Boothe HW, Simpson RB, et al. Effect of tympanic cavity evacuation and flushing on microbial isolates during total ear canal ablation with lateral bulla osteotomy in dogs. J Am Vet Med Assoc 2005;227(5):748–55.

ELSEVIER
SAUNDERS

Vet Clin Small Anim 36 (2006) 1061–1085

VETERINARY CLINICS
SMALL ANIMAL PRACTICE

The Clinical Pharmacology of Cyclooxygenase-2–Selective and Dual Inhibitors

Terrence P. Clark, DVM, PhD

Department of Biology Research and Technology Acquisitions, Elanco Animal Health, A Division of Eli Lilly and Company, 2001 West Main Street, GL14, Greenfield, IN 46140, USA

BIOLOGY OF CYCLOOXYGENASE

As mediators of biologic processes, prostaglandins were first extracted from tissues in the 1930s and were demonstrated to exert an effect on blood pressure and smooth muscle contraction [1]. Much later, arachidonic acid (AA) was identified as the common precursor to prostaglandins [2,3], followed by the identification of cyclooxygenase (COX) as the enzyme that cyclized and oxygenated AA to yield prostaglandin [4]. The first purification of a COX enzyme from tissue was later achieved in sheep [5] and bovine seminal vesicles [6]. It is now well established that a variety of isomerases and oxidoreductases produce an array of biologically important prostaglandins from a COX-derived common intermediate. The collision between prostaglandin research and pharmacology occurred in 1971, when Vane [7] demonstrated that aspirin, indomethacin, and salicylate, common nonsteroidal anti-inflammatory drugs (NSAIDs), exerted their effect by inhibiting COX. Before this time, NSAIDs were commonly used in clinical medicine to alleviate pain, inflammation, and fever without an understanding of the underlying mechanism.

Shortly after the recognition that NSAIDs work through COX inhibition, it was proposed that there existed more than one COX enzyme. In particular, an acetaminophen-inhibitable form of COX was hypothesized to exist in canine brain that was not present in other tissues or species [8]. The most compelling evidence that more than one COX existed was the timing of prostaglandin appearance in various tissues after mitogen stimulation. For example, Habenicht and colleagues [9] demonstrated early (10 minutes) and late (2–4 hours) peak inductions in prostaglandin synthesis in a fibroblast cell line. It was only the late peak induction that required protein synthesis, and thus was considered inducible. Finally, in 1991, two laboratories independently reported a gene sequence that coded a new inducible COX enzyme [10,11]. It is now clear that the original

E-mail address: clarktp@lilly.com

0195-5616/06/$ – see front matter
doi:10.1016/j.cvsm.2006.07.001

vetsmall.theclinics.com

COX isolated from seminal vesicles was noninducible, identified as COX-1, whereas the newly identified isoform was inducible and referred to as COX-2.

More recently, a brain-specific splice variant of COX-1 has been identified in dogs, termed COX-3 by the authors [12]. This enzyme results from the COX-1 gene that retains an additional 90 nucleotides from intron-1. Thus, unlike COX-2, which is encoded from a unique gene, COX-3 is considered a variant of COX-1. It is, however, biologically different from COX-1; COX-3 contains less prostaglandin synthesis activity. and the analgesic and antipyretic drugs acetaminophen and dipyrone preferentially inhibit its activity.

COX enzymes have important biologic and pathophysiologic roles. A common adverse reaction observed with classic NSAIDs is gastrointestinal (GI) ulceration, which can now be better explained with a fuller understanding of COX. Prostaglandin synthesis generally attributable to COX-1 has been documented in all portions of the GI tract, with a rank order from highest to lowest synthesis being gastric muscle, gastric mucosa, colon, rectum, ileum, cecum, duodenum, jejunum, and esophagus [13]. Prostaglandins are considered cytoprotective, and insults to the gastric mucosa can be reduced or eliminated by coadministration with various prostaglandins [14]. This cytoprotective effect is brought about by three general mechanisms. First, prostaglandins reduce the secretion of gastric acid by the parietal cells of the stomach [15]. Second, prostaglandins exert a direct vasodilatory effect on the gastric mucosa, thereby increasing mucosal blood flow and maintaining the integrity of the gastric tissue [16]. Finally, prostaglandins stimulate the production of viscous mucus and bicarbonate by the epithelial and smooth muscle cells of the stomach, which likely plays a defensive role in mucosal injury [17]. These observations have led to the general notion that preserving the function of COX-1 should minimize GI adverse reactions attributable to NSAIDs.

In addition to their cytoprotective effect on the gastric mucosa, prostaglandins play an important physiologic role in the kidney, central nervous system (CNS), reproductive system, and cardiovascular system. In the kidney, vasodilatory prostaglandins play a key role in regulating renal blood flow, diminishing vascular resistance, dilating renal vascular beds, and enhancing organ perfusion [18]. In the CNS, COX-1 is found in neurons throughout the brain, where it may be involved in complex integrative functions [19]. COX-1 is also expressed in fetal, amniotic, and uterine tissues, where it establishes implantation, maintains pregnancy, and contributes to placental development [20,21]. Blood platelets contain only COX-1, which converts AA to the potent proaggregatory and vasoconstrictor prostaglandin thromboxane (TBX) A_2; this is the rationale for using COX-1–selective compounds (eg, aspirin) in human beings to prevent myocardial infarction. A special note regarding the cardiovascular safety of COX-2–selective drugs should be considered. Recent regulatory and legal action has been taken for some COX-2–selective drugs in human health as the result of apparent adverse cardiovascular events. The concern in human medicine is that the use of COX-2 inhibitors can lead to heart ailments or strokes [22]. Whereas this continues to be examined in human health, the US Food and Drug Administration (FDA) Center for Veterinary Medicine (CVM) does not believe there is compelling data to merit concern for cardiovascular events in dogs or cats [23]. Therefore, in addition to improved GI safety, NSAIDs that preserve COX-1 activity may presumably spare other important organ system functions.

A primary reason for the clinical use of NSAIDs in veterinary medicine is to treat inflammation, pain, and fever by reducing prostaglandin synthesis brought about by inducible COX-2. Proinflammatory cytokines and mitogens elaborated as the result of noxious stimuli induce COX-2. A key role for COX-2 in joint inflammation was demonstrated through the induction of COX-2 expression in chondrocytes, osteoblasts, and synovial microvessel endothelial cells [24]. Taken together, it has been proposed that selective inhibition of COX-2 should result in anti-inflammatory activity, whereas sparing COX-1 should minimize GI, renal, and other toxicities associated with NSAIDs [25].

CYCLOOXYGENASES AND DRUG DISCOVERY AND DEVELOPMENT

Even before the discovery of COX-2, pharmaceutical companies were searching for NSAIDs with a more favorable GI safety profile. This work resulted in the development of three drugs intended for human health that were later developed for veterinary medicine: carprofen, etodolac, and meloxicam. After the discovery of COX-2 in 1991, these new NSAIDs with greater GI safety were shown to selectively inhibit COX-2, thus accounting for their improved GI safety profile. After these early introductions, screens for drugs with even higher selectivity toward COX-2 were developed, with the presumption being that a higher safety profile could be achieved by further minimizing COX-1 inhibition. As a result of this work, newer compounds were introduced to veterinary medicine, including deracoxib and firocoxib. Importantly, each of these drugs is approved by the FDA for use in dogs or cats and should be considered safe and effective when used according to the label. Since their introduction, however, some new information and concerns have been raised.

On the basis of experimental information and clinical data, the correlation of COX-2 selectivity with safer NSAIDs was widely supported. Emerging information supports a role for COX-2 in the stomach that may have an impact on the GI safety of COX-2–selective NSAIDs, however. For example, COX-2 induction has been documented in *Helicobacter pylori* gastritis, inflammatory bowel disease, and bacterial infections of the gastric mucosa; thus, administration of a COX-2 inhibitor may become harmful in the presence of GI inflammation. This is supported in studies in which transgenic animals lacking the COX-1 gene did not develop gastric ulcers spontaneously [26] and administration of a COX-2–selective inhibitor exacerbated mucosal injury [27]. In another study in a rat model of colitis, administration of a selective COX-2 inhibitor at doses that do not inhibit COX-1 resulted in significant inhibition of mucosal prostaglandin synthesis and a marked increase in colonic damage [28]. When treatment continued with a COX-2–selective drug for 1 week in these rats, colonic injury was exacerbated to perforation, resulting in 100% death. Taken together, COX-2 may also be required for GI defense, and ulcers may result from the inhibition of COX-2 and COX-1.

This pathophysiology may have played a role in recent results that examined GI tract perforation reported in dogs administered deracoxib, a highly selective COX-2 inhibitor [29]. In a retrospective evaluation of the records of 29 dogs treated with deracoxib in which GI tract perforation was documented, 20 dogs died or were euthanized and 9 survived. Sixteen (55%) of the 29 dogs had received deracoxib at a dosage higher than that approved by the FDA for the particular indication being treated. Seventeen (59%) dogs had received at least one other NSAID or a glucocorticoid in close temporal association (within 24 hours) with deracoxib administration (ie, immediately before or after). Altogether, 26 (90%) dogs had received deracoxib at a higher than approved dosage or had received at least one other NSAID or glucocorticoid in close temporal association with deracoxib administration. Perforation and death seemed to be related to higher than approved doses of deracoxib or coadministration with other NSAIDs or glucocorticoids. The authors concluded that deracoxib should only be used at approved dosages and that glucocorticoids and other less selective NSAIDs should not be coadministered in close temporal association with selective COX-2 inhibitors.

Subsequent to the discovery of COX-2–selective NSAIDs, it has been established that COX-2 plays a role in the maintenance of renal function. Consequently, another concern that has been raised is the safety of COX-2–selective NSAIDs in relation to renal function and ischemia [30]. To date, the evidence does not support the notion that COX-2–selective NSAIDs raise the risk of renal injury when used chronically for osteoarthritis. In addition, renal safety is further supported when they are used to control perioperative pain in otherwise healthy animals in conjunction with standard intraoperative supportive care. For example, in a blind multicenter study of 454 dogs undergoing various soft tissue procedures, dogs were administered carprofen (2 mg/lb) approximately 2 hours before surgery and then once daily after surgery as needed [31]. Relevant renal clinical pathologic variables evaluated included, in part, clinical chemistries, urinalysis, and urinary gamma glutamyl transpeptidase (GGT)/creatinine ratio. None of the dogs developed renal impairment. These results have been repeated in numerous small and large studies using laboratory Beagles and client-owned dogs with several different COX-2–selective NSAIDS. The safety of hypotensive or volume-depleted dogs undergoing surgery that were treated with a COX-2–selective drug has not been reported.

Importantly, greater inhibition of COX-2 over COX-1 has been linked to greater GI safety. Therefore, as a drug discovery tool, compounds with limited COX-1 inhibition (COX-1 sparing) in in vitro screens are brought forward for further evaluation by pharmaceutical companies. Although it is tempting to equate an in vitro COX-2/COX-1 inhibition ratio to overall in vivo safety, the data do not support this approach. The true overall safety for any individual compound is based on its evaluation in laboratory margin-of-safety studies, reproductive safety studies and blind multicenter field studies in client-owned animals. Therefore, when choosing a COX-2–selective compound for clinical use, all in vivo data must be taken into account to understand comparative safety and continued use must be based on the drug's performance in the individual being treated. Therefore, to support a full understanding of NSAID selection and continued use in a clinical setting, the following discussion on the individual drugs focuses on evidence-based medicine supporting their safe and effective use in companion animals.

INDIVIDUAL CYCLOOXYGENASE-2–SELECTIVE DRUGS

Carprofen

Carprofen was the first COX-2–selective NSAID approved for use in dogs new animal drug application ([NADA] 141-053). Its selective inhibition of COX-2 has been demonstrated in vitro and ex vivo [32,33]. Carprofen is indicated for the relief of pain and inflammation associated with osteoarthritis and for the control of postoperative pain associated with soft tissue and orthopedic procedures in dogs. It is available as caplets, chewable tablets, or a solution for subcutaneous injection. The approved dose is 2 mg/lb (4.4 mg/kg) administered once daily or 1 mg/lb (2.2 mg/kg) administered twice daily. When used for postoperative pain, the dose should be given 2 hours before surgery.

As stated previously, early development of carprofen preceded the discovery of COX-2. Therefore, shortly after its introduction, the notion that carprofen does not work through COX inhibition was put forth, based on studies using in vivo models of inflammation. First, it was observed in early data that carprofen had no effect on prostaglandin synthesis in mice [34]. We now know, however, that data from murine systems must not be extrapolated to potency and efficacy in dogs for two reasons: there can be inherent differences between species in potency and selectivity against COX-1 and COX-2 enzymes, and there are significant differences in metabolism between mice and dogs that make interpretation of in vivo data difficult. Second, carprofen did not inhibit ex vivo platelet TBX B_2 synthesis at a dose of 0.7 mg/kg (1.54 mg/lb) in dogs [35]. Since the discovery of COX-2, ex vivo synthesis of TBX B_2 is now considered an accepted assay for COX-1 inhibition, and given carprofen's COX selectivity [32], these data are consistent with carprofen's mechanism. Third, in cats, whereas 0.7 mg/kg did not inhibit TBX B_2 synthesis, 4.0 mg/kg reduced ex vivo synthesis of TBX B_2 for up to 24 hours when administered subcutaneously [36]. In cats, carprofen has a similar potency and selectivity against COX-1 and COX-2 but is not metabolized as efficiently compared with dogs. The lower dose of 0.7 mg/kg likely resulted in blood levels below the COX-1 inhibitory concentration, whereas the 4.0-mg/kg dose likely exceeded the COX-1 inhibitory concentration for an extended period. Taken together, these data do not refute activity against COX-2 but rather support it in light of the fact that ex vivo prostaglandin E_2 (PGE_2) levels were not determined.

The effectiveness of carprofen for the treatment of osteoarthritis was established in a multicenter study in dogs diagnosed with osteoarthritis [37]. Safety studies in healthy, laboratory dogs have demonstrated that carprofen has a high safety margin according to the US prescribing information label. When administered at 1, 3, and 5 times the recommended total daily dose for 6 weeks, no significant adverse reactions were reported. When 10 times the recommended total daily dose was administered for 14 days, hypoalbuminemia was reported in two of eight dogs, but there was no GI ulceration. In separate safety studies lasting approximately 2 weeks and 1 year, dogs were administered orally up to 5.7 times the recommended total daily dose. No gross or histologic changes were reported in any of the treated animals, with the primary finding being an increase in serum alanine aminotransferase (ALT) of approximately 20 IU in dogs receiving the highest doses.

In field studies, anorexia, vomiting, and diarrhea are the most commonly reported adverse reactions, affecting 8.9 cases per 10,000 treated dogs [38]. In contrast to the apparent high safety margin described in laboratory and field studies, however, idiosyncratic hepatic toxicity has also been reported [39]. Pharmacovigilance information from the manufacturer has further described liver involvement into two categories: elevated enzymes without hepatic dysfunction affecting 4.2 cases per 10,000 treated dogs and liver insufficiency or failure affecting 1.7 cases per 10,000 dogs treated [38]. As a result, it is recommended that pretreatment blood samples be obtained to establish a baseline. Posttreatment blood samples should be obtained at regular intervals or if an adverse reaction is suspected. Anorexia seems to be associated with hepatopathy as well as with elevation of ALT and aspartate aminotransferase (AST) within the first few days. If encountered, carprofen should be discontinued and supportive care initiated. It should be noted that with the addition of other approved NSAIDs, pharmacovigilance has shown that hepatic toxicity is not limited to carprofen.

There have been limited head-to-head comparisons with other drugs. In one study, carprofen was compared with meloxicam in dogs presented with osteoarthritis [40]. A total of 16 dogs were each treated with meloxicam (0.2 mg/kg once and then 0.1 mg/kg daily thereafter) or carprofen (1 mg/lb twice daily) for 60 days. Subjective improvement was not noted by the owners of carprofen-treated dogs but was noted in dogs treated with meloxicam, which contradicted the previously reported findings [36]. Orthopedic surgeons noted subjective improvement in both groups, and objective ground reaction force improvements via a force plate were documented in both groups. The inability of the owners to identify an improvement in carprofen-treated dogs may be the result of large variability in subjective assessments in untrained observers and of the small number of animals participating in the study.

In another study [41], 575 dogs diagnosed with osteoarthritis were treated with firocoxib (5 mg/kg/d), carprofen (4 mg/kg/d), or etodolac (10–15 mg/kg/d) for 30 days. There were 292 dogs treated with firocoxib, 132 with carprofen, and 151 with etodolac. There was no report of comparative effectiveness; however, fewer dogs experienced diarrhea with firocoxib (3.1%) than with carprofen (6.8%). In addition, the incidence of at least one health-related event was less with firocoxib (1.0%) compared with carprofen (6.1%). There was no difference in the number of dogs that dropped out of the study. To assign greater safety, data from larger numbers of dogs are needed via pharmacovigilance.

The effectiveness of carprofen to control postoperative pain was established in a study in which it was compared with the opioid pethidine [42]. Forty dogs undergoing a variety of orthopedic surgical procedures were randomly assigned to pethidine (2 mg/kg administered before surgery and 3 mg/kg after surgery) or carprofen (4 mg/kg administered before surgery). Carprofen provided slightly better pain relief than pethidine, produced less sedation, and provided good analgesia during the 18 hours the dogs were in the hospital. Subsequently, it was demonstrated that better analgesia was provided when carprofen was given before surgery compared with postoperative administration [31,43,44].

The safety of carprofen in association with anesthesia and surgery has been extensively examined in healthy dogs. A safety summary was reported in 628 dogs that were randomly allocated to administration of placebo (312 dogs) or carprofen (316 dogs) orally or subcutaneously at a dose of 2 mg/lb (4.4 mg/kg) approximately 2 hours before surgery and then daily after surgery as needed [45]. Study subjects were client-owned dogs presented to veterinary practices for one of the following surgery types: ovariohysterectomy (262 dogs), aural surgery (192 dogs), or cruciate repair (174 dogs). There were no clinically significant differences in mean clinical pathologic variables evaluated, including hematology, clinical chemistries, coagulation profile, urinalysis, urinary GGT/creatinine ratio, and fecal occult blood. In addition, instances of abnormal health were mild and infrequent, with similar distributions for the placebo- and carprofen-treated dogs. Carprofen has also been shown to have no effect on bleeding time in conscious dogs [46] and dogs undergoing orthopedic surgery [47]. In addition, when administered to normal dogs undergoing anesthesia, carprofen did not cause clinically important alterations in renal function [48–51]. Finally, carprofen has no effect on the minimum alveolar concentration of halothane when administered to dogs [52].

Carprofen is not approved for use in cats in the United States or Canada, but the injectable solution has been approved in Europe at a dose of 4 mg/kg administered intravenously or subcutaneously. In addition, several independent publications have supported its safe use in cats primarily for soft tissue and orthopedic postoperative pain. In a double-blind, randomized, placebo-controlled study, carprofen administered after surgery was compared with pethidine in 60 cats undergoing ovariohysterectomy [53]. Cats administered carprofen were in less pain after surgery overall, with 4.0 mg/kg being the most effective dose and superior to pethidine from 2 to 20 hours after extubation. In addition, none of the analgesic regimens seemed to affect renal function adversely, as measured by urea and creatinine levels. A subsequent study in which carprofen was administered in a preemptive manner confirmed the previous findings [54]. In addition, carprofen seems to provide analgesia superior to butorphanol [55] and equivalent to other NSAIDs [56] when examined on the day of surgery.

For orthopedic pain, an additional dosage regimen has been evaluated over a 5-day period [57]. In a placebo-controlled, randomized, blind study, carprofen was administered on extubation at an initial dose of 4 mg/kg of body weight, followed by one third of that dose three times daily on days 2 to 5. This was compared with buprenorphine (0.01 mg/kg administered on extubation and subsequently every 8 hours) and levomethadone (0.3 mg/kg administered on extubation and subsequently every 8 hours). Carprofen was found to have better antinociceptive efficacy when compared with the two opioid analgesics but showed greater pain variability on the first postoperative day. Nevertheless, it was noted that none of the tested analgesics produced sufficient analgesia in the postoperative phase. From a safety perspective, there were no clinically elevant adverse reactions or any undesired renal, GI, or hepatic effects.

Whereas clinical data may support the safe use of carprofen for postoperative pain in cats, caution must be exercised. There are no published reports of chronic use; therefore, the true safety profile and margin of safety are unknown. In addition, compared with dogs, the pharmacokinetics in cats are markedly different [58]. The mean half-life in cats is approximately 20 hours, whereas carprofen has a mean half-life of approximately 8 hours in dogs [59]. Given the lack of a clear pharmacokinetic-pharmacodynamic relation for carprofen, additional dose titration work in cats is necessary to understand its safe use in that species. Such caution is exemplified in a 1-year-old, female, domestic short-hair cat that developed septic peritonitis secondary to a perforated duodenum after a routine ovariohysterectomy and subsequent oral administration of carprofen [60].

Etodolac

Etodolac is approved in dogs for the management of pain and inflammation associated with osteoarthritis (NADA 141-108). It should be noted that etodolac has not been evaluated in cats for any clinical use. It is available in scored tablets and is approved at the flexible dose of 10 to 15 mg/kg administered once daily based on the responsiveness of the disease condition and individual tolerance to the drug. Etodolac has been reported to inhibit COX-2 preferentially as evaluated in a canine whole-blood assay [61]. This seems to be corroborated based on its reported GI safety. In healthy laboratory dogs administered etodolac at the approved dose over a 1-month period, gastric lesions were minor when observed endoscopically and were equivalent to those caused by carprofen and placebo [62,63]. Nevertheless, there are opposing data suggesting that etodolac may not selectively inhibit COX-2. For example, in dogs with osteoarthritis administered etodolac at the approved dose for 10 days, PGE_2 concentrations in blood at days 3 and 10 were not suppressed compared with baseline [33]. In contrast, carprofen and deracoxib significantly suppressed PGE_2 concentrations in blood. In this same study, none of the drugs suppressed TBX B_2 in blood or gastric prostaglandin E_1 (PGE_1) synthesis, whereas all three drugs significantly decreased gastric and synovial synthesis of PGE_2. This differential effect on prostaglandin synthesis suggests that etodolac may be COX-1 sparing but also has variable effects on COX-2, depending on the tissue. Moreover, in a different in vitro assay, etodolac was reported to be COX-1 selective [64].

The effectiveness of etodolac for the treatment of osteoarthritis was established in a multicenter study in client-owned dogs diagnosed with osteoarthritis [65]. According to the US prescribing information label, etodolac was well tolerated when given at the approved dose for periods as long as 1 year. In a study of healthy laboratory dogs, oral administration at the approved dose for up to 12 months resulted in some dogs showing a mild weight loss; loose, mucoid, mucosanguineous feces or diarrhea; and hypoproteinemia. Erosions in the small intestine were observed in one of eight dogs receiving 15 mg/kg after 6 months of daily dosing. At elevated doses of 40 mg/kg/d or greater (2.7 times the maximum daily dose), etodolac caused GI ulceration, emesis, fecal occult blood, and weight loss. At a dose of 80 mg/kg/d or greater (5.3 times the maximum daily dose), six of eight treated dogs died or became moribund as a result of GI ulceration. One dog died within 3 weeks of treatment initiation, whereas the other five died after 3 to 9 months of daily treatment. Death was preceded by clinical signs of emesis, fecal abnormalities, decreased food intake, weight loss, and pale mucous membranes. Renal tubular nephrosis was also found in one dog treated with 80 mg/kg for 12 months. Taken together, it seems that etodolac has a comparatively narrower margin of safety, as demonstrated by severe adverse events and death at doses greater than the approved dose.

When evaluating thyroid function tests in dogs administered etodolac, caution should be exercised when interpreting the results [66] In client-owned dogs with orthopedic disorders that received etodolac at the approved dose, there was a significant decrease in thyroxine (T_4) values, with 21% of values falling below the reference range. In conjunction, a significant increase in canine thyroid-stimulating hormone (cTSH) was reported, but none of the values was above the reference range. There was no significant change in the mean free thyroxine (fT_4) values; however, 10% of the values fell below the reference range. These results were not observed when etodolac was administered for 1 month to random-source mixed-breed dogs, although significant decreases in plasma total protein, albumin, and globulin concentrations were detected on days 14 and 28 of administration [67].

Keratoconjunctivitis sicca (KCS) has been reported in dogs receiving etodolac. According to the adverse drug event reports by the FDA CVM, complaints of KCS comprised 78 of 1169 total etodolac-associated adverse event reports during a 28-month period from 1999 to 2001 [68]. The mean age of dogs was 10.2 years, and the range of onset times after first drug administration was from 6 days to 18 months, with most incidents occurring between 3 months and 1 year after first administration. Although the exact mechanism is not defined, anecdotal evidence suggests that when KCS attributable to etodolac administration develops, it is severe and usually irreversible [69]. This may be because dogs continue to receive etodolac after KCS develops. Accordingly, signs of KCS, such as blepharospasm, conjunctival hyperemia, and mucoid ocular discharge, should be monitored.

Should clinical signs of KCS be observed, tear production should be evaluated before continuing therapy.

Etodolac has also been evaluated for the control of postoperative pain associated with ovariohysterectomy in dogs [70]. In laboratory 1-year-old, healthy, mixed-breed, hound-type dogs, etodolac administered at 12 to 14 mg/kg 1 hour before surgery resulted in reduced measures of pain alone or in combination with butorphanol (0.4 mg/kg administered intravenously). Isoflurane concentration over time (area under the curve), buccal mucosal bleeding time, and indices of renal function were not significantly different among the treatment groups.

Meloxicam

Dogs

Meloxicam is approved in dogs for the control of pain and inflammation associated with osteoarthritis (NADA 141-213). It is available as a 1.5-mg/mL flavored suspension intended for oral administration. On the first day of dosing, a 0.2 mg/kg loading dose should be administered once, followed by 0.1 mg/kg given once daily on all subsequent days. A 5-mg/mL injectable solution that is indicated for the control of pain and inflammation associated with osteoarthritis (NADA 141-219) is also approved for dogs. It should be noted that it is not approved for postoperative pain. The injectable form should be administered initially as a single dose at 0.2 mg/kg intravenously or subcutaneously, followed by the oral suspension, if needed, beginning 24 hours after the injection.

Preferentially, inhibition of COX-2 by meloxicam has been established through in vitro assays [61,71,72]. This observation has been further confirmed in vivo by demonstrated GI safety in healthy dogs [73,74] and dogs with osteoarthritis [75]. In addition, decreased GI safety was demonstrated when meloxicam was coadministered with dexamethasone over 3 days (0.25 mg/kg given subcutaneously every 12 hours), and like all NSAIDs, caution should be exercised when it is used in conjunction with glucocorticoids.

The effectiveness of the meloxicam oral suspension formulation for the control of pain and inflammation associated with osteoarthritis was demonstrated in an induced synovitis model in dogs [76,77] and in multicenter trials in client-owned dogs [40,78,79]. Interestingly, in acute synovitis induced by intra-articular injection of monosodium urate, meloxicam was less effective than carprofen and etodolac, as measured by ground reaction forces applied on a force plate [77]. This result needs confirmation in large, randomized, head-to-head studies, which are currently lacking in the veterinary literature. The more recently introduced injectable solution has also been evaluated in dogs with osteoarthritis in a randomized, controlled, multicenter clinical trial [80]. In this study, dogs were randomly assigned to meloxicam ($n = 105$, 0.2 mg/kg administered subcutaneously once on day 1 and then 0.1 mg/kg administered orally every 24 hours for 13 days) or placebo ($n = 112$). Dogs treated with meloxicam had significantly greater improvement in general clinical scores assigned by a veterinarian blinded to treatment, compared with baseline scores, on days 8 and 15 than did dogs treated with placebo.

Meloxicam demonstrates a wide margin of safety when evaluated in healthy laboratory dogs. As reported on the US prescribing information label, meloxicam was administered orally at one, three, and five times (8 dogs per group) the recommended dose with no clinically significant adverse reactions. Some treatment-related changes seen in hematology and chemistry were observed, including decreased red blood cell counts in 4 dogs given three times the recommended dose and 3 dogs given five times the recommended dose; decreased hematocrit in 18 of 24 dogs (including 3 control dogs); dose-related neutrophilia in 1 dog given one time the recommended dose, 2 dogs given three times the recommended dose, and 3 dogs give five times the recommended dose; evidence of regenerative anemia in 2 dogs given three times the recommended dose and 1 dog given five times the recommended dose; increased blood urea nitrogen (BUN) in 2 dogs given five times the recommended dose; and decreased albumin in 1 dog given five times the recommended dose. No macroscopic or microscopic renal changes were observed in any dogs receiving meloxicam. The primary adverse reactions observed in field studies as reported on the US prescribing information label are vomiting, diarrhea, and inappetence, which are similar to those of other NSAIDs. Additional adverse reactions reported in the literature include hepatotoxicity and death [81], perforating duodenal ulcer [82], and peritonitis secondary to ulceration [83]. As with other NSAIDs, appropriate laboratory testing to establish hematologic and serum biochemical baseline data is recommended before and periodically during administration.

Although not approved for use, there are numerous reports on the use of meloxicam for the control of pain associated with soft tissue surgery. In an assessment limited to the day of surgery, 15 dogs were each administered meloxicam (0.2 mg/kg subcutaneously) or butorphanol (0.2 mg/kg intramuscularly) 30 minutes before anesthetic induction, followed by ovariohysterectomy [84]. Over the first 12 hours after surgery, animals administered meloxicam were in significantly less pain than those administered butorphanol based on various pain assessment methods. In another study evaluating various soft tissue abdominal operations in healthy dogs, 12 dogs were each administered meloxicam (0.2 mg/kg intravenously), ketoprofen (2 mg/kg intravenously), or butorphanol (0.2 mg/kg intravenously) after anesthetic induction [85]. At the end of the operation, dogs in the butorphanol group were administered a second dose (0.2 mg/kg intravenously). Using subjective pain assessments, overall efficacy was rated as good or excellent in 9 of the 12 dogs that received meloxicam compared with 9 of the 12 dogs that received ketoprofen and only 1 of the 12 dogs that received butorphanol. It was concluded that the analgesic effects of meloxicam were comparable to those of ketoprofen and superior to those of butorphanol over the 20-hour observation period. In a final study evaluating postoperative soft tissue pain, treatment and observations were extended beyond the day of surgery [86]. Over 72 hours, 13 dogs were each administered meloxicam (0.2 mg/kg subcutaneously) or carprofen (4 mg/kg subcutaneously) 30 minutes before anesthetic induction, followed by ovariohysterectomy. Beginning the day after surgery, treatment was continued and dogs were administered an oral meloxicam suspension (0.1 mg/kg once daily with food) or carprofen (2 mg/kg twice daily). Carprofen and meloxicam provided satisfactory analgesia for 72 hours, supporting the idea that therapy can be extended beyond the day of surgery.

The safety of administering meloxicam to control pain associated with soft tissue surgery is also supported. In a study to evaluate primary hemostasis, 10 healthy female dogs undergoing elective ovariohysterectomy were administered meloxicam (0.2 mg/kg intravenously) and control dogs received an equivalent volume of saline solution administered intravenously [87]. There was no measured effect on platelet aggregation, buccal mucosa bleeding time, platelet count, or hematologic indices when evaluated at 0, 1, 6, and 24 hours after the administration of meloxicam. Other studies have demonstrated that meloxicam given during surgery has no effect on bleeding time [84,85], packed cell volume (PCV), total solids, ALT, BUN, or creatinine [85]. Although not evaluated in animals undergoing surgery, the renal safety of meloxicam was evaluated in healthy dogs that were anesthetized and subjected to painful electrical stimulation [49]. Meloxicam (0.2 mg/kg intravenously) was administered to 12 female, healthy, young-adult Beagles 1 hour before anesthetic induction, and the dogs were then subjected to intermittent electrical stimulation for 30 minutes. There was no effect on glomerular filtration rate or serum concentrations of urea and creatinine compared with values for the saline treatment.

Again, although not approved for use, there are several reports on the use of meloxicam for the control of pain associated with orthopedic surgery on the day of surgery. In a double-blind, prospective, randomized clinical trial, 60 client-owned dogs with surgical orthopedic disorders were randomly assigned to meloxicam (0.2 mg/kg administered intravenously immediately before induction) or ketoprofen (2 mg/kg administered intravenously 30 minutes before the end of surgery) [88]. No significant differences in pain were observed, supporting the use of meloxicam for surgical orthopedic pain for 24 hours. Moreover, there was no effect on buccal bleeding time and whole-blood clotting. Alkaline phosphatase (ALP) and ALT were significantly elevated compared with baseline in both groups, but this was thought to be attributable to anesthesia. Vomiting and subcutaneous hematoma were the only adverse events reported in meloxicam-treated dogs. In a second study that corroborates the results of the first, 32 dogs undergoing orthopedic surgery were randomly assigned to carprofen (4 mg/kg subcutaneously) or meloxicam (0.2 mg/kg subcutaneously) administered 30 minutes before anesthetic induction [89]. As in the previous study, both drugs were effective in alleviating pain for up to 24 hours in all the dogs. Supporting safety, there were no significant changes in the concentrations of urea and creatinine, and no adverse effects were reported during the postoperative period.

Meloxicam has also been evaluated in conjunction with other analgesics. The analgesic efficacy of an epidural morphine-mepivacaine combination alone versus epidural morphine-mepivacaine in combination with meloxicam administered before the onset of anesthesia was assessed in 20 dogs undergoing cranial cruciate ligament repair [90]. Pain scores tended to be lower in dogs receiving meloxicam, and no meloxicam-treated dogs required rescue analgesia compared with 3 of 10 dogs in the epidural-only group. Administration of meloxicam thus seems to provide improved analgesia as compared with epidural morphine-mepivacaine alone. In another study, the combination of meloxicam and butorphanol was compared with butorphanol alone for control of postoperative pain in dogs undergoing surgical repair of a cranial cruciate ligament rupture [91]. In this blind randomized study, 40 client-owned dogs were assigned to receive butorphanol (0.2 mg/kg administered intravenously) and meloxicam (0.2 mg/kg administered intravenously) just before surgery or butorphanol alone just before surgery (0.2 mg/kg administered intravenously) and at incision closure (0.1 mg/kg administered intravenously). Subjective pain assessments were improved in dogs that were treated with the meloxicam-butorphanol combination. In addition, the total serum cortisol concentration was significantly lower in meloxicam-butorphanol–treated dogs compared with dogs treated with butorphanol alone. Taken together, these data support the idea that a single dose of meloxicam-butorphanol is equivalent to or slightly better than the administration of two perioperative doses of butorphanol for the control of pain associated with orthopedic surgery.

Cats

Unique to currently available NSAIDs, meloxicam is approved for use in cats (NADA 141-219). A 5-mg/mL solution for injection is indicated in cats for the control of postoperative pain and inflammation associated with orthopedic surgery, ovariohysterectomy, and castration. For this use, a single subcutaneous dose of 0.3 mg/kg of body weight should be administered before surgery. Use of additional meloxicam or any other NSAIDs is contraindicated.

A recent in vitro method of testing the COX selectivity of NSAIDs in cats has been published that concluded that meloxicam is only slightly preferential for COX-2 [92]. This may be the reason why meloxicam is not approved for chronic use, in that chronic use or elevated doses are associated with unacceptable adverse events. According to the US prescribing information label, in a 3-day safety study, subcutaneous administration of up to 1.5 mg/kg (five times the recommended dose) resulted in vomiting, loose stools, and fecal occult blood. Clinically significant hematologic changes described included increased prothrombin time, increased activated partial thromboplastin time, and elevated white blood cell counts in cats having renal or GI tract lesions. Serum chemistry changes observed included decreased total protein and increased BUN and creatinine levels. Histologic examination revealed GI lesions ranging from inflammatory cell infiltration of the mucosa of the GI tract to erosions. Renal changes ranged from dilated medullary and cortical tubules and inflammation or fibrosis of the interstitium to necrosis of the tip of the papilla. These adverse events seemed to increase in severity when treatment was extended out to 9 days.

Again, according to the US prescribing information label, when meloxicam was given as a single subcutaneous injection of 0.3 or 0.6 mg/kg on day 0 and meloxicam oral suspension was then administered orally once daily at the same dose (0.3 or 0.6 mg/kg, respectively) for 8 consecutive days, clinical adverse reactions included vomiting, diarrhea, lethargy, and decreased food consumption. Necropsy revealed reddened GI mucosa in three of four cats in the 0.3-mg/kg group and in one of four cats in the 0.6-mg/kg group. By day 9, one cat in the 0.3-mg/kg group and one cat in the 0.6-mg/kg group died, and another cat in the 0.3-mg/kg group was moribund. The cause of death for these cats could not be determined, although the pathologist reported pyloric or duodenal ulceration in the cats in the 0.6-mg/kg group. These safety studies demonstrate a narrow margin of safety; thus, repeat injections or follow-up with oral NSAIDs is contraindicated. One study contradicts this conclusion, where meloxicam suspension was administered at a dose of 0.3 mg/kg orally on day 1 followed by 0.1 mg/kg daily for 4 more consecutive days in cats with chronic locomotor disorders [93]. This treatment resulted in a significant improvement in demeanor, feed intake, and weight bearing as well as a significant reduction in lameness, pain on palpation, and inflammation and was associated with minimal observed side effects.

Evidence that meloxicam is effective for the control of postoperative pain in cats was provided in a study in which cats underwent onychectomy or onychectomy plus neutering (castration or ovariohysterectomy) [94]. In this study, cats were randomized to meloxicam (0.3 mg/kg administered subcutaneously) or butorphanol (0.4 mg/kg administered subcutaneously) 15 minutes after premedication and before anesthesia. Meloxicam-treated cats were less lame, had lower pain scores, and had better general impression scores compared with butorphanol-treated cats. As an objective measurement, cortisol concentrations were lower at 1, 5, and 12 hours in the meloxicam-treated cats and fewer meloxicam-treated cats required rescue analgesia compared with butorphanol-treated cats. Safety was supported by the fact that there was no treatment effect on buccal bleeding time; PCV and BUN concentrations decreased in both groups, and glucose concentration decreased in meloxicam-treated cats.

Additional work has concluded that meloxicam is equivalent to carprofen in controlling pain associated with ovariohysterectomy in cats [56,95]. Meloxicam has also been compared with buprenorphine for the control of postoperative pain associated with ovariohysterectomy in cats [96]. In a randomized controlled study of 51 cats, oral and subcutaneous meloxicam (0.3 mg/kg) was compared with oral and subcutaneous buprenorphine (0.01 mg/kg) administered at the time of anesthetic induction. Cats receiving meloxicam orally or subcutaneously had significantly lower pain scores compared with cats receiving buprenorphine orally. Moreover, rescue analgesia was not required by any of the cats receiving meloxicam compared with 3 of 10 cats receiving buprenorphine orally and 2 of 10 cats receiving buprenorphine subcutaneously. Taken together, cats receiving meloxicam orally or subcutaneously seemed to have less pain after surgery than those receiving oral buprenorphine but not less pain than those receiving subcutaneously administered buprenorphine.

Dericoxib

Deracoxib is approved in dogs for the control of pain and inflammation associated with osteoarthritis (NADA 141-203). It is commercially available as chewable tablets and should be administered at a dose of 1 to 2 mg/kg as a single daily dose as needed based on the responsiveness of the disease condition and individual tolerance to the drug. It is also approved for the control of postoperative pain and inflammation limited to orthopedic surgery. For this indication, 3 to 4 mg/kg/d should be administered before surgery and the same dose given on subsequent days as needed, not to exceed 7 days of administration.

Preferential inhibition of COX-2 by deracoxib has been established through in vitro and ex vivo assays in laboratory dogs with unilateral osteoarthritis treated with deracoxib for 10 days [33]. Like carprofen, deracoxib decreased synovial fluid and blood PGE_2 concentrations but did not suppress blood TBX B_2 concentrations or gastric PGE_1 synthesis. GI safety is consistent with these results, as demonstrated by the administration of deracoxib to healthy dogs over 28 days [97]. Endoscopic lesion scores and days of vomiting were superior compared those in with dogs receiving aspirin and equivalent to those in dogs receiving placebo.

The use of deracoxib in dogs with osteoarthritis was demonstrated in two studies. In a dose titration study conducted in dogs with intra-articular urate crystal–induced synovitis, the minimum effective dose of deracoxib (1 mg/kg) was established to treat joint inflammation and was equivalent to carprofen (2.2 mg/kg) [98]. There are no published multicenter controlled studies on the effectiveness of deracoxib on the treatment of pain and inflammation associated with osteoarthritis. The US prescribing information label describes a placebo-controlled blind study in 209 client-owned dogs with clinical and radiographic signs of osteoarthritis, however. Deracoxib was administered by the owner at a dosage of approximately 1 to 2 mg/kg/d for 43 consecutive days. Although details are limited, an improvement in force plate parameters and owner evaluations was reported. As with other NSAIDs, vomiting and diarrhea were the most common adverse reactions reported in this study.

There are no published multicenter controlled studies on the effectiveness of deracoxib on the treatment of pain with orthopedic surgery. The US prescribing information label describes a placebo-controlled study in 207 dogs admitted to veterinary hospitals for repair of a cranial cruciate injury, however. Placebo or deracoxib was administered at a dose of 3 to 4 mg/kg beginning the evening before surgery and continued once daily for 6 days after surgery. Significant improvement was reported for lameness at the walk and trot as well as for pain on palpation values at all postsurgical time points compared with placebo. The most frequent adverse reactions were vomiting, diarrhea, hematochezia, and draining or oozing at the incision site. There are no published reports on the effectiveness of deracoxib for the control of pain associated with soft tissue surgery.

When administered chronically, deracoxib seems to have a wide safety margin, with some evidence of reduced renal safety with increasing doses. As described on the US prescribing information label, in a 6-month study, where dogs were dosed at 0, 2, 4, 6, 8, and 10 mg/kg, there were no clinical abnormalities observed and buccal bleeding time was not altered. Urinalysis results showed hyposthenuria (specific gravity < 1.005) and polyuria in one male dog and one female dog in the 60-mg/kg group after 6 months of treatment, however. After 6 months of treatment, the mean BUN values for dogs treated with 6, 8, or 10 mg/kg/d were above normal and were 30.0, 35.3, and 48.2 mg/dL, respectively. Moreover, dose-dependent focal renal tubular degeneration or regeneration was seen in some dogs treated at a dose of 6, 8, or 10 mg/kg/d, and focal renal papillary necrosis was seen in dogs dosed at 8 or 10 mg/kg/d. In a second study at doses of 0, 4, 6, 8, and 10 mg/kg of body weight for 21 consecutive days, a dose-dependent trend toward increased levels was observed. Taken together, although no renal lesions were seen at the label doses of 2 and 4 mg/kg/d, appropriate precautions should be taken in dogs with preexisting renal disease and overdosing should be avoided.

As stated previously, it has been generally established that selective inhibition of COX-2 results in anti-inflammatory activity, whereas sparing COX-1 minimizes GI, renal, and other toxicities associated with NSAIDs. Recently reported GI tract perforation in dogs administered deracoxib may add a caveat to this notion [29]. Perforation and death seemed to be related to higher than approved doses of deracoxib or coadministration with other NSAIDs or glucocorticoids. It was concluded that deracoxib should only be used at approved dosages and that glucocorticoids and other less selective NSAIDs should not be coadministered in close temporal association with selective COX-2 inhibitors. Therefore, although COX-2–selective NSAIDs have demonstrated GI safety in normal laboratory dogs, in clinical cases, coadministration of other NSAIDs or glucocorticoids should be avoided, and when there are preexisting GI pathologic findings, caution should be exercised.

The safety and effectiveness of deracoxib in cats have not been evaluated at any dose or for any indication. The pharmacokinetics of deracoxib have been described in seven cats administered a single oral dose of 1 mg/kg using a compounded liquid formula, however [99]. The terminal half-life ($t_{1/2}$) was 7.9 hours, and the time to reach maximum plasma concentration (T_{max}) was 3.64 hours, which are slightly longer than those reported in dogs ($t_{1/2} = 3$ hours and $T_{max} = 2$ hours according to the US prescribing information label in dogs). Although no adverse effects were observed in this small study, treatment in cats should be avoided until margin-of-safety studies are completed and demonstrated effectiveness is achieved in clinical field studies.

Firocoxib

Firocoxib is the most recently approved COX-2–selective NSAID introduced in the United States. It is approved in dogs and is indicated for the control of pain and inflammation associated with osteoarthritis in dogs (NADA 141-230). It is available as a chewable tablet and should be administered at a dose of 5 mg/kg once daily. The selectivity of firocoxib to inhibit COX-2 was demonstrated using an in vitro assay [100]. The effectiveness of firocoxib to treat joint inflammation was demonstrated in a dose titration study conducted in dogs with intra-articular urate crystal–induced synovitis [100]. Confirmation of this effect in a multicenter, active, controlled study in 249 client-owned dogs with osteoarthritis is described on the US prescribing information label. Dogs treated with firocoxib were reported to show a level of improvement in veterinarian-assessed lameness, pain on palpation, range of motion, and owner-assessed improvement that was comparable to the active control. In addition, the level of improvement in firocoxib-treated dogs in limb weight bearing on the force plate gait analysis assessment was comparable to the active control. The most frequent adverse reactions in this study were vomiting and decreased appetite.

In a target animal safety study, firocoxib was administered orally to healthy adult Beagle dogs (eight dogs per group) at 5, 15, and 25 mg/kg (one, three, and five times the recommended total daily dose) for 180 days. At the indicated dose of 5 mg/kg, there were no treatment-related adverse events. Decreased appetite, vomiting, and diarrhea were seen in dogs in all dose groups, including unmedicated controls, although vomiting and diarrhea were seen more often in dogs in the group give five times the recommended dose. One dog in the group given three times the recommended dose was diagnosed with juvenile polyarteritis of unknown etiology after exhibiting recurrent episodes of vomiting and diarrhea, lethargy, pain, anorexia, ataxia, proprioceptive deficits, decreased albumin levels, decreased and then elevated platelet counts, increased bleeding times, and elevated liver enzymes. On histopathologic examination, a mild ileal ulcer was found in one dog given five times the recommended dose. This dog also had decreased serum albumin, which returned to normal by study completion. One control and three dogs given five times the recommended dose had focal areas of inflammation in the pylorus or small intestine. Vacuolization without inflammatory cell infiltrates was noted in the thalamic region of the brain in three control dogs, one dog given three times the recommended dose, and three dogs given five times the recommended dose. Mean ALP was within the normal range for all groups but was greater in the groups given three times and five times the recommended dose than in the control group. Transient decreases in serum albumin were seen in multiple animals in the groups given three times and five times the recommended dose and in one control animal.

The margin of safety, as demonstrated in healthy laboratory dogs, seems to be narrow in young dogs. A specific warning is included on the US prescribing information label that states the use of this product at doses greater than the recommended 5.0 mg/kg in puppies less than 7 months of age has been associated with serious adverse reactions, including death. The results supporting this are as follows. In a separate safety study, firocoxib was administered orally to healthy juvenile (10–13 weeks of age) Beagle dogs at 5, 15, and 25 mg/kg (one, three, and five times the recommended total daily dose) for 180 days. At the indicated recommended dose of 5 mg/kg, on histopathologic examination, 3 of 6 dogs had minimal periportal hepatic fatty change. On histopathologic examination, 1 control dog, 1 dog given the recommended dose, and 2 dogs given five times the recommended dose had diffuse slight hepatic fatty change. These animals showed no clinical signs and had no liver enzyme elevations. In the group given three times the recommended dose, 1 dog was euthanized because of poor clinical condition (day 63). This dog also had mildly decreased serum albumin. At study completion, of 5 surviving and clinically normal dogs given three times the recommended dose, 3 had minimal periportal hepatic fatty change. Of 12 dogs in the group given five times the recommended dose, 1 died (day 82) and 3 moribund dogs were euthanized (days 38, 78, and 79) because of anorexia, poor weight gain, depression, and, in 1 dog, vomiting. One of the euthanized dogs had ingested a rope toy. Two of these dogs in the group given five times the recommended dose had mildly elevated liver enzymes. At necropsy, all 5 of the dogs that died or were euthanized had moderate periportal or severe panzonal hepatic fatty change, 2 had duodenal ulceration, and 2 had pancreatic edema. Of 2 other clinically normal dogs given five times the recommended dose (of 4 dogs euthanized as comparators to the clinically affected dogs), 1 had slight and 1 had moderate periportal hepatic fatty change. Drug treatment was discontinued for 4 dogs in the group given five times the recommended dose. These dogs survived during the remaining 14 weeks of the study. On average, the dogs in the groups given three and five times the recommended dose did not gain as much weight as control dogs. The rate of weight gain was measured (instead of weight loss), because these were young growing dogs. Thalamic vacuolation was seen in 3 of 6 dogs in the group given three times the recommended dose, 5 of 12 dogs in the group given five times the recommended dose, and to a lesser degree in 2 unmedicated controls. Diarrhea was seen in all dose groups, including unmedicated controls.

As stated previously, comparative field safety has been reported [41]. Five hundred seventy-five dogs diagnosed with osteoarthritis were treated with firocoxib (5 mg/kg/d), carprofen (4 mg/kg/d), or etodolac (10–15 mg/kg/d) for 30 days. There were 292 dogs treated with firocoxib, 132 with carprofen, and 151 with etodolac. There was no report of comparative effectiveness; however, fewer dogs experienced diarrhea with firocoxib (3.1%) than with carprofen (6.8%). In addition, the incidence of at least one health-related event was less with firocoxib (1.0%) compared with carprofen (6.1%). There was no difference in the number of dogs that dropped out of the study. To assign greater safety accurately, data from larger numbers of dogs are needed via pharmacovigilance.

Although not approved for the control of postoperative pain, firocoxib has been evaluated in dogs undergoing ovariohysterectomy [101]. In a negative-control double-blind study of 20 client-owned female dogs, firocoxib was administered orally approximately 3 hours before surgery at a dose of 5 mg/kg and then once daily for 4 additional days. Pain scores were lower for the firocoxib-treated group at 2 hours and 4 hours after surgery as well as on day 1. On days 2, 3, and 4, pain scores were not statistically different between treatments. Treatment of orthopedic pain has not been evaluated.

The safety and effectiveness of firocoxib in cats has not been evaluated at any dose or for any indication. The COX selectivity, pharmacokinetics, and effect on lipopolysaccharide (LPS)-induced fever have been accepted in laboratory cats, however [102]. In vitro evaluation confirmed that firocoxib is COX-2 selective in cats. In addition, pharmacokinetic properties were determined after intravenous (2 mg/kg) and oral (3 mg/kg) administration showed moderate to high oral bioavailability (54%–70%), low plasma clearance (4.7–5.8 mL/min/kg), and an elimination $t_{1/2}$ of 8.7 to 12.2 hours. When administered 1 or 14 hours before LPS-induced pyrexia in female cats, firocoxib attenuated fever at doses ranging from 0.75 to 3 mg/kg. Although no adverse effects were observed in this small study, treatment in cats should be avoided until margin-of-safety studies are completed and demonstrated effectiveness is achieved in clinical field studies.

DUAL INHIBITORS

The alternative metabolic pathway of AA is the leukotriene pathway. The enzyme 5-lipoxygenase (5-LOX) converts AA into leukotrienes that are potent chemotactic agents involved in inflammation. Dual COX/5-LOX inhibitors constitute a valuable alternative to classic NSAIDs and selective COX-2 inhibitors for the treatment of pain and inflammation. It remains to be seen if balanced inhibition of COX and 5-LOX provides superior effectiveness and reduced adverse reactions compared with COX-2–selective NSAIDs. Presently, the recently introduced tepoxalin is the only dual inhibitor available in veterinary medicine.

Tepoxalin

Tepoxalin is approved in dogs for the control of pain and inflammation associated with osteoarthritis. The safety and effectiveness of tepoxalin have not been evaluated at any dose or for any indication in cats. It is available as a rapidly dissolving oral tablet and should be administered with food at an initial dose of 10 or 20 mg/kg on the first day of treatment, followed by 10 mg/kg once daily thereafter as needed based on the responsiveness of the disease condition and individual tolerance to the drug.

The dual action of tepoxalin has been established by an in vitro assay [103]. Selectivity against COX isoforms and 5-LOX has also been evaluated in vivo [104]. In mixed-breed adult dogs with chronic unilateral arthritis in a stifle joint, the dogs were administered placebo, meloxicam, or tepoxalin for 10 days at the approved doses. Consistent with dual inhibition, tepoxalin decreased leukotriene B_4 concentrations in the blood and gastric mucosa and PGE_2 in the synovial fluid. Interestingly, tepoxalin also inhibited TBX B_2 in blood, which is supportive of COX-1 inhibition, an effect not observed in meloxicam- or placebo-treated dogs. Therefore, although tepoxalin may be a dual inhibitor, it may also inhibit COX-1 in a tissue-dependent manner.

Effectiveness in the control of pain and inflammation associated with osteoarthritis has been demonstrated in dogs. There are no published reports;

however, as described on the US prescribing information label, 62 dogs were evaluated in a 7-day, controlled, blind field study. On the seventh day of treatment, improvements in ambulation, weight bearing, pain, forced movement, general improvement, and overall improvement were reported. In a separate uncontrolled field safety study of 107 client-owned dogs, the most frequent adverse reactions included diarrhea, vomiting, and inappetence. Laboratory safety evaluation supports a wide margin of safety. When administered for 1 year at doses of 0, 10, 30, and 100 mg/kg/d, the primary findings were increased emesis and gastric ulceration in 2 of 8 dogs in the highest dose group.

Although not approved for use in postoperative pain, tepoxalin has been evaluated in an experimental pain model [105]. Twelve laboratory dogs were randomized to placebo or tepoxalin (10 mg/kg) administered 2 hours before anesthetic induction, followed by a full-thickness thoracic skin incision. Tepoxalin had no effect on buccal mucosal bleeding when assessed out to 24 hours. In addition, when measured out to 48 hours, tepoxalin had no effect on hematology, renal parameters (BUN, creatinine, creatinine clearance, and GGT/creatinine ratio) and hepatic parameters (ALT, AST, and GGT). Although this pilot study supports its safe use in soft tissue surgery, larger multicenter studies in client-owned dogs should more closely gauge true safety and effectiveness.

SUMMARY

The discovery of COX isoforms as the target for NSAIDs led to a greater understanding of the mechanism and clinical use of NSAIDs. Later, COX-2 was targeted in drug discovery efforts, resulting in the introduction of highly selective COX-2 inhibitors. As a result, over the past decade, there have been several NSAIDs introduced in veterinary medicine with an increased GI safety profile consistent with a COX-1–sparing effect. More recently, an NSAID with additional 5-LOX activity has also been approved for use. Although it is tempting to equate in vitro COX-2/COX-1 and 5-LOX inhibition to overall in vivo safety, the data do not support this approach. The true overall safety for any individual compound is based on its evaluation in laboratory margin-of-safety studies, reproductive safety studies, and blind multicenter field studies in client-owned animals. Therefore, when choosing a COX-2–selective or dual-inhibitor NSAID for clinical use, all in vivo data must be taken into account to understand comparative safety, and continued use must be based on the drug's performance in the individual being treated. Until head-to-head trials in multicenter blind studies are published, comments on comparative safety and effectiveness must be reserved.

References

[1] Goldblatt MW. A depressor substance in seminal fluid. Journal of the Society of Chemistry 1933;52:1056–7.

[2] van Dorp DA, Beerthuis RK, Nugteren DH, et al. Enzymatic conversion of all-cis-polyunsaturated fatty acids into prostaglandins. Nature 1964;203:839–41.

[3] Bergstrom S, Danielsson H, Samuelsson B. The enzymatic formation of prostaglandin E2 from arachidonic acid prostaglandins and related factors. Biochim Biophys Acta 1964;90:207–10.
[4] Hamberg M, Svensson J, Samuelsson B. Prostaglandin endoperoxides. A new concept concerning the mode of action of prostaglandins. Proc Natl Acad Sci USA 1974;71:3824–8.
[5] Hemler M, Lands WE. Purification of the cyclooxygenase that forms prostaglandins: demonstration of two forms of iron in the holoenzyme. J Biol Chem 1976;251:5575–9.
[6] Miyamoto T, Ogino N, Yamamoto S, et al. Purification of prostaglandin endoperoxide synthetase from bovine vesicular gland microsomes. J Biol Chem 1976;251:2629–36.
[7] Vane JR. Inhibition of prostaglandin synthesis as a mechanism of action for aspirin-like drugs. Nature 1971;231:232–5.
[8] Flower RJ, Vane JR. Inhibition of prostaglandin synthetase in brain explains the anti-pyretic activity of paracetamol 94-acetamidophenol. Nature 1972;240:410–1.
[9] Habenicht AJ, Goerig M, Grulich J, et al. Human platelet-derived growth factor stimulates prostaglandin synthesis by activation and by rapid de novo synthesis of cyclooxygenase. J Clin Invest 1985;75:1381–7.
[10] Simmons DL, Xie W, Chipman JG, et al. Multiple cyclooxygenases: cloning of an inducible form. In: Baily IM, editor. Prostaglandins, leukotrienes, lipoxins and PAF. New York: Plenum Press; 1919. p. 67–78.
[11] Kujubu DA, Fletcher BS, Varnum BC, et al. TIS 10, a phorbol ester tumor promoter-inducible mRNA from Swiss 3T3 cells, encodes a novel prostaglandin synthase/cyclooxygenase homologue. J Biol Chem 1991;266:12866–72.
[12] Chandrasekharan NV, Dai H, Ross KL, et al. COX 3, a cyclooxygenase-1 variant inhibited by acetaminophen and other analgesic/antipyretic drugs: cloning, structure, and expression. Proc Natl Acad Sci USA 2002;99:13926–31.
[13] Whittle BJR, Salmon JA. In: Turnberg LA, editor. Intestinal secretion. Welwyn Garden City (UK): Smith Kline and French Publications; 1983. p. 69–73.
[14] Miller TA. Protective effects of prostaglandins against gastric mucosal damage: current knowledge and proposed mechanisms. Am J Physiol 1983;245:G601–23.
[15] Gerkens JF, Gerber JC, Shand DG, et al. Effect of PGI2, PGE2 and 6-keto-PGF1α on canine gastric blood flow and acid secretion. Prostaglandins 1978;16:815–23.
[16] Whittle BJ, Boughton-Smith NK, Moncada S, et al. Actions of prostacyclin (PGI2) and its product 6-oxo-PGF1α on the rat gastric mucosa in vivo and in vitro. Prostaglandins 1978;15:955–68.
[17] Allen A, Garner A. Mucous and bicarbonate secretion in the stomach and their possible role in mucosal protection. Gut 1980;21:249–62.
[18] Whelton A. Nephrotoxicity of nonsteroidal anti-inflammatory drugs: physiologic foundations and clinical implications. Am J Med 1999;106(Suppl):13S–24S.
[19] Yamagata K, Andreasson KI, Kaufman WE, et al. Expression of a nitrogen-inducible cyclooxygenase in brain neurons. Regulation by synaptic activity and glucocorticoids. Neuron 1993;11:371–8.
[20] Troutman MS, Edwin SS, Collmer D, et al. Prostaglandin H synthase-2 in human gestational tissues. Regulation in amnion. Placenta 1996;17:239–45.
[21] Chakraborty I, Das SK, Wang J, et al. Development expression of the cyclooxygenase-1 and cyclooxygenase-2 genes in the peri-implantation mouse uterus and their differential regulation by the blastocyst and ovarian steroids. J Mol Endocrinol 1996;16:107–22.
[22] Krotz F, Schiele TM, Klauss V, et al. Selective COX-2 inhibitors and risk of myocardial infarction. J Vasc Res 2005;42(4):312–24.
[23] FDA Veterinarian Newsletter. November/December 2004; XIX (VI). Available at: http://www.fda.gov/cvm/November2004.htm#5074. Accessed August 21, 2006.
[24] Szezepansky A, Moatter T, Carley WW, et al. Induction of cyclooxygenase II in human synovial microvessel endothelial cells by interleukin-I. Arthritis Rheum 1994;198:955–60.

[25] Vane JR, Botting R. Mechanism of action of nonsteroidal anti-inflammatory drugs. Am J Med 1998;104(Suppl):2S–8S.
[26] Lanenbach R, Morham SG, Tiano HF, et al. Prostaglandin synthase 1 gene disruption in mice reduces arachidonic acid-induced inflammation and indomethacin-induced gastric ulceration. Cell 1995;83:483–92.
[27] Morteau O, Morham SG, Sellon R, et al. Impaired mucosal defense to acute colonic injury in mice lacking cyclooxygenase-1 or cyclooxygenase-2. J Clin Invest 2000;105:469–78.
[28] Reuter BK, Asfaha S, Buret S, et al. Exacerbation of inflammation-associated colonic injury in rat through inhibition of cyclooxygenase-2. J Clin Invest 1996;98:2067–85.
[29] Lascelles BD, Blikslager AT, Fox SM, et al. Gastrointestinal tract perforation in dogs treated with a selective cyclooxygenase-2 inhibitor: 29 cases (2002–2003). J Am Vet Med Assoc 2005;227(7):1112–7.
[30] Van Ryn J, Pairet M. Clinical experience with cyclooxygenase-2 inhibitors. Inflamm Res 1999;48:247–54.
[31] Clark TP, Curto M, Huhn JC, et al. The effect of perioperative carprofen administration on the alleviation of pain associated with soft tissue surgery. In: Programs and Abstracts of the American College of Veterinary Anesthesia Annual Forum. New Orleans (LA): American College of Veterinary Internal Medicine, 2001.
[32] Ricketts AP, Lundy KM, Seibel SB, et al. Evaluation of selective inhibition of canine cyclooxygenase 1 and 2 by carprofen and other nonsteroidal anti-inflammatory drugs. Am J Vet Res 1998;59:1441–6.
[33] Sessions JK, et al. In vivo effects of carprofen, deracoxib and etodolac on prostanoid production in blood, gastric mucosa, and synovial fluid in dogs with chronic osteoarthritis. Am J Vet Res 2005;66(5):812–7.
[34] Straub KM, et al. Pharmacological properties of carprofen. Eur J Rheum Inflamm 1982;5:478–87.
[35] McKellar QA, et al. Pharmacokinetics, tolerance and serum thromboxane inhibition of carprofen in the dog. J Small Anim Pract 1990;31:443–8.
[36] Taylor PM, et al. Pharmacodynamic and enantioselective pharmacokinetics of carprofen in the cat. Res Vet Sci 1996;60:144–51.
[37] Vasseur PB, et al. Randomized, controlled trial of the efficacy of carprofen, a nonsteroidal anti-inflammatory drug, in the treatment of osteoarthritis in dogs. J Am Vet Med Assoc 1995;206(6):807–11.
[38] Fox SM, Campbell S. Update: two years (1997–1998) clinical experience with Rimadyl (carprofen). Pfizer Animal Health Technical Bulltin. New York: Pfizer Animal Health; 1999.
[39] MacPhail CM, et al. Hepatocellular toxicosis associated with administration of carprofen in 21 dogs. J Am Vet Med Assoc 1998;212(12):1895–901.
[40] Moreau M, et al. Clinical evaluation of a nutraceutical, carprofen and meloxicam for the treatment of dogs with osteoarthritis. Vet Rec 2003;152:323–9.
[41] Hanson PD, Romano D, Fleishman C, et al. Health events recorded from 575 dogs treated for osteoarthritis with firocoxib, carprofen or etodolac. In: Programs and Abstracts of the 22nd Annual Forum of the American College of Veterinary Internal Medicine Annual Forum. Minneapolis (MN), 2004.
[42] Lascelles BD, Butterworth SJ, Waterman AE. Postoperative analgesic and sedative effects of carprofen and pethidine in dogs. Vet Rec 1994;134(8):187–91.
[43] Welsh EM, et al. Beneficial effects of administering carprofen before surgery in dogs. Vet Rec 1997;141:251–3.
[44] Lascelles BD, et al. Efficacy and kinetics of carprofen, administered preoperatively or postoperatively, for the prevention of pain in dogs undergoing ovariohysterectomy. Vet Surg 1998;27:568–82.

[45] Curto M, Clark TP, Russo S, et al. Clinical pathology results in dogs administered carprofen (Rimadyl) perioperatively. Presented at the American College of Veterinary Internal Medicine, Annual Veterinary Medicine Forum. Denver, May 24, 2001.
[46] Hickford FH, Barr SC, Erb HN. Effect of carprofen on hemostatic variables in dogs. Am J Vet Res 2001;62(10):1642–6.
[47] Grisneaux E, Pibarot P, Dupuis J, et al. Comparison of ketoprofen and carprofen administered prior to orthopedic surgery for control of postoperative pain in dogs. J Am Vet Med Assoc 1999;215(8):1105–10.
[48] Bergmann HM, Nolte IJ, Kramer S. Effects of preoperative administration of carprofen on renal function and hemostasis in dogs undergoing surgery for fracture repair. Am J Vet Res 2005;66(8):1356–63.
[49] Forsyth SF, Guilford WG, Pfeiffer DU. Effect of NSAID administration on creatinine clearance in healthy dogs undergoing anaesthesia and surgery. J Small Anim Pract 2000;41(12):547–50.
[50] Lobetti RG, et al. Effect of administration of nonsteroidal anti-inflammatory drugs before surgery on renal function in clinically normal dogs. Am J Vet Res 2000;61: 1501–6.
[51] Crandell DE, et al. Effect of meloxicam and carprofen on renal function when administered to healthy dogs prior to anesthesia and painful stimulation. Am J Vet Res 2004;65: 1384–90.
[52] Alibhai HIK, Clarke KW. Influence of carprofen on minimum alveolar concentration of halothane in dogs. J Vet Pharmacol Ther 1996;19:320–1.
[53] Lascelles BD, Cripps P, Mirchandani S, et al. Carprofen as an analgesic for postoperative pain in cats: dose titration and assessment of efficacy in comparison to pethidine hydrochloride. J Small Anim Pract 1995;36(12):535–41.
[54] Balmer TV, Irvine D, Jones RS, et al. Comparison of carprofen and pethidine as postoperative analgesics in the cat. J Small Anim Pract 1998;39(4):158–64.
[55] Al-Gizawiy MM, Rude PE. Comparison of preoperative carprofen and postoperative butorphanol as postsurgical analgesics in cats undergoing ovariohysterectomy. Vet Anaesth Analg 2004;31(3):164–74.
[56] Slingsby LS, Waterman-Pearson AE. Postoperative analgesia in the cat after ovariohysterectomy by use of carprofen, ketoprofen, meloxicam or tolfenamic acid. J Small Anim Pract 2000;41(10):447–50.
[57] Mollenhoff A, Nolte I, Kramer S. Anti-nociceptive efficacy of carprofen, levomethadone and buprenorphine for pain relief in cats following major orthopaedic surgery. J Vet Med A Physiol Pathol Clin Med 2005;52(4):186–98.
[58] Parton K, Balmer TV, Boyle J, et al. The pharmacokinetics and effects of intravenously administered carprofen and salicylate on gastrointestinal mucosa and selected biochemical measurements in healthy cats. J Vet Pharmacol Ther 2000;23(2):73–9.
[59] Clark TP, Chieffo C, Huhn JC, et al. The steady-state pharmacokinetics and bioequivalence of carprofen administered orally and subcutaneously in dogs. J Vet Pharmacol Ther 2003;26(3):187–92.
[60] Runk A, Kyles AE, Downs MO. Duodenal perforation in a cat following the administration of nonsteroidal anti-inflammatory medication. J Am Anim Hosp Assoc 1999;35(1): 52–5.
[61] Wilson JE, Chandrasekharan NV, Westover KD, et al. Determination of expression of cyclooxygenase-1 and -2 isozymes in canine tissues and their differential sensitivity to nonsteroidal anti-inflammatory drugs. Am J Vet Res 2004;65(6):810–8.
[62] Reimer ME, et al. The gastroduodenal effects of buffered aspirin, carprofen, and etodolac in healthy dogs. J Vet Intern Med 1999;13:472–7.
[63] Nishihara K, Kikuchi H, Kanno T, et al. Comparison of the upper gastrointestinal effects of etodolac and aspirin in healthy dogs. J Vet Med Sci 2001;63(10):1131–3.

[64] Streppa HK, Jones CJ, Budsberg SC. Cyclooxygenase selectivity of nonsteroidal anti-inflammatory drugs in canine blood. Am J Vet Res 2002;63(1):91–4.
[65] Budsberg SC, Johnston SA, Schwarz PD, et al. Efficacy of etodolac for the treatment of osteoarthritis of the hip joints in dogs. J Am Vet Med Assoc 1999;214(2):206–10.
[66] Ness TA, Torres SM, Kramek EA, et al. Effect of dosing and sampling time on serum thyroxine, free thyroxine, and thyrotropin concentrations in dogs following multidose etodolac administration. Vet Ther 2003;4(4):340–9.
[67] Panciera DL, Johnston SA. Results of thyroid function tests and concentrations of plasma proteins in dogs administered etodolac. Am J Vet Res 2002;63(11):1492–5.
[68] Hampshire VA, Doddy FM, Post LO, et al. Adverse drug event reports at the United States Food and Drug Administration Center for Veterinary Medicine. J Am Vet Med Assoc 2004;225(4):533–6.
[69] Stiles J. Warning of an adverse effect of etodolac. J Am Vet Med Assoc 2004;225(4):503.
[70] Inoue T, Ko JC, Mandsager RE, et al. Efficacy and safety of preoperative etodolac and buttorphanol administration in dogs undergoing ovariohysterectomy. J Am Anim Hosp Assoc 2006;42(3):178–88.
[71] Kay-Mugford P, et al. In vitro effects of nonsteroidal anti-inflammatory drugs on cyclooxygenase activity in dogs. Am J Vet Res 2000;61:802–10.
[72] Brideau C, et al. In vitro effects of cyclooxygenase inhibitors in whole blood of horses, dogs and cats. Am J Vet Res 2001;62:1755–60.
[73] Boston SE, et al. Endoscopic evaluation of the gastroduodenal mucosa to determine the safety of short-term concurrent administration of meloxicam and dexamethasone in healthy dogs. Am J Vet Res 2003;63:1369–75.
[74] Forsyth SF, et al. Endoscopy of the gastroduodenal mucosa after carprofen, meloxicam and ketoprofen administration in dogs. J Small Anim Pract 1998;39:421–4.
[75] Jones CJ, et al. In vivo effects of meloxicam and aspirin on blood, gastric mucosal, and synovial fluid prostanoid synthesis in dogs. Am J Vet Res 2002;63:1527–31.
[76] Cross AR, Budsberg SC, Keefe TJ. Kinetic gait analysis assessment of meloxicam efficacy in a sodium urate-induced synovitis model in dogs. Am J Vet Res 1997;58(6):626–31.
[77] Borer LR, Peel JE, Seewald W, et al. Effect of carprofen, etodolac, meloxicam, or butorphanol in dogs with induced acute synovitis. Am J Vet Res 2003;64(11):1429–37.
[78] Doig PA, et al. Clinical efficacy and tolerance of meloxicam in dogs with chronic arthritis. Can Vet J 2000;41:296–300.
[79] Nell T, Bergman J, Hoeijmakers M, et al. Comparison of vedaprofen and meloxicam in dogs with musculoskeletal pain and inflammation. J Small Anim Pract 2002;43(5):208–12.
[80] Peterson KD, Keefe TJ. Effects of meloxicam on severity of lameness and other clinical signs of osteoarthritis in dogs. J Am Vet Med Assoc 2004;225(7):1056–60.
[81] Nakagawa K, Yamagami T, Takemura N. Hepatocellular toxicosis associated with the alternate administration of carprofen and meloxicam in a Siberian husky. J Vet Med Sci 2005;67(10):1051–3.
[82] Duerr FM, Carr AP, Bebchuk TN, et al. Challenging diagnosis—icterus associated with a single perforating duodenal ulcer after long-term nonsteroidal antiinflammatory drug administration in a dog. Can Vet J 2004;45(6):507–10.
[83] Reed S. Nonsteroidal anti-inflammatory drug-induced duodenal ulceration and perforation in a mature rottweiler. Can Vet J 2002;43(12):971–2.
[84] Caulkett N, Read M, Fowler D, et al. A comparison of the analgesic effects of butorphanol with those of meloxicam after elective ovariohysterectomy in dogs. Can Vet J 2003;44(7): 565–70.
[85] Mathews KA, Pettifer G, Foster R, et al. Safety and efficacy of preoperative administration of meloxicam, compared with that of ketoprofen and butorphanol in dogs undergoing abdominal surgery. Am J Vet Res 2001;62(6):882–8.
[86] Leece EA, Brearley JC, Harding EF. Comparison of carprofen and meloxicam for 72 hours following ovariohysterectomy in dogs. Vet Anaesth Analg 2005;32(4):184–92.

[87] Fresno L, Moll J, Penalba B, et al. Effects of preoperative administration of meloxicam on whole blood platelet aggregation, buccal mucosal bleeding time, and haematological indices in dogs undergoing elective ovariohysterectomy. Vet J 2005;170(1):138–40.
[88] Deneuche AJ, Dufayet C, Goby L, et al. Analgesic comparison of meloxicam or ketoprofen for orthopedic surgery in dogs. Vet Surg 2004;33(6):650–60.
[89] Laredo FG, Belda E, Murciano J, et al. Comparison of the analgesic effects of meloxicam and carprofen administered preoperatively to dogs undergoing orthopaedic surgery. Vet Rec 2004;155(21):667–71.
[90] Fowler D, Isakow K, Caulkett N, et al. An evaluation of the analgesic effects of meloxicam in addition to epidural morphine/mepivacaine in dogs undergoing cranial cruciate ligament repair. Can Vet J 2003;44(8):643–8.
[91] Budsberg SC, Cross AR, Quandt JE, et al. Evaluation of intravenous administration of meloxicam for perioperative pain management following stifle joint surgery in dogs. Am J Vet Res 2002;63(11):1557–63.
[92] Giraudel JM, Toutain PL, Lees P. Development of in vitro assays for the evaluation of cyclooxygenase inhibitors and predicting selectivity of nonsteroidal anti-inflammatory drugs in cats. Am J Vet Res 2005;66(4):700–9.
[93] Lascelles BD, Henderson AJ, Hackett IJ. Evaluation of the clinical efficacy of meloxicam in cats with painful locomotor disorders. J Small Anim Pract 2001;42(12):587–93.
[94] Carroll GL, Howe LB, Peterson KD. Analgesic efficacy of preoperative administration of meloxicam or butorphanol in onychectomized cats. J Am Vet Med Assoc 2005;226(6):913–9.
[95] Slingsby LS, Waterman-Pearson AE. Comparison between meloxicam and carprofen for postoperative analgesia after feline ovariohysterectomy. J Small Anim Pract 2002;43(7):286–9.
[96] Gassel AD, Tobias KM, Egger CM, et al. Comparison of oral and subcutaneous administration of buprenorphine and meloxicam for preemptive analgesia in cats undergoing ovariohysterectomy. J Am Vet Med Assoc 2005;227(12):1937–44.
[97] Sennello KA, Leib MS. Comparison of the effects of deracoxib, buffered aspirin, and placebo on the gastric mucosa of healthy dogs. In: Programs and Abstracts of the American College of Veterinary Internal Medicine Annual Forum. 2004.
[98] Millis DL, Weigel JP, Moyers T, et al. Effect of deracoxib, a new COX-2 inhibitor, on the prevention of lameness induced by chemical synovitis in dogs. Vet Ther 2002;3(4):453–64.
[99] Gassel AD, Tobias KM, Cox SK. Disposition of deracoxib in cats after oral administration. J Am Anim Hosp Assoc 2006;42(3):212–7.
[100] McCann ME, Andersen DR, Zhang D, et al. In vitro effects and in vivo efficacy of a novel cyclooxygenase-2 inhibitor in dogs with experimentally induced synovitis. Am J Vet Res 2004;65(4):503–12.
[101] Lever D, Gogolewski R, Larsen D, et al. Management of peri-operative pain associated with soft tissue surgery in dogs treated with firocoxib. In: Programs and Abstracts of the American College of Veterinary Internal Medicine Annual Forum. 2004.
[102] McCann ME, Rickes EL, Hora DF, et al. In vitro effects and in vivo efficacy of a novel cyclooxygenase-2 inhibitor in cats with lipopolysaccharide induced pyrexia. Am J Vet Res 2005;66(7):1278–84.
[103] Argentieri DC, Ritchie DM, Ferro MP, et al. Tepoxalin: a dual cyclooxygenase/5-lipoxygenase inhibitor of arachidonic acid metabolism with potent anti-inflammatory activity and a favorable gastrointestinal profile. J Pharmacol Exp Ther 1994;271(3):1399–408.
[104] Agnello KA, Reynolds LR, Budsberg SC. In vivo effects of tepoxalin, an inhibitor of cyclooxygenase and lipoxygenase, on prostanoid and leukotriene production in dogs with chronic osteoarthritis. Am J Vet Res 2005;66(6):966–72.
[105] Kay-Mugford PA, Grimm KA, Weingarten AJ, et al. Effect of preoperative administration of tepoxalin on hemostasis and hepatic and renal function in dogs. Vet Ther 2004;5(2):120–7.

ELSEVIER
SAUNDERS
Vet Clin Small Anim 36 (2006) 1087–1105
VETERINARY CLINICS
SMALL ANIMAL PRACTICE

Update on Drugs Used to Treat Endocrine Diseases in Small Animals

Ellen N. Behrend, VMD, MS, PhD
Department of Clinical Sciences, College of Veterinary Medicine, Auburn University, Auburn, AL 36849, USA

Drug therapy for the endocrine system is implemented to replace a hormone deficiency or to prevent or reduce the formation or effects of excess hormone. Ideally, a deficient hormone itself can be replaced (eg, giving insulin to a patient with diabetes mellitus [DM]) or a tumor oversecreting a hormone is removed. This is not always possible or necessary, however. For example, for treatment of hypoparathyroidism, therapy requires administration of vitamin D, because no commercially available preparation of parathyroid hormone exists. In hyperthyroidism, surgical removal or ablation of the tumor with radioactive iodine can be performed; alternatively, medical management can be used to decrease thyroid hormone synthesis.

Treatment of endocrine disorders covers diseases of the pituitary, adrenal, parathyroid, and thyroid glands as well as the endocrine pancreas. Discussing all diseases is beyond the scope of this article. This article focuses on new therapies currently available for specific diseases. Administration of trilostane for treatment of hyperadrenocorticism (HAC) and use of insulin glargine, PZI insulin, and porcine Lente insulin for DM are discussed. In addition, transdermal methimazole therapy for treatment of feline hyperthyroidism and administration of progestins for pituitary dwarfism are considered.

HYPERTHYROIDISM

Feline hyperthyroidism may be medically controlled with methimazole and ipodate. Both can be used as the sole drug to manage hyperthyroidism or in preparation for surgery or radioiodine administration. In general, methimazole blocks synthesis of thyroid hormones. As a result, thyroid hormones (T_3 and T_4) are not secreted. Carbimazole is a methimazole prodrug currently used in Europe but not available in the United States. It seems to be equal in efficacy but safer than methimazole. Ipodate is a cholecystographic agent that acts primarily by inhibiting conversion of T_3 to T_4 but also has some direct inhibitory effects on thyroid hormone secretion. In comparison to feline thyroidal tumors, which are 99% benign, canine thyroidal tumors causing hyperthyroidism are

E-mail address: behreen@vetmed.auburn.edu

0195-5616/06/$ – see front matter
doi:10.1016/j.cvsm.2006.05.007

vetsmall.theclinics.com

almost always, if not always, malignant. Therefore, medical therapy for canine hyperthyroidism is not recommended–the tumor should be addressed directly with surgery, chemotherapy, or radiation therapy.

Relation of Treatment for Feline Hyperthyroidism to Renal Disease

Treatment of hyperthyroidism can lead to decreases in glomerular filtration rate (GFR) and unmask chronic renal disease. Unfortunately, however, a question that remains is how best to assess cats before definitive therapy for hypherthyroidism (ie, ^{131}I or surgery). Although a GFR value of 2.25 mL/kg/min may represent a cutoff for deciding if renal failure is a possibility with resolution of the hyperthyroid state [1], measurement of GFR is not easily obtained and, unfortunately, no readily available clinical indicators exist [2]. Another option is to treat cats transiently with methimazole until the serum T_4 concentration is adequately controlled and to maintain euthyroidism for 30 days. When the serum T_4 concentration is maintained within the normal range, renal function and the effect of definitive therapy can be assessed. Many cats have an increase in serum blood urea nitrogen (BUN) or creatinine concentration with therapy, but the clinical result must be assessed. Most cats are clinically improved despite the increased renal parameters when their hyperthyroidism is treated, and if they are improved, the hyperthyroidism can be definitively treated. If trial therapy unmasks clinically relevant kidney disease that causes adverse clinical signs, definitive therapy should not be undertaken. Instead, methimazole should be administered at a dose that maintains serum T_4 concentrations as low as possible with acceptable renal function, which is a hard balance to preserve.

Whether all cats that are to undergo ^{131}I treatment or thyroidectomy need to have their kidney function evaluated like this also should be determined. If there is any question about the adequacy of renal function, trial therapy with methimazole is warranted. This author recommends a methimazole trial, if possible, in all cats to undergo definitive therapy. Alternatively, if renal failure does become overt after definitive correction of hyperthyroidism, exogenous thyroid hormone can be supplemented to support the kidneys. A balance must then be struck between creating iatrogenic hyperthyroidism and maintaining renal function.

Methimazole Therapy

Overall, methimazole is highly effective at reversing thyrotoxicosis and maintaining euthyroidism. In 262 spontaneously hyperthyroid cats, oral methimazole treatment lowered the serum T_4 in more than 99% [3]. A small percentage of cats may be truly methimazole-resistant. Clinical side effects occur, unrelated to the dose of methimazole used, in 18% of treated cats, including anorexia (11%), vomiting (11%), lethargy (9%), excoriation of the face and neck (2%), bleeding (2%), and icterus (2%) [3]. Myasthenia gravis has been reported after treatment with methimazole in 4 cats. In 2 cats, prednisone was used to control the myasthenia [4].

On hematologic screening, eosinophilia, lymphocytosis, leukopenia, thrombocytopenia, and agranulocytosis may be noted in cats receiving methimazole.

The milder adverse effects, including eosinophilia, lymphocytosis and leukopenia, are usually noted within 1 to 2 months of initiation of treatment and are transient despite continued therapy. The more serious complications, including thrombocytopenia and agranulocytosis, occur in a few cats ($\leq$3%) within the first 3 months of therapy and necessitate permanent discontinuation of methimazole administration [3]. The mechanism of hematologic disorders induced by methimazole is not understood. Interestingly, bleeding occurred in one cat without a decrease in platelet number; thus, thrombocytopenia is not the only mechanism that can cause a bleeding tendency. In human patients receiving propylthiouracil, a medication similar to methimazole, vitamin K therapy has reduced bleeding caused by hypoprothrombinemia; however, the benefits of vitamin K therapy have not been studied in cats on methimazole therapy [5]. Immunologic effects, including induction of positive antinuclear antibodies (ANAs), can occur. The risk of developing positive ANAs seems to increase with the length of therapy and dose. Despite the presence of these abnormalities, however, clinical signs of lupus-like syndrome (ie, dermatitis, polyarthritis, glomerulonephritis, thrombocytopenia, fever) or hemolysis do not occur [3].

A starting dose of 10 to 15 mg/d divided into two or three doses depending on the severity of the hyperthyroid state has been recommended. The goal for cats on methimazole is to have the serum T_4 concentration in the lower half of the reference range. A serum sample to assess therapeutic efficacy can be drawn at any time after pill administration as long as a normal dosing routine is maintained. For example, if a cat is receiving twice-daily therapy, the sample can be drawn any time within the 12 hours after pill administration before the next dose is due. Although some cats only require methimazole once daily for adequate control, overall, methimazole is more effective twice daily [6]. For the first 3 months of drug administration, the period during which most adverse effects develop, cats receiving methimazole should be evaluated every 2 to 3 weeks with a complete physical examination, determination of serum T_4 concentration, and complete blood cell count (CBC). Renal parameters should also be monitored to assess kidney function. Although cats with a subnormal serum T_4 concentration typically are not clinically hypothyroid, development of a positive ANA titer may be related to dose. Thus, the minimal dose necessary to maintain a serum T_4 concentration in the lower half of the reference range (and not below) should be used. If the serum T_4 concentration remains high and poor compliance or difficulty in giving the medication has been ruled out as the cause of persistent hyperthyroidism, the methimazole dose should be increased in 2.5- to 5-mg increments to a maximum of 20 mg/d. If hepatopathy, facial excoriation, a bleeding tendency, or serious hematologic consequences occur, the medication should be halted and alternative therapy used. After the first 3 months, the serum T_4 concentration should be determined every 3 to 6 months to evaluate the adequacy of therapy. Because blood dyscrasias are unlikely but not impossible after 3 months of therapy, a CBC need only be performed if clinical signs suggest agranulocytosis, hemolysis, or thrombocytopenia [3].

To try to avoid development of adverse effects, other authors have recommended an initial dose of 2.5 mg twice daily for 2 weeks [7]. If an owner observes no untoward side effects after this period, the physical examination reveals no new problems, and a CBC (including platelets) is within normal limits, the dosage should be increased to 2.5 mg three times daily for an additional 2 weeks. A similar recheck should then be completed, including measurement of a serum T_4 concentration. If the serum T_4 concentration is within or near the reference range, the dose may be maintained for a period of 2 to 6 weeks to determine the need for any further dosage adjustments. The dose should continue to be increased by 2.5 mg/d increments to a maximum of 20 mg/d (assuming correct administration of methimazole) or until the hyperthyroidism is controlled [7]. Monitoring for adverse effects should be done as discussed previously.

Because of the relation between hyperthyroidism and renal disease, a third protocol has been advocated if abnormal renal parameters are present. Methimazole should be administered at a dose of 2.5 mg twice daily for 2 weeks, then at 2.5 mg three times daily for 2 weeks, then at 5.0 mg twice daily for 2 weeks and, finally, at 5.0 mg three times daily as needed. The serum T_4, BUN, creatinine, and phosphate concentrations and a CBC should be evaluated at the end of each 2-week period. The dose escalation should stop once the serum T_4 concentration has normalized. If the serum T_4 concentration can be decreased to within the reference range and the renal parameters remain stable or improve, continued antithyroid medications or permanent therapy can be considered. If the renal parameters and clinical signs of renal disease worsen with therapy, treatment of the hyperthyroidism needs to be re-evaluated. Some cats may be healthier without treatment [7]. Alternatively, the dose of methimazole can be titrated to achieve as good a control as possible of the hyperthyroidism while maintaining adequate renal function.

Methimazole can be given transdermally. Although methimazole in pleuronic lecithin organogel (PLO) is absorbed poorly in healthy cats after a single dose [8], it is likely that chronic dosing leads to improved absorption and resolution of hyperthyroidism. Serum T_4 concentration decreased in hyperthyroid cats treated transdermally with 2.5 to 10 mg of methimazole dissolved in PLO once or twice daily [9]. The transdermal route may take longer, however, to achieve remission. In a randomized prospective study of hyperthyroid cats, owners dosed their cats with methimazole orally (tablets) or transdermally (in PLO; 50 mg/mL) at a rate of 2.5 mg every 12 hours [10]. Fifty-six percent of cats treated by the transdermal route were euthyroid at 2 weeks, which was significantly fewer cats than the control rate in response to oral administration (88%); by 4 weeks the difference was no longer statistically significant (67% control with transdermal methimazole versus 82% for oral methimazole), but the lack of difference may have been attributable to a small number of cats remaining in the study at 4 weeks. Whether transdermal administration for a longer period would have controlled the hyperthyroidism in more cats was not evaluated. An advantage of transdermal methimazole is a significantly decreased rate of gastrointestinal adverse effects. The incidence of hepatopathy, facial excoriation, and blood dyscrasias is similar for the transdermal and oral routes, however. Some cats develop erythema at the transdermal dosing site, but it is typically not severe enough to require drug discontinuation [10].

Methimazole administration does not affect tumor size. Clinical signs recur if and when the drug is discontinued. Methimazole can be used before surgery to decrease serum T_4 concentrations to within the reference range to stabilize a patient. Discontinuation of methimazole 2 weeks before radionuclide scanning or therapy has been recommended. Radionuclide uptake is increased in normal tissue for 9 days after discontinuation of methimazole therapy [11], so treatment within that window may increase the risk of iatrogenic hypothyroidism with radioiodine administration.

DIABETES MELLITUS

Dietary Therapy

Dietary therapy is important for treatment of DM. Through unknown mechanisms, dietary fiber can delay gastrointestinal glucose absorption, reducing postprandial fluctuations in blood glucose concentration and enhancing glycemic control. High-fiber diets have been traditionally recommended for diabetic patients, but this is now being questioned. Insoluble fiber can be beneficial in diabetic dogs [12,13]. The response of diabetic dogs to fiber can vary between individuals, however, and a recent study showed that diets with high fiber and moderate starch were not advantageous for dogs with stabilized DM compared with a moderate-fiber and low-starch diet [14]. Insoluble fiber, the type present in commercial feline high-fiber diets, can improve glycemic control in diabetic cats [15]. Recent theories suggest that high-carbohydrate diets may lead to DM in cats, however, and that high protein may be beneficial instead. A number of cats on a high-protein and low-carbohydrate diet had their DM resolve or experienced a marked reduction in insulin dose [16,17]. Thus, diets like Purina DM (Nestle Purina Pet Care Company, St. Louis, Missouri) and Hill's M/d (Hills Pet Products, Topeka, Kansas) are now recommended for diabetic cats; caution should be used in cats with renal disease, however, because of the high protein content.

Drug Therapy

For treatment of DM, insulin can be used in dogs or cats or oral hypoglycemic agents can be used in cats. For a complete discussion of therapeutic considerations and options, the reader is referred elsewhere [18,19]. This article focuses on three insulin preparations that have recently been assessed or become available for use in veterinary medicine.

A purified pork Lente insulin (Vetsulin, Intervet, Millsboro, Delaware) was recently approved by the US Food and Drug Administration (FDA) for use in dogs and is the only insulin approved for dogs. It has been available for many years in other countries. Because the amino acid sequences of pork and canine insulin are identical, porcine insulin does not stimulate an immune response in dogs. Whether the lack of antibody formation is desirable is unclear. Although anti-insulin antibodies can cause insulin resistance, this seems to be rare, at least in cats. Conversely, anti-insulin antibodies may decrease the rate of insulin metabolism and prolong its duration of action, which is a beneficial effect.

A study has recently been completed in which 53 dogs with uncomplicated diabetes were treated with Vetsulin for 60 days after a variable initial dose determination period. Therapy was started once daily and was changed to twice daily as needed. The starting dose used was the one recommended in the product insert: 1 U/kg, with a supplemental dose depending on body weight (dogs weighing <10 kg received a 1-U supplement, those weighing 10–11 kg received a 2-U supplement, those weighing 12–20 kg received a 3-U supplement, and those weighing >20 kg received a 4-U supplement). Efficacy and safety were evaluated at the end of the dose determination period (time 0) and 30 (time 1) and 60 (time 2) days later. With treatment, 80% to 96% of dogs had resolution of polyuria, polydipsia, and ketonuria. The mean blood glucose concentration was 370 mg/dL before treatment but was 151 to 185 mg/dL while receiving pork Lente insulin. At times 0, 1, and 2, 100%, 66%, and 75% of the dogs were judged to be adequately controlled based on blood glucose concentrations and clinical signs, respectively. At the end of the dose determination period, 57% were receiving Vetsulin twice daily (43% were receiving once-daily injections), and by day 60, 66% were receiving twice-daily injections. Overall, the median number of days to achieve adequate glycemic control was 35 (range: 5–151 days). No unexpected side effects were observed, but 22 dogs had signs at some time that could have been caused by hypoglycemia and 2 dogs died of presumed hypoglycemia. Owners of 7 dogs reported swelling or pain at the injection site, but nothing was noted by investigators on physical examination [20]. Thus, pork Lente insulin seems to be a good option for use in diabetic dogs.

The starting dose of insulin deserves consideration. Although some authors recommend a starting dose of insulin in general of 0.25 U/kg twice daily for dogs [18], others recommend using 0.5 U/kg if the blood glucose concentration is greater than 360 mg/dL and 0.25 U/kg if it is less than 360 mg/dL [21]. This author uses the former recommendation. Thus, the starting dose given in the package insert may be high, and a lower dose may be more appropriate. Furthermore, in one study of dogs, 94% of dogs required twice-daily dosing regardless of the insulin type used for adequate control [22]. Thus, initiating therapy twice daily should also be considered.

In cats, good options are Lente, PZI, and glargine insulins. Ultralente was used frequently at one time but is no longer available. For PZI, one article reported use in 67 cats studied for 45 days. The initial dose of PZI ranged from 0.2 to 0.6 U/kg twice daily. At the end of the 45 days, the mean dose was 0.9 U/kg (range: 0.2–1.8 U/kg). The mean blood glucose nadir occurred approximately 5 to 7 hours after insulin injection but ranged from 1 to 9 hours [23]. Overall, 90% of owners believed their cat improved. Clinical hypoglycemia occurred in 5 cats, and hypoglycemia without clinical signs occurred in another 21 (31%). Ten cats were not controlled by day 45. Whether longer treatment and more dosage adjustment would have achieved control is unknown. In general, cats with newly diagnosed DM had a better response than those cats with previously treated DM; perhaps the cats that failed previous treatment had an underlying cause of insulin resistance. Most diabetic cats require PZI twice daily for adequate control, but once-daily injections may suffice in up to 25% of diabetic cats. The initial PZI dose should be low (eg, 1 U per injection) to avoid hypoglycemia [23].

"Designer" recombinant insulins are now being made in which the amino acid structure of the insulin is being altered slightly to change the pharmacokinetic profile. One of these products, insulin glargine, has been used in veterinary medicine. Glargine differs from human insulin by substitution of glycine for asparagine at position 21 in the α-chain of insulin and by the addition of two arginine residues to the β-chain. Glargine is a clear aqueous solution with a pH of 4 until injected subcutaneously. The interaction of the acidic insulin and the relatively neutral pH of subcutaneous tissues forms microprecipitates, and thus gives a relatively constant systemic absorption profile. The formation of microprecipitates and slow absorption are dependent on the acidity of glargine; thus, glargine cannot be mixed or diluted [24].

In diabetic cats, the use of glargine seems to be extremely promising, and, currently, this author's first-choice insulin in cats. Glargine has a long duration of action and a predictable blood glucose lowering effect. In eight newly diagnosed cats treated with a high-protein and low-carbohydrate diet, the DM resolved in all cats within 4 months [25]. It should be noted that at least four of the cats were of the Burmese breed. The pathophysiology of DM in this breed may differ from that in most cats, and resolution of DM may be more likely in Burmese cats. In any case, glargine seems to be a good insulin to use in any cat, giving reliable control of blood glucose concentrations throughout most of the day. Long-term diabetic cats have been switched to and treated with glargine as well with good success, but the DM has not resolved.

Recommendations are to start cats on glargine at a dose of 0.5 U/kg if the blood glucose concentration is greater than 360 mg/dL and at 0.25 U/kg if the blood glucose concentration is less than 360 mg/dL. In either case, twice-daily administration is recommended. Because the doses are small, 0.3-mL syringes should be used for accurate dosing.

Lente insulin can be used in cats. Although Vetsulin is not approved for cats in the United States, an identical product has been available for years in Europe and used for treatment of feline diabetics. Porcine Lente insulin has a shorter duration of action in cats than in dogs and needs to be administered twice daily [26]. A recommended starting dose is 0.25 U/kg twice daily if the blood glucose concentration is between 216 and 342 mg/dL and 0.5 U/kg twice daily if the blood glucose concentration is greater than 360 mg/dL [27]. Alternatively, a dose of 1 U per cat twice daily for cats weighing less than 4 kg and 1.5 to 2.0 U per cat twice daily for cats weighing greater than 4 kg can be used to initiate therapy [28].

Serial glucose curves are recommended to establish time to peak effect and duration of effect of any administered insulin. When performing a curve, the blood glucose concentration should be established at 2-hour intervals. A curve should be performed on the first day insulin is given. Glucose concentrations may be lower than expected after the first 24 to 48 hours of insulin therapy, especially in cats as stress hyperglycemia resolves [29]. This first curve is done solely to ensure that hypoglycemia does not occur. If hypoglycemia is found, the insulin dose should be decreased 25% and another curve should be done the following day with the same goal in mind–to check for hypoglycemia. The insulin dose should not be increased based on the first day's curve. A patient requires 5 to 7 days on a dose of insulin to equilibrate and reach maximal effect. Another blood glucose curve should be performed 7 days after discharge; based on assessment of this curve, the insulin dose can be increased or decreased as deemed necessary.

The goals of therapy for DM are to maintain blood glucose concentrations between 100 and 250 mg/dL in dogs and between 100 and 300 mg/dL in cats during a 24-hour period and for clinical signs to improve. The symptoms of DM can largely be avoided if blood glucose concentrations are kept below 180 to 200 mg/dL in dogs and below 300 mg/dL in cats. Maximum improvement may take up to 6 months (eg, mean time to improvement for PZI in cats was 3 months). Fine-tuning of the exact dose should not be expected during a single hospitalization.

The pattern of insulin effect should be used to determine the dose, interval, and feeding schedule. Ideally, glucose concentrations should reach a nadir of 80 to 150 mg/dL. The actual nadir and peak concentrations in a patient are probably lower or higher, respectively, than measured, because the exact time of nadir and peak effects of insulin are not known. Changes in the dose of insulin can usually be made without affecting the duration of effect. The glucose differential is the difference between the nadir and the blood glucose concentration before the next dose and can be a measurement of insulin effectiveness [30]. If the curve is relatively flat (eg, differential of 50–100 mg/dL), the insulin may not be having the desired effect. The absolute blood glucose concentration must also be taken into consideration.

If all blood glucose concentrations are less than 200 mg/dL, the administered insulin is effective. If all blood glucose concentrations are between 350 and 400 mg/dL, however, the insulin is ineffective at that dose or stress hyperglycemia is present. In assessing a glucose curve, whether it is the first curve performed on a patient or the last of many, two basic questions need to be asked. First, has the insulin succeeded in lowering the blood glucose? Second, how long has the insulin lasted? By answering these questions, logical changes in the dosing regimen, if necessary, can be made. Results of a serial glucose curve should always be interpreted in light of clinical signs. Curves in dogs can vary from day to day [31] and do so in cats as well [32]. Stress hyperglycemia can also falsely elevate results. If a patient is not polyphagic, polydipsic, or polyuric and body weight is stable or increasing, diabetic control is likely good.

For all insulins, except glargine, the first aim in regulating a diabetic patient is to achieve an acceptable nadir. (For guidelines on how to adjust the glargine dose, see the discussion elsewhere in this article.) In general, if an acceptable nadir is not achieved, the insulin dose should be adjusted depending on the size of the animal and the degree of hyperglycemia. Usually, changes of approximately 10% are appropriate. Obtaining an acceptable glucose nadir may not be possible in some animals, however, if insulin with a short duration of activity is used. In these patients, the blood glucose concentration is typically quite high in the morning, because there has been inadequate control for most of the previous day. Even if an insulin injection is capable of lowering blood glucose, it does not have a long enough effective period to lower the glucose into an acceptable range. In other words, a blood glucose curve in this situation shows a noticeable but brief decrease in serum glucose concentration after the insulin injection.

Hypoglycemia should always be avoided. No matter what other blood glucose concentrations are during the day, if the blood glucose concentration is less than 80 mg/dL at any time, a reduction in insulin dose is indicated. Decrease the dose 25%, and then do another curve to ensure that hypoglycemia does not recur.

Once an acceptable nadir is accomplished, duration of action, which is roughly defined as the time from the insulin injection through the lowest glucose concentration and until the blood glucose concentration exceeds 200 to 250 mg/dL, can be determined by a blood glucose curve. If the insulin dose is inadequate and the target glucose nadir has not yet been achieved, the dose must be increased until the nadir is acceptable before duration of effect of the insulin can be determined. Duration and nadir cannot be assessed at the same time if one or the other is insufficient.

Based on the length of action, the following general recommendations can be made. If the duration of action is 22 to 24 hours, once-daily therapy is adequate. If the duration of action is 16 to 20 hours, a shorter acting insulin should be used twice daily. If the duration is 12 to 16 hours, twice-daily insulin therapy can be tried but the evening dose may need to be lower than the morning dose. If the duration of action is 10 to 12 hours, the patient should receive the same insulin dose twice daily. If the duration of action seems to be less than 8 hours, a blood glucose nadir of greater than 80 mg/dL must be ensured. If blood glucose drops to less than 60 mg/dL at any time, the Somogyi phenomenon can occur. In this scenario, the body tries to correct the hypoglycemia through release of counterregulatory hormones, such as epinephrine or glucagon, and the blood glucose concentration quickly increases to high levels, falsely decreasing the apparent interval of effect. The appropriate response to this occurrence is to decrease the insulin dose so that the nadir is greater than 80 mg/dL; counterregulatory hormones then do not interfere with the action of the exogenous insulin and the true duration of effect becomes apparent. If the duration is truly less than 8 hours, adequate therapy with that type of insulin may require injections more frequently than twice daily, which is impractical. Accordingly, the type of insulin should be changed to a longer acting insulin if one is available or to another type or species of origin of insulin. In cats, human insulin can be substituted for beef or pork insulin. A switch between different types of intermediate-acting insulin can also be beneficial. For example, a dog or cat may metabolize neutral protamine Hagedorn (NPH) insulin quickly, resulting in too short an effect, but Lente insulin may have a longer duration.

Once control has been achieved, blood glucose curves should be performed to assess adequacy of glycemic control every 3 to 6 months or earlier if clinical signs suggest that control has been lost. The more precarious the control, the more frequently rechecks should be done. As during the initial curves, if the nadir is unacceptable, the insulin dose must be lowered or raised accordingly. If the duration of action seems to have changed, the same modifications as discussed previously can be made.

If using insulin glargine in cats, interpretation of blood glucose curves and dose adjustment are different than for other insulin types. For the first 3 days after initiating therapy, 12-hour blood glucose curves should be performed (ie, the curve should be performed for the interval between the morning and evening dose). The purpose of the blood glucose curve is to detect hypoglycemia, if present, and to lower the dose of glargine as needed. Many cats require dose reduction within the first 3 days. The insulin dose should not be increased for the first week no matter what the curves look like. After the first 3 days, the cat should be sent home and then return for performance of a curve 7 days later (week 1). Subsequent blood glucose curves should be performed at weeks 2 and 4 and then as required.

Recommendations for dose adjustment are based on the preinsulin blood glucose level (compared with other insulins, where the dose is altered based on the nadir). If the preinsulin blood glucose concentration is greater than 290 mg/dL at recheck, increase the glargine dose by 1.0 U per cat. The dose should not be changed if the preinsulin blood glucose concentration is 220 to 290 mg/dL. In either of these first two scenarios, a curve should be done the following day to make sure that hypoglycemia is not occurring. The dose should be decreased 0.5 to 1.0 U per cat if the preinsulin blood glucose concentration is 80 to 180 mg/dL. If biochemical hypoglycemia is present (ie, blood glucose concentration is <80 mg/dL, but no clinical signs of hypoglycemia are present), the dose should be decreased by 1.0 U per cat. If clinical signs of hypoglycemia are present, the glargine dose should be decreased by 50% [33].

Interestingly, cats may alternate between being insulin-dependent and not, and the DM can go into remission for weeks to years with appropriate therapy. Persistent hyperglycemia can profoundly reduce insulin secretion, ultimately causing permanent DM in cats that had a normal β-cell mass at one point [34], a situation referred to as "glucose toxicity." These effects occur within 2 days of persistent hyperglycemia, and the impact on β cells increases with the magnitude of hyperglycemia. The impact of glucose toxicity is also more severe in the presence of a reduced β-cell mass, underscoring the importance of effective control and preservation of β cells. Control of blood glucose with insulin or oral hypoglycemic therapy may allow β cells to regain insulin secretory capacity. As a result, the diabetic state is transient in up to 20% to 40% of cats [34–37]. If treating a cat with glargine, administration should not be discontinued within 2 weeks of starting treatment even if normoglycemia is present; decrease the dose if needed, but do not stop the insulin [33] because 2 weeks are required to allow complete recovery of β cells from glucose toxicity.

To determine if a cat is in remission, insulin glargine administration should be continued until the cat is receiving 1 U twice daily. Then, if the preinsulin blood glucose concentration is less than 180 mg/dL, go to once-daily administration. If the preinsulin blood glucose concentration is still less than 180 mg/dL the next day, do not administer insulin and do a complete curve. If the preinsulin blood glucose concentration is greater than 180 mg/dL when receiving once-daily insulin, go back to twice-daily administration. An attempt to wean the cat can again be made in a couple of weeks. Diabetic cats in remission should stay on a low-carbohydrate diet [33].

If performance of a curve is impossible because of temperament or financial issues, start insulin glargine at a dose of 2 U per cat administered subcutaneously twice daily and have the owner monitor urine glucose concentration or water intake. A cat well regulated on glargine should have trace urine glucose at most, and urine glucose should be negative most of the time. If urine glucose is greater than trace after 2 weeks of receiving glargine, the dose should be increased 1 U per cat per week until urine glucose is negative or water intake is less than 20 mL/kg every 24 hours if eating canned food and less than 70 mL/kg every 24 hours if eating dry food. At this point, keep the cat on the same dose for 2 weeks and then start decreasing the dose by 1 U per cat per week until urine glucose is positive or the insulin has been discontinued (J. Rand, BVSc, DVSc, personal communication, 2004).

Performance of blood glucose curves has become controversial because they are certainly not perfect. Blood glucose curves can be affected by the stress of hospitalization, especially in cats, and deviation from normal routine and can vary significantly from day to day. Other monitoring can be done, including performance of curves at home [38–42], continuous monitoring of glucose concentrations [32,43,44], measurement of serum glycosylated hemoglobin or fructosamine concentrations [45–48], and home monitoring of clinical signs alone [49]. Home glucose curves may be ideal, because the situation most closely mimics a patient's normal routine. Measure of glycosylated proteins or monitoring of clinical signs by themselves is inadequate in this author's opinion; periods of hypoglycemia may go unnoticed until severe complications occur. In addition, if a patient's control is inadequate, the only way to know how to adjust insulin administration is by performance of a curve.

HYPERADRENOCORTICISM

Canine and feline HAC can be pituitary or adrenal dependent. The pituitary form is more common in dogs and cats than the adrenal form, accounting for approximately 80% to 85% of cases of HAC. In pituitary-dependent hyperadrenocorticism (PDH), a corticotrophic tumor secretes corticotropin or ACTH. The excess corticotropin secretion leads to increased release of cortisol from the adrenal glands. In adrenal-dependent HAC, an adrenal tumor (AT) autonomously secretes cortisol. In dogs and cats, corticotropin-secreting pituitary tumors are almost 100% benign, whereas cortisol-secreting ATs are approximately 50% benign and 50% malignant. In either form of the disease, most of the clinical signs are caused by hypercortisolemia. The pathophysiology leading to the clinical sequelae is complex because of the large number of body tissues influenced by glucocorticoids. Large tumors, adrenal or pituitary, can also lead to clinical signs attributable to space-occupying effects.

Surgical and medical options exist for treatment of canine and feline HAC. By whatever means, the ultimate goal of therapy is to eliminate hypersecretion of cortisol. For PDH, medical therapy is most often used for dogs in the United States. In Europe, hypophysectomy is available and has been successful [50]. Currently, this operation is only offered at one academic center in the United States. For cats with PDH, because of the limited success of medical therapy, bilateral adrenalectomy is the treatment of choice, followed by lifelong therapy for hypoadrenocorticism [51]. For dogs and cats with an AT, surgery is recommended.

Currently, there is no drug therapy that cures PDH. Lifelong therapy should be anticipated. Mitotane, or o,p′-DDD, has long been the mainstay of medical therapy for canine PDH and still remains a good option. A chlorinated hydrocarbon, mitotane, is adrenocorticolytic, causing selective necrosis of the zona fasciculata and zona reticularis, the adrenocortical zones that secrete cortisol and sex hormones. The toxin is specific for the adrenal glands, particularly hyperplastic glands, with the exception that mitotane can cause fatty degeneration and centrilobular atrophy of the liver. Mitotane can be used to treat cortisol-secreting ATs as well if surgery is not an option. The reader is referred elsewhere for discussion of treatment protocols using mitotane [51,52].

Ketoconazole is a triazole antifungal drug widely used for treatment of disseminated fungal diseases. The drug inhibits cytochrome P450 enzymes responsible for the synthesis of gonadal and adrenal steroids and has been used to treat HAC in human patients [53,54]. In addition, ketoconazole may antagonize glucocorticoid receptors. The efficacy of ketoconazole, however, is less than that of mitotane. After ketoconazole therapy, basal and postcorticotropin cortisol concentrations may even be higher than pretreatment levels in some dogs [51]. Of 132 veterinary internists and dermatologists surveyed, who were specialists likely to treat Cushing's syndrome, 52% considered ketoconazole to be effective in less than 25% of cases, 19% reported effectiveness in 25% to 49% of cases, and 14% each believed ketoconazole to be efficacious in 50% to 74% and 75% to 100% of cases. Ketoconazole does seem to be relatively safe, with a low incidence of adverse effects, including anorexia, vomiting, elevated liver enzymes, diarrhea, and icterus [55].

Selegiline (L-deprenyl) is a monoamine oxidase B inhibitor, and thus inhibits degradation of biogenic amines, most notably dopamine. Elevated dopamine levels and dopamine agonism suppress corticotropin secretion, at least from the intermediate lobe of the pituitary. Thus, increasing dopamine concentrations may inhibit oversecretion of corticotropin and be useful for treatment of PDH. Selegiline can only be effective for PDH. Because endogenous corticotropin secretion is suppressed in patients with an AT, dopamine agonism or alteration of dopamine metabolism would have little if any further effect on corticotropin release. Moreover, because ATs function autonomously of corticotropin, lowering corticotropin levels would not alter cortisol secretion.

A crucial question is whether dopamine's corticotropin-lowering effect is on the anterior or intermediate lobe of the pituitary. If dopamine only inhibits intermediate lobe corticotropin secretion, as is generally believed, selegiline use would be efficacious only in cases of PDH attributable to intermediate lobe tumors (ie, approximately 20% of canine PDH cases). Indeed, one study of 10 dogs suggested only a 20% response rate [56]. A more recent study found selegiline to be ineffective for treatment of PDH [57].

In Europe, trilostane is now being used to treat HAC. Trilostane inhibits the adrenal enzyme 3β-hydroxysteroid dehydrogenase, thereby suppressing production of progesterone and its end products, including cortisol and aldosterone. Overall, trilostane seems to be highly effective in suppressing cortisol secretion. Polyuria and polydipsia resolved over the first 6 months (mainly within the first 1–2 months) in 91% of dogs with PDH treated with trilostane, whereas polyphagia resolved in 81%. In 62% of dogs with dermatologic abnormalities, there was marked improvement that took up to 3 months. A small proportion of dogs with PDH are not well controlled, however, with trilostane [58–60].

The recommended starting dose of trilostane is 2 to 10 mg/kg once daily. Because trilostane is available as 30-, 60-, and 120-mg capsules, the exact dose is related to the patient's size and may need to be compounded for smaller dogs. In approximately 50% of dogs, dosage adjustments, either up or down, are required. Authors of one study noted that in most dogs, there was an initial sensitivity to the drug, followed by a need for an increase in dose. After time, the dose required hit a plateau [60]. Interestingly, the final dose required for control has varied greatly between studies. In one study, the median final dose was 6.1 mg/kg [59], whereas another study found the therapeutic dose for most dogs is likely to be 16 to 19 mg/kg [60]. Part of the discrepancy may relate to the differences in what was considered the ideal postcorticotropin serum cortisol concentration. In any case, the point remains that each dog should be started on the recommended dose, with the dose adjusted according to corticotropin stimulation test results. The survival rate is at least as good as that achieved with mitotane therapy [61].

For the most part, reported adverse effects are relatively mild, including lethargy and vomiting, but death has occurred [59,60,62]. Although some studies found a relatively low incidence of side effects, one non-peer-reviewed report states that mild self-limiting side effects, such as diarrhea, vomiting, and lethargy, occur in 63% of treated dogs [63]. Trilostane can affect aldosterone secretion as well as cortisol; thus, an Addisonian crisis can ensue [60,62]. Excess adrenal suppression can occur at any time during therapy. One dog died despite appropriate treatment for hypoadrenocorticism, and the true cause of death remained undetermined [58].

As with mitotane therapy, excess adrenal gland suppression can occur and warrants discontinuing medication temporarily and lowering the dose. Although, in theory, the effects of trilostane as an enzyme inhibitor should be rapidly reversible within a couple of days, suppression can last weeks to months. In a few cases, trilostane was discontinued when cortisol secretion was noted to be too low, and cortisol secretion remained low for 6 weeks to 4 months but eventually returned to pretherapy levels [60]. In two additional cases, signs of glucocorticoid and mineralocorticoid deficiency occurred in dogs being treated with trilostane and bilateral adrenal necrosis was documented. The cause of the necrosis was undetermined [64]. The hypoadrenocorticism lasted for at least 3 months but is likely to be permanent for the life of the dogs. How often acute iatrogenic hypoadrenocorticism occurs in dogs treated with trilostane is unknown.

A few questions still need to be answered. First, the optimal postcorticotropin serum cortisol concentration should be determined. Second, the ideal timing of postpill sampling also needs to be elucidated. Postcorticotropin cortisol may vary with the interval between dosing and testing. Third, the appropriate starting dose and interval (once or twice daily) needs clarification. How long control must be maintained throughout the day needs to be elucidated. The exact length of trilostane's duration of action is unknown, but it is less than 24 hours. If the effects only last 12 hours in some dogs, is that adequate for control of HAC?

Currently, recommendations are to start trilostane therapy at a dose of 2 to 10 mg/kg once daily. If minor side effects are seen, drug administration should be stopped for 3 to 5 days and then restarted, giving trilostane every other day for 1 week before continuing with the initial dosing scheme. A corticotropin stimulation test should be performed beginning at 4 to 6 hours after administration of a pill at 10 to 14, 30, and 90 days after being on a full dose of trilostane. (It should be noted that postpill timing of corticotropin stimulation testing is important in dogs receiving trilostane, which is different from evaluation of dogs on mitotane, when testing can occur at any time.) If the postcorticotropin cortisol concentration is less than 20 nmol/L, trilostane administration should cease for 48 to 72 hours [63]. Although trilostane could then be safely reinitiated at a lower dose in most dogs, given the long-term suppression seen in some cases, a corticotropin stimulation test should ideally be performed and trilostane should not be reinstituted until the cortisol secretion has recovered. If the postcorticotropin cortisol level is greater than 200 nmol/L, the trilostane dose should be increased. The exact increment depends on a patient's weight and available capsule sizes. If the postcorticotropin serum cortisol concentration is between 20 and 200 nmol/L and the dog is doing well, therapy should continue as is. Conversely, if the postcorticotropin serum cortisol concentration is between 20 and 200 nmol/L but clinical signs are continuing, twice-daily therapy should be used. The same dose that was given once daily should be given twice daily (eg, if giving 30 mg once daily, then double it to 30 mg twice daily). Once the clinical condition of the dog and the dose has stabilized, a corticotropin stimulation test should be performed every 3 to 6 months to evaluate ongoing control. Serum potassium concentration should also be measured to check for hyperkalemia [63].

Trilostane has been used to treat a few dogs with an AT. Not enough information is available to ascertain whether the treatment protocol or efficacy varies if treating dogs with PDH versus those with an AT. Clinical signs were controlled, at least transiently, and survival was prolonged [63,65]. In dogs with an AT, however, mitotane is the preferred treatment. Mitotane is truly a chemotherapeutic drug in this instance, killing primary neoplastic cells and perhaps metastatic cells as well. Trilostane simply would control tumoral secretion and not tumor growth. In fact, in dogs with PDH treated with trilostane, adrenal gland size increases [66].

A few disadvantages exist for using trilostane. The largest is availability. At the current time, trilostane is not approved for use in the United States. To obtain trilostane in the United States, a compassionate use form must be filed with the FDA. Second, the cost of trilostane is two to three times that of mitotane, depending on the size of the dog [60]. Because repeat corticotropin stimulation testing is needed with mitotane or trilostane, the cost of repeat evaluation would be the same for either drug. Finally, until the questions about required duration of action are answered, this author recommends use of mitotane in dogs with serious complications of HAC when breaks in control could be detrimental (eg, dogs with pulmonary thromboembolism).

DISORDERS OF GROWTH HORMONE

Therapy for pituitary dwarfism (ie, congenital growth hormone [GH] deficiency) relies on obtaining adequate serum GH concentrations, but no effective GH product is readily available for use in dogs. Recombinant human GH is expensive and can induce antibody formation that interferes with its effectiveness [67]. Although porcine and canine GH is identical, the availability of porcine GH is variable. If available, the recommended initial dose of porcine GH is 0.1 IU/kg administered subcutaneously three times weekly. Subsequent adjustments in dosage and frequency of administration should be based on clinical response and plasma insulin-like growth factor-1 (IGF-1) concentrations; IGF-1 concentrations are a marker of GH activity. The goal of treatment is to have the plasma IGF-1 concentration within the reference range for the breed. Hypersensitivity reactions, carbohydrate intolerance, and DM are the primary adverse effects; DM may become permanent if not detected early and the GH administration is discontinued [68].

Because progestins can cause mammary gland production and secretion of GH in dogs, their administration may be a potential therapy for canine GH deficiency. Two pituitary dwarves treated with medroxyprogesterone acetate (2.5–5 mg/kg initially at 3-week intervals and then at 6-week intervals) had an increased body size and growth of a complete adult hair coat. Pruritic pyoderma, cystic endometrial hyperplasia with mucometra, and signs of acromegaly were noted in one or both dogs, however. The dogs were alive and healthy for at least 3 years after starting therapy [69]. Another three dogs were treated with proligestone (10 mg/kg administered subcutaneously every 3 weeks), and growth, increases in IGF-1 levels, and improvement in hair coat were seen, but complications included development of clinical features of acromegaly, mammary development, and vulvar discharge in one intact female dog [70]. The dose of progestin used to treat GH deficiency needs to be altered to avoid side effects while maintaining a clinical response. Progestins can cause DM, however, as can GH, so appropriate monitoring must be done to avoid this complication.

In conclusion, new options are available for treatment of endocrine diseases. Methimazole remains the mainstay of medical therapy for feline hyperthyroidism. Transdermal formulations provide an efficacious way of controlling hyperthyroidism that may be more convenient for owners. Trilostane seems to be equally as effective as mitotane for treatment of canine PDH, but questions on the optimal dosing and testing protocols remain to be determined. PZI and pork Lente insulins are good options to treat diabetic animals; insulin glargine seems to be extremely promising in cats and has been associated with a high remission rate. Finally, progestogens can be used to treat canine congenital GH deficiency.

References

[1] Adams WH, Daniel GB, Legendre AM, et al. Changes in renal function in cats following treatment of hyperthyroidism using ^{131}I. Vet Radiol Ultrasound 1997;38:231–8.

[2] Rogers KS, Burkholder WJ, Slater MR, et al. Development and predictors for renal disease and clinical outcomes in hyperthyroid cats treated with 131-I [abstract]. J Vet Intern Med 2000;14:343.

[3] Peterson ME, Kintzer PP, Hurvitz AI. Methimazole treatment of 262 cats with hyperthyroidism. J Vet Intern Med 1988;2:150–7.

[4] Shelton GD, Joseph R, Richter K, et al. Acquired myasthenia gravis in hyperthyroid cats on tapazole therapy [abstract]. J Vet Intern Med 1997;11:120.

[5] Graves TK. Complications of treatment and concurrent illness associated with hyperthyroidism in cats. In: Bonagura JD, editor. Kirk's current veterinary therapy XII: small animal practice. Philadelphia: WB Saunders; 1996. p. 369–72.

[6] Trepanier LA, Hoffman SB, Kroll M, et al. Efficacy and safety of once versus twice daily administration of methimazole in cats with hyperthyroidism. J Am Vet Med Assoc 2003;222:954–8.

[7] Feldman EC, Nelson RW. Feline hyperthyroidism (thyrotoxicosis). In: Feldman EC, Nelson RW, editors. Canine and feline endocrinology and reproduction. St. Louis (MO): WB Saunders; 2004. p. 152–218.

[8] Hoffman SB, Yoder AR, Trepanier LA. Bioavailability of transdermal methimazole in pluronic lecithin organogel (PLO) in healthy cats. J Vet Pharmacol Ther 2002;25:189–93.

[9] Hoffman G, Marks SL, Taboada J, et al. Transdermal methimazole treatment in cats with hyperthyroidism. J Feline Med Surg 2003;5:77–82.

[10] Sartor LL, Trepanier LA, Kroll MM, et al. Clinical efficacy of transdermal methimazole in cats with hyperthyroidism. J Vet Intern Med 2004;18:651–5.

[11] Nieckarz JA, Daniel GB. The effect of methimazole on thyroid uptake of pertechnetate and radioiodine in normal cats. Vet Radiol Ultrasound 2001;42:448–57.

[12] Nelson RW, Duesberg CA, Ford SL, et al. Effect of dietary insoluble fiber on control of glycemia in dogs with naturally acquired diabetes mellitus. J Am Vet Med Assoc 1998;212:380–6.

[13] Kimmel SE, Michel KE, Hess RS, et al. Effects of insoluble and soluble dietary fiber on glycemic control in dogs with naturally occurring insulin-dependent diabetes mellitus. J Am Vet Med Assoc 2000;216:1076–82.
[14] Fleeman LM, Rand JS, Markwell PJ. Diets with high fiber and moderate starch are not advantageous for dogs with stabilized diabetes compared to a commercial diet with moderate fiber and low starch [abstract]. J Vet Intern Med 2003;17:433.
[15] Nelson RW, Scott-Moncrieff C, Feldman EC, et al. Effect of dietary insoluble fiber on control of glycemia in cats with naturally acquired diabetes mellitus. J Am Vet Med Assoc 2000;216:1082–8.
[16] Mazzaferro EM, Greco DS, Turner AS, et al. Treatment of feline diabetes mellitus using an α-glucosidase inhibitor and a low-carbohydrate diet. J Feline Med Surg 2003;5: 183–9.
[17] Frank G, Anderson W, Pazak H, et al. Use of a high-protein diet in the management of feline diabetes mellitus. Vet Ther 2001;2:238–46.
[18] Feldman EC, Nelson RW. Canine diabetes mellitus. In: Feldman EC, Nelson RW, editors. Canine and feline endocrinology and reproduction. St. Louis (MO): WB Saunders; 2004. p. 486–538.
[19] Feldman EC, Nelson RW. Feline diabetes mellitus. In: Feldman EC, Nelson RW, editors. Canine and feline endocrinology and reproduction. St. Louis (MO): WB Saunders; 2004. p. 539–79.
[20] Monroe WE, Laxton D, Fallin EA, et al. Efficacy and safety of a purified porcine insulin zinc suspension for managing diabetes mellitus in dogs. J Vet Intern Med 2005;19:675–82.
[21] Fleeman LM, Rand JS. Management of canine diabetes. Vet Clin North Am Small Anim Pract 2001;31:855–80.
[22] Hess RS, Ward CR. Effect of insulin dosage on glycemic response in dogs with diabetes mellitus: 221 cases (1993–1998). J Am Vet Med Assoc 2000;216:217–21.
[23] Nelson RW, Lynn RC, Wagner-Mann CC, et al. Efficacy of protamine zinc insulin for treatment of diabetes mellitus in cats. J Am Vet Med Assoc 2001;218:38–42.
[24] Rand JS, Marshall RD. Insulin glargine and the treatment of feline diabetes mellitus. In: Proceedings of the 22nd Annual American College of Veterinary Internal Medicine Forum, Minneapolis, MN, 2004. p. 584–6.
[25] Marshall RD, Rand JS. Insulin glargine and a high protein-low carbohydrate diet are associated with high remission rates in newly diagnosed diabetic cats [abstract]. J Vet Intern Med 2004;18:401.
[26] Martin GJ, Rand JS. Pharmacology of a 40 IU/ml porcine lente insulin preparation in diabetic cats: findings during the first week and after 5 or 9 weeks of therapy. J Feline Med Surg 2001;3:23–30.
[27] Rand JS. Management of feline diabetes. Aust Vet Pract 1997;27:68–76.
[28] Reusch CE. Monitoring and treatment of the diabetic cat. In: Proceedings of the European College of Veterinary Internal Medicine-Companion Animal 15th Annual Congress, Glasgow, Scotland, 2005. p. 125–7.
[29] Rand JS. Understanding feline diabetes. In: Proceedings of the 14th Ann American College of Veterinary Internal Medicine Forum, San Antonio, TX, 1996. p. 82–3.
[30] Nelson RW. Disorders of the endocrine pancreas. In: Nelson RW, Couto CG, editors. Essentials of small animal internal medicine. Philadelphia: Mosby Year Book; 1998. p. 734–74.
[31] Fleeman LM, Rand JS. Evaluation of day-to-day variability of serial blood glucose concentration curves in diabetic dogs. J Am Vet Med Assoc 2003;222:317–21.
[32] Ristic JME, Herrtage ME, Walti-Lauger SMM, et al. Evaluation of a continuous glucose monitoring system in cats with diabetes mellitus. J Feline Med Surg 2005;7:153–62.
[33] Rand JS, Marshall RD. Update on insulin glargine use in diabetic cats. In: Proceedings of the 23rd Annual American College of Veterinary Internal Medicine Forum, Baltimore, MD, 2005. p. 483–4.

[34] Rand JS. Pathogenesis of feline diabetes. In: Reinhart GA, Carey DP, editors. Recent advances in canine and feline nutrition: 1998 Iams Nutrition Symposium Proceedings. Wilmington (OH): Orange Frazer Press; 1998. p. 83–95.
[35] Nelson RW, Griffey SM, Feldman EC, et al. Transient clinical diabetes mellitus in cats: 10 cases (1989–1991). J Vet Intern Med 1999;13:28–35.
[36] Nelson RW, Feldman EC, Ford SL, et al. Effect of an orally administered sulfonylurea, glipizide, for treatment of diabetes mellitus in cats. J Am Vet Med Assoc 1993;203:821–7.
[37] Feldman EC, Nelson RW, Feldman MS. Intensive 50-week evaluation of glipizide administration in 50 cats with previously untreated diabetes mellitus. J Am Vet Med Assoc 1997;210:772–7.
[38] Reusch CE, Wess G, Casella M. Home monitoring of blood glucose concentration in the management of diabetes mellitus. Compend Contin Educ Pract Vet 2001;23:544–56.
[39] Casella M, Wess G, Reusch CE. Measurement of capillary blood glucose concentrations by pet owners: a new tool in the management of diabetes mellitus. J Am Anim Hosp Assoc 2002;38:239–45.
[40] Maele VD, Daminet R. Retrospective study of owners' perceptions on home monitoring of blood glucose in diabetic dogs and cats. Can Vet J 2005;46:718–23.
[41] Casella M, Wess G, Hassig M, et al. Home monitoring of blood glucose concentration by owners of diabetic dogs. J Small Anim Pract 2003;44:298–305.
[42] Casella M, Hassig M, Reusch CE. Home-monitoring of blood glucose in cats with diabetes mellitus: evaluation over a 4-month period. J Feline Med Surg 2005;7:163–71.
[43] Wiedmeyer CE, Johnson PJ, Cohn LA, et al. Evaluation of a continuous glucose monitoring system for use in dogs, cats, and horses. J Am Vet Med Assoc 2003;223:987–92.
[44] Davison LJ, Slater LA, Herrtage ME, et al. Evaluation of continuous glucose monitoring system in diabetic dogs. J Small Anim Pract 2003;44:435–42.
[45] Elliott DA, Nelson RW, Feldman EC, et al. Glycosylated hemoglobin concentrations in the blood of healthy dogs and dogs with naturally developing diabetes mellitus, pancreatic B-cell neoplasia, hyperadrenocorticism, and anemia. J Am Vet Med Assoc 1997;211(6):723–7.
[46] Elliott DA, Nelson RW, Reusch CE, et al. Comparison of serum fructosamine and blood glycosylated hemoglobin concentrations for assessment of glycemic control in cats with diabetes mellitus. J Am Vet Med Assoc 1999;214:1794–8.
[47] Plier ML, Grindem CB, MacWilliams PS, et al. Serum fructosamine concentration in nondiabetic and diabetic cats. Vet Clin Pathol 1998;27:34–9.
[48] Elliott DA, Nelson RW, Feldman EC. Glycosylated hemoglobin concentration for assessment of glycemic control in diabetic cats. J Vet Intern Med 1997;11:161–5.
[49] Briggs CE, Nelson RW, Feldman EC, et al. Reliability of history and physical examination findings for assessing control of glycemia in dogs with diabetes mellitus: 53 cases (1995–1998). J Am Vet Med Assoc 2000;217:48–53.
[50] Meij B, Voorhout G, Rijnberk A. Progress in transsphenoidal hypophysectomy for treatment of pituitary-dependent hyperadrenocorticism in dogs and cats. Molec Cell Endocrin 2002;197:89–96.
[51] Feldman EC, Nelson RW. Canine hyperadrenocorticism (Cushing's syndrome). In: Feldman EC, Nelson RW, editors. Canine and feline endocrinology and reproduction. St. Louis (MO): WB Saunders; 2004. p. 252–357.
[52] Behrend EN, Kemppainen RJ. Medical therapy of canine Cushing's syndrome. Compend Contin Educ Pract Vet 1998;20(6):679–97.
[53] Sonino N, Boscaro M, Paoletta A. Ketoconazole treatment in Cushing's syndrome: experience in 34 patients. Clin Endocrinol (Oxf) 1991;35:347–52.
[54] West JR. Ketoconazole in Cushing's syndrome. Ann Pharmacol 1987;21:972–3.
[55] Behrend EN, Kemppainen RJ, Clark TP, et al. Treatment of hyperadrenocorticism in dogs: a survey of internists and dermatologists. J Am Vet Med Assoc 1999;215:938–43.

[56] Reusch C, Steffen T, Hoerauf A. The efficacy of L-deprenyl in dogs with pituitary-dependent hyperadrenocorticism. J Vet Intern Med 1999;13:291–301.
[57] Braddock JA, Church DB, Robertson ID, et al. Inefficacy of selegiline in treatment of canine pituitary-dependent hyperadrenocorticism. Aust Vet J 2004;82:272–7.
[58] Neiger R, Ramsey IK, O'Conner J, et al. Trilostane treatment of 78 dogs with pituitary-dependent hyperadrenocorticism. Vet Rec 2002;150:799–804.
[59] Ruckstuhl NS, Nett CS, Reusch C. Results of clinical examinations, laboratory tests, and ultrasonography in dogs with pituitary-dependent hyperadrenocorticism treated with trilostane. Am J Vet Res 2002;63:506–12.
[60] Braddock JA, Church DB, Robertson ID, et al. Trilostane treatment in dogs with pituitary-dependent hyperadrenocorticism. Aust Vet J 2003;81:600–7.
[61] Barker EN, Campbell S, Tebb AJ, et al. A comparison of the survival times of dogs treated with mitotane or trilostane for pituitary-dependent hyperadrenocorticism. J Vet Intern Med 2005;19:810–5.
[62] Neiger R, Ramsey IK. Trilostane therapy of canine hyperadrenocorticism. In: Proceedings of the 20th Annual American College of Veterinary Internal Medicine Forum, Dallas, TX, 2002. p. 544–6.
[63] Neiger R. Hyperadrenocorticism: the animal perspective—comparative efficacy and safety of trilostane. In: Proceedings of the Annual Veterinary Medical Forum, Minneapolis, MN, 2004. p. 699–701.
[64] Chapman PS, Kelly DF, Archer J, et al. Adrenal necrosis in a dog receiving trilostane for the treatment of hyperadrenocorticism. J Small Anim Pract 2004;45:307–10.
[65] Eastwood JM, Elwood CM, Hurley KJ. Trilostane treatment of a dog with functional adrenocortical neoplasia. J Small Anim Pract 2003;44:126–31.
[66] Mantis P, Lamb CR, Witt A, et al. Changes in ultrasonographic appearance of adrenal glands in dogs with pituitary-dependent hyperadrenocorticism treated with trilostane. Vet Radiol Ultrasound 2003;44:682–5.
[67] van Herpen H, Rijnberk A, Mol JA. Production of antibodies to biosynthetic human growth hormone in the dog. Vet Rec 1994;134:171.
[68] Feldman EC, Nelson RW. Disorders of growth hormone. In: Feldman EC, Nelson RW, editors. Canine and feline endocrinology and reproduction. St. Louis (MO): WB Saunders; 2004. p. 45–84.
[69] Kooistra HS, Voorhout G, Selman PJ, et al. Progestin-induced growth hormone (GH) production in the treatment of dogs with congenital GH deficiency. Domest Anim Endocrinol 1998;15:93–102.
[70] Knottenbelt CM, Herrtage ME. Use of proligestone in the management of three German shepherd dogs with pituitary dwarfism. J Small Anim Pract 2002;43:164–70.

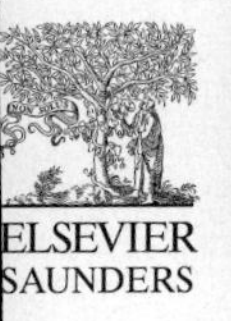
ELSEVIER
SAUNDERS

Vet Clin Small Anim 36 (2006) 1107–1127

VETERINARY CLINICS
SMALL ANIMAL PRACTICE

Anticonvulsant Therapy in Dogs and Cats

Curtis W. Dewey, DVM, MS

Department of Clinical Sciences, Cornell University, College of Veterinary Medicine, Ithaca, NY 14853, USA

Seizure disorders are commonly encountered in small animal practice and may be attributable to a variety of brain disorders [1,2]. Dealing with a patient afflicted with seizures is particularly challenging for the small animal practitioner for a number of reasons. These reasons include owner perceptions and expectations, the natures of the seizure disorders themselves, and differing opinions and guidelines concerning treatment options. In addition to these concerns, the inability to extrapolate knowledge concerning canine anticonvulsant drugs to the treatment of feline seizure disorders safely is a constant impediment to developing new anticonvulsant therapies for cats.

Because of the unpredictable and often violent nature of seizures, pet owners are often emotionally distraught when seeking veterinary advice and guidance. Naturally, many such owners want and expect the veterinarian to make the seizures cease entirely. It is important for the attending clinician to explain early on that reduction of seizure frequency and duration is likely but that cessation of seizure activity is unlikely. Despite this, attaining a seizure-free status for a particular patient is always a clinical goal, but it is sought within the confines of drug side effects. It has been estimated that attaining a seizure-free status without unacceptable side effects of drug therapy is likely in less than half of patients [3]; however, this estimation predates the introduction of several of the newer anticonvulsant agents discussed in this article.

Because seizures are always a manifestation of an underlying brain disorder, the veterinarian is often faced with simultaneously treating the pet for seizures while trying to elucidate and sometimes treat the cause of the seizures. In patients highly suspected of having idiopathic epilepsy as the causative disorder for seizure activity, treatment concerns are limited to controlling seizures. When seizures are secondary to a structural (eg, brain tumor, encephalitis) or metabolic (eg, hepatic encephalopathy) disorder, treatment options for the primary disease as well as for the effects that particular anticonvulsant drugs may have on that disease must be considered.

E-mail address: cwd27@cornell.edu

0195-5616/06/$ – see front matter
doi:10.1016/j.cvsm.2006.05.005

vetsmall.theclinics.com

The ultimate goal of anticonvulsant therapy is to reduce the frequency and duration of seizure activity as much as possible while avoiding excessive drug-induced side effects. With the recent introduction of several new anticonvulsant drugs over the past 5 to 10 years for use in dogs and cats, there are more opportunities to improve seizure control in these species with minimal adverse side effects. In the author's experience, dogs and cats with recurrent seizure activity that is not treated or is treated with subtherapeutic doses of anticonvulsant drugs tend to experience an increase in seizure frequency or duration over time. Seizure control tends to be more successful if initiated before such an increase. In light of these factors, the concept of an arbitrary number of "acceptable" seizures per month (eg, one seizure per month) for patients holds little meaning. Similarly, basing the success or failure of individual anticonvulsant drugs on such an absolute goal is not realistic. A more realistic measure of success of an anticonvulsant drug is a reduction in seizure frequency by at least 50%, with minimal drug side effects [4].

This article reviews anticonvulsant therapies in current use for dogs and cats and briefly describes new modes of anticonvulsant therapy that are being investigated or pending publication. Most of the information contained within the article is based on published literature. Some of the information, however, is based on the author's clinical experience and is identified as such.

MAINTENANCE ANTICONVULSANT THERAPY

Phenobarbital

Phenobarbital (PB) remains one of the first-choice drugs for use in dogs with seizures and is also the preferred anticonvulsant drug for cats [1–3]. PB is an effective anticonvulsant drug in both of these species. PB has been reported to be effective as a sole agent in 60% to 80% of epileptic dogs; specific efficacy data are not available for epileptic cats, but PB has been shown to be generally effective in controlling feline seizures [2,5–7]. The proposed mechanisms of action of PB include increasing neuronal responsiveness to gamma-aminobutyric acid (GABA), antiglutamate effects, and decreasing calcium inflow into neurons [1–3]. PB is metabolized by hepatic microsomal enzymes, with a serum half-life ($t_{1/2}$) of elimination between 40 and 90 hours in the dog, and approximately 40 to 50 hours in the cat after oral administration. It takes approximately 10 to 15 days to reach steady-state kinetics with oral dosing at a maintenance level [1–3,8]. PB is a potent inducer of hepatic microsomal enzyme activity (eg, cytochrome P450), and can thus lead to accelerated elimination of itself as well as other hepatically metabolized drugs [2,3,9]. PB use in dogs at standard anticonvulsant doses has also been shown to cause an increase in plasma concentrations of α_1-acid glycoprotein, which is the major binding protein for circulating basic drugs [9]. Through this mechanism, PB may also affect the unbound or available fraction of other concurrently administered drugs.

The maintenance dose range used by the author for PB in dogs is 3 to 5 mg/kg of body weight administered orally every 12 hours. In cats, a similar dose range is used, but the initial dose is 2.5 mg/kg of body weight administered orally every

12 hours. Serum levels should be obtained 2 to 3 weeks after instituting therapy or changing dose regimens [1–3]. Timing of blood draw does not affect the level in 91% of canine cases; therefore, obtaining a trough serum level in dogs receiving PB is probably unnecessary [10]. Serum separator tubes should not be used, because the silicone binds the PB. The therapeutic range used by the author is between 20 and 35 μg/mL. Although the published ranges are between 15 and 45 μg/mL, the author has found that most dogs administered a dose below 20 μg/mL are not well controlled and that most reported cases of hepatotoxicity occurred in dogs with levels above 35 μg/mL [1–3,11].

Commonly reported side effects of PB in dogs and cats include sedation, polyuria/polydipsia (PU/PD), polyphagia (PP) with weight gain, and ataxia. These side effects usually subside dramatically within the first several weeks of treatment [1–3,5,6]. The author has had many clients complain that some of the side effects, although lessened from the time of treatment initiation, are a constant problem (eg, weight gain, sedation). The author has found that dogs with brain tumors often experience an unacceptable level of sedation with PB use, even at low doses. In the author's experience, cats are resistant to developing PU/PD and PP in comparison to dogs. Provided that seizure control is adequate, most owners seem to be tolerant of PB side effects. An uncommon but potentially life-threatening consequence of PB use is hepatic failure [1–3,11,12]. Because of this, patients receiving PB therapy should be monitored on a regular basis for evidence of hepatic damage. Less commonly reported side effects attributable to PB use in dogs include bone marrow necrosis (with attendant blood dyscrasias) and superficial necrolytic dermatitis (SND) [1,2,13–16]. Bone marrow necrosis is suspected to be an idiosyncratic reaction to PB. Blood dyscrasias (eg, leukopenia, thrombocytopenia, anemia) are likely to resolve after PB discontinuation [2,13–15]. SND is thought to be related to a low level of plasma amino acids, which, in turn, is suspected to be attributable to PB effects on the liver. Dogs with SND are unlikely to have evidence of hepatic failure; it has been theorized that chronic PB administration leads to accelerated hepatic catabolism of amino acids, ultimately leading to SND. Unfortunately, SND is not likely to resolve simply by discontinuing PB therapy [16]. Uncommon PB-associated side effects reported in cats include facial pruritus, generalized pruritus with distal limb edema, thrombocytopenia, and leukopenia; these disorders resolved after discontinuation of PB [6]. There is one report of a cat with severe cutaneous eruptions and lymphadenopathy associated with PB use; the suspected hypersensitivity reaction resolved shortly after discontinuing PB therapy [17]. Chronic (>3 weeks) PB administration at standard therapeutic doses has been shown to cause a significant decrease in total (TT4) and free (FT4) serum thyroxine levels. Serum thyroid-stimulating hormone (TSH) levels are often increased in dogs receiving chronic PB therapy; however, the increases tend to be relatively small and often remain within the reference range. It is believed that decreased serum levels of thyroid hormone (TT4 and FT4) in dogs receiving PB may be attributable to enhanced hepatic clearance of these hormones [1,2,18,19]. Whether or not dogs on chronic PB therapy with serum thyroid hormone levels below the normal reference range are truly hypothyroid is debatable. Many such patients have no clinical signs attributable to hypothyroidism. Alternatively, some clinical signs potentially attributable to hypothyroidism (eg, lethargy, weight gain) may simply be side effects of PB [1,2,18–20]. If clinical signs support hypothyroidism in a dog with subnormal serum thyroid hormone levels, supplementation with thyroid replacement therapy is warranted. PB has no measurable effect on adrenal function tests in dogs [3,20–22].

Serum chemistry values should be checked every 6 months in patients receiving PB. Increased serum alkaline phosphatase (ALP) is expected in dogs receiving PB. Increases in serum alanine aminotransferase (ALT) are cause for concern [1,2]. It is generally thought that serum ALT increases represent hepatocellular damage, whereas serum ALP elevations reflect PB-induced hepatic enzyme production [2,11,23]. Recent evidence suggests that serum elevations of both these enzymes may be attributable to subclinical hepatocellular damage rather than to PB induction [24,25]. If there is any concern over hepatic dysfunction, serum bile acids should also be evaluated. It is also advisable to check the serum PB level every 6 months because it decreases as a result of hepatic enzyme stimulation in some dogs [1,3].

Bromide

Bromide (Br) is a halide salt that has been used primarily as a second-line (ie, add-on to PB) drug in dogs but is gaining popularity as a first-choice anticonvulsant in this species [1–3,26–28]. Br has been shown to be an effective add-on therapy for dogs receiving PB; most dogs on PB that receive Br as an add-on therapy experience at least a 50% reduction in seizure frequency [28]. In addition, reduction or eventual discontinuation of PB can be achieved in some dogs after the addition of Br therapy, without loss of seizure control [1–3,28]. Br has been shown to be effective as a sole anticonvulsant agent in epileptic dogs but is not as effective as PB. With the exception of effects on the liver, side effects of Br therapy are similar to those of PB when compared as sole anticonvulsant agents [29]. Br is usually administered as the potassium salt (KBr). The sodium salt form (NaBr) contains more Br per gram of drug; therefore, the dose should be approximately 15% less than that calculated for KBr [1,26]. The anticonvulsant mechanism of Br is thought to be attributable to its competition with chloride ions; the Br ion is thought to hyperpolarize neuronal membranes after traversing neuronal chloride channels [1–3,26–28]. Br is renally excreted, and is thus a good choice for patients with hepatic disease (eg, portosystemic shunt). Br ions compete with chloride ions for reabsorption by the renal tubules [1,2,26]. The $t_{1/2}$ of elimination for KBr is 24 days in dogs; therefore, steady-state kinetics are not reached for 80 to 120 days with a maintenance dose [1,2,26,28]. The author's initial maintenance dose for oral KBr is 35 mg/kg of body weight divided into two daily doses. A loading dose is often administered over a 5-day period to dogs to attain steady-state kinetics sooner. The loading dose used by the author is 125 mg/kg of body weight divided into two daily doses. Liquid Br is used to load (it is easy to decrease the dose if side effects are unacceptable), and capsules are used for maintenance. In emergency situations (eg, status epilepticus), KBr can be loaded over 24 hours. This can be done rectally if the patient is not able to take oral drugs. A 24-hour loading protocol is 100 mg/kg administered every 4 hours [30]. A sterile NaBr solution can also be used for intravenous loading. A 3% NaBr solution in sterile water administered as a continuous rate infusion (CRI) over 24 hours at a dose of 900 mg/kg has been suggested [31].

Serum Br levels should be obtained within 1 week of loading, 1 month after loading, and 3 months after administration of a maintenance dose. If the 1-month Br level is more than 10% lower than the postloading level, the maintenance dose should be increased accordingly [2]. The therapeutic range for Br is 1 to 3 mg/mL [1–3,26]. For dogs already receiving PB, the therapeutic range for Br is somewhat less (0.8–2.4 mg/mL) than for dogs in which Br is being used as a sole anticonvulsant drug (0.9–3.0 mg/mL) [32]. Diets high in chloride have been shown to decrease the elimination $t_{1/2}$ for Br in dogs significantly and to increase the dose necessary to maintain serum concentrations within the therapeutic range; this phenomenon is believed to be attributable to competition between the Br and chloride ions for renal reabsorption [33]. Chloride levels are often falsely elevated on serum chemistry analyses because the assays cannot distinguish between chloride and Br ions [1,2,26].

Side effects of KBr include pelvic limb stiffness and ataxia, sedation, vomiting, PU/PD, PP with weight gain, hyperactivity, and skin rash. Less commonly, aggressive behavior and pancreatitis have been associated with KBr use [1–3,26–28,34]. Pancreatitis has been suggested to be more likely when KBr is used in conjunction with PB [34]. In dogs with Br toxicity (eg, profound sedation, ataxia), diuresis with chloride containing intravenous fluids (eg, 0.9% NaCl) can be used to hasten renal elimination of Br [3,26].

Because of lack of hepatic metabolism, Br has been investigated as a potential anticonvulsant drug for cats [35]. At a dosing schedule of 15 mg/kg administered orally every 12 hours, the elimination $t_{1/2}$ for Br in cats is approximately 11 days and steady state is achieved within 6 weeks; cats are generally in the low end of the therapeutic range with this dosing protocol [35]. In addition to being less effective an anticonvulsant drug for cats as compared with dogs, Br has been associated with a severe bronchial asthma-like condition in 35% to 42% of cats administered the drug [35,36]. Because of questionable efficacy and the potential for life-threatening side effects, the author does not consider Br a viable anticonvulsant option for cats.

The author has encountered several canine seizure cases in which the dogs developed a persistent cough that seemed to be associated with Br therapy. Coughing activity resolved shortly after Br discontinuation in these dogs. If a bronchial asthma-like condition is a potential side effect of Br therapy in dogs, it is likely a comparatively rare development in comparison with cats. Development of a persistent cough in a dog receiving Br therapy should alert the clinician to the possibility of a Br-associated side effect, however, especially if other diagnostic tests do not elucidate a cause for the cough.

Benzodiazepines

Benzodiazepine drugs used in dogs and cats with seizure disorders include diazepam, clonazepam, clorazepate, midazolam, and lorazepam. Benzodiazepines exert their anticonvulsant effects by enhancing GABA activity in the brain. Diazepam is ineffective as an oral maintenance anticonvulsant in dogs because of its short $t_{1/2}$ of elimination (2–4 hours) and the tendency for dogs to develop tolerance to its anticonvulsant effect. In contrast, diazepam is an effective oral anticonvulsant in cats [1–3]. Unfortunately, acute fatal hepatic necrosis has been associated with oral diazepam use in cats [1–3,37,38]. Because of this potential side effect of oral diazepam use in cats, the author does not consider diazepam to be a viable maintenance oral anticonvulsant option for this species. Clonazepam is an oral anticonvulsant drug of limited use in dogs because of the rapid development of tolerance to the drug's anticonvulsant effects. There is an intravenous form of clonazepam for use in status epilepticus; unfortunately, this form of the drug is not available in the United States [2]. Clorazepate has an elimination $t_{1/2}$ between 3 and 6 hours in dogs after oral administration, and the dose range is 0.5 to 1 mg/kg of body weight administered every 8 hours. Although development of tolerance to the anticonvulsant effects of clorazepate is less of a problem in dogs than with diazepam or clonazepam, it is still a potential drawback of this drug. Other potential difficulties associated with clorazepate use in dogs include decreasing serum level of the active metabolite (nordiazepam) over time, elevated serum levels of concurrently administered PB, decreased serum nordiazepam levels associated with concurrent PB use, and hepatotoxicity [1–3,39–43]. Clinical use of clorazepate in cats has been suggested [3], but there are no studies regarding efficacy or long-term tolerability of clorazepate in this species. The author has found clorazepate to be only moderately effective as an anticonvulsant, and maintaining the correct dosage can be difficult. In the author's experience, the main indication for oral clorazepate use is as a short-term at-home treatment for dogs having cluster seizures. Midazolam and lorazepam are injectable benzodiazepine drugs that are discussed, along with injectable diazepam, in the section regarding cluster seizures and status epilepticus.

Felbamate

Felbamate is a dicarbamate drug that has demonstrated efficacy for focal (partial) and generalized seizures in experimental animal studies and human clinical trials [1–3,39,44]. Proposed mechanisms of action include blocking of *N*-methyl-D-aspartate (NMDA)–mediated neuronal excitation, potentiation of GABA-mediated neuronal inhibition, and inhibition of voltage-sensitive neuronal sodium and calcium channels [1–3,39,44–46]. Felbamate may also offer some protection to neurons from hypoxic or ischemic damage [3,39,44]. Approximately 70% of the orally administered dose of felbamate in dogs is excreted in the urine unchanged; the remainder undergoes hepatic metabolism. The $t_{1/2}$ of felbamate in adult dogs is typically between 5 and 6 hours (range: 4–8 hours) [1–3,39,45,47]. Felbamate is well absorbed after oral administration in adult dogs, but bioavailability in puppies may be only 30% that of adults. The $t_{1/2}$ of elimination in puppies has also been shown to be much shorter than in adult dogs (approximately 2.5 hours) [48,49]. For adult dogs, the author recommends an initial felbamate dose regimen of 15 mg/kg of body weight administered every 8 hours. Felbamate has a wide margin of safety in dogs, with serious toxic effects usually not apparent below a daily dose of 300 mg/kg of body weight [1–3,39,46,50]. If the initial dose of felbamate is ineffective, the dose is increased by 15-mg/kg increments every 2 weeks until efficacy is achieved, unacceptable side effects are evident, or the drug becomes cost-prohibitive. The therapeutic range for serum felbamate concentration in dogs is believed to be similar to that in people (20–100 μg/mL) [2,39,46]. Serum felbamate assays are typically costly. In addition, the wide therapeutic range and low toxicity potential of felbamate make routine serum drug monitoring of questionable clinical value. The author does not routinely check felbamate levels in dogs.

Side effects are infrequently associated with felbamate use in dogs. A major advantage of felbamate over more standard anticonvulsant drugs is that it does not cause sedation. Because felbamate does undergo some hepatic metabolism, liver dysfunction is a potential side effect [1–3,39,46]. In one study, 4 of 12 dogs receiving felbamate as an add-on therapy developed liver disease; however, all these patients were also receiving high doses of PB [51]. In people, felbamate has been shown to increase serum phenobarbital concentrations in some patients receiving combination therapy [2,52]. It is unclear whether felbamate, PB, or the combination of the two drugs is responsible for the reported hepatotoxicity in dogs. In people, serious hepatotoxicity is rarely associated with felbamate use and usually occurs in patients concurrently receiving other anticonvulsant drugs [2,44,53]. Aplastic anemia (caused by bone marrow suppression) has been reported to occur in people receiving felbamate at a rate of 10 per 100,000 patients; this uncommon side effect is also usually encountered with patients receiving combination anticonvulsant drug therapy [2,53]. Fortunately, this severe side effect does not seem to occur in dogs receiving the drug. In one report, however, reversible bone marrow suppression was suspected in 2 dogs receiving felbamate: the first dog developed mild thrombocytopenia, and the other dog developed mild leukopenia. Both of these abnormalities resolved after discontinuation of felbamate. One patient in this report developed bilateral keratoconjunctivitis sicca (KCS); it is unknown whether or not this was related to felbamate use [54]. The author has encountered several patients being given felbamate that developed KCS. Generalized tremor activity in small-breed dogs receiving high doses of felbamate has also been reported as a rarely encountered side effect [39,46].

The limited published material regarding the clinical efficacy of felbamate is similar to the author's experience. In one report of refractory epileptic dogs, 12 of 16 patients experienced a reduction of seizure frequency after initiation of felbamate therapy [51]. In another report of 6 dogs with suspected focal seizure activity, all dogs experienced a substantial reduction in seizure frequency when felbamate was used as a sole anticonvulsant drug; 2 of these dogs became seizure-free [54].

The author has used felbamate extensively in the treatment of dogs with seizure disorders. Felbamate seems to be effective as an add-on therapy and as a sole anticonvulsant agent for patients with focal and generalized seizures. Because of its lack of sedative effect, felbamate is particularly useful as monotherapy in dogs exhibiting obtunded mental status because of their underlying neurologic disease (eg, brain tumor, cerebral infarct). The author has found side effects from felbamate to be infrequent, especially when it is used as a sole anticonvulsant drug. Hepatic dysfunction associated with felbamate use tends to resolve after discontinuation of the drug. In dogs with evidence of preexisting hepatic disease, felbamate should be avoided. Because of the potential for hepatoxicity, it is recommended that serum biochemistry analysis be performed every 6 months for dogs receiving felbamate, especially if it is given concurrently with PB. It may also be advisable to evaluate complete blood cell counts (CBCs) every few months in the unlikely event that blood dyscrasia develops.

To the author's knowledge, there is no clinical information regarding the use of felbamate in cats. Because of the potential for felbamate-associated hepatotoxicity and blood dyscrasias in dogs, felbamate is not likely to become a viable anticonvulsant option for cats.

Gabapentin

Gabapentin, a structural analogue of GABA, has been suspected to exert its antiseizure effects via enhancing the release and action of GABA in the brain as well as by inhibiting neuronal sodium channels [1–3,39,46,52,53]. More recent evidence, however, suggests that gabapentin's anticonvulsant activity is due primarily to inhibition of voltage-gated calcium channels in the brain [55]. Gabapentin is well absorbed in dogs and people, with peak serum concentrations occurring within 1 to 3 hours after ingestion. In people, absorption is somewhat dose dependent, relying on a saturable amino acid transport mechanism in the gastrointestinal tract; this saturable transport process is thought to be the reason why anticonvulsant effects may last longer than would be expected based on the serum elimination $t_{1/2}$ of the drug [2,39,52]. In people, virtually all the orally administered dose of gabapentin is excreted unchanged in the urine (ie, no hepatic metabolism). In dogs, however, 30% to 40% of the orally administered dose of gabapentin undergoes hepatic metabolism to *N*-methyl-gabapentin [1–3,39,46,56,57]. Despite undergoing some hepatic metabolism in dogs, there is no appreciable induction of hepatic microsomal enzymes in this species. The $t_{1/2}$ of elimination for gabapentin in dogs is between 3 and 4 hours. The recommended dose range of gabapentin for dogs is 25 to 60 mg/kg of body weight divided into doses administered every 6 to 8 hours [1,2,39,46,56,57].

The author recommends an initial dose regimen of 10 mg/kg of body weight administered every 8 hours. The suspected therapeutic range for dogs is 4 to 16 mg/L [39,53]. As is the case with felbamate, serum gabapentin concentrations are seldom pursued in dogs.

Long-term toxicity trials for gabapentin have not been reported in dogs. Nevertheless, the drug seems to be well tolerated by this species, usually with few to no side effects. Sedation does not seem to be a major problem with gabapentin use in dogs. The author has had many clients report that their dogs experienced mild sedation or mild polyphagia and weight gain associated with gabapentin use, however. In one prospective study evaluating gabapentin as an add-on therapy for dogs with refractory seizures, there was no significant decrease in overall seizure frequency over a 4-month evaluation period; however, 3 of 17 dogs were seizure-free during this time period, and 4 others had at least a 50% decrease in seizure frequency [58]. In a similar study of 11 dogs, 5 dogs experienced a 50% or more reduction in seizure frequency after instituting gabapentin, and there was an overall significant decrease in seizure frequency [59]. For both of these studies, sedation and pelvic limb ataxia were the only reported side effects [58,59]. In the author's experience, gabapentin is occasionally helpful as an anticonvulsant drug in dogs. In people, gabapentin seems to be much more effective in the treatment of focal seizure disorders compared with its efficacy for the treatment of generalized seizures [53]. Because of its short $t_{1/2}$ in dogs, gabapentin probably needs to be administered at least every 8 hours, and possibly every 6 hours, to maintain serum gabapentin concentrations within the therapeutic range. The potential need for every 6-hour dosing can make it difficult for some pet owners to administer gabapentin reliably.

There exists only anecdotal information regarding gabapentin use in cats. An oral dose of 5 to 10 mg/kg of body weight administered every 8 to 12 hours has been suggested but is not based on any published data. To the author's knowledge, there is no information regarding the safety or efficacy of chronic gabapentin administration to cats.

Levetiracetam

Levetiracetam is a new piracetam anticonvulsant drug that has demonstrated efficacy in the treatment of focal and generalized seizure disorders in people as well as in several experimental animal models [1,39,52,53,60–66]. Although generally recommended as an add-on anticonvulsant drug [39,63–66], levetiracetam has been used successfully as monotherapy in people [67]. In human patients with refractory epilepsy, levetiracetam has manifested antiseizure effects within the first day of therapy [68]. The mechanism of action for levetiracetam's anticonvulsant effects is unknown; unlike other anticonvulsant drugs, levetiracetam does not seem to affect common neurotransmitter pathways (eg, GABA, NMDA) or ion channels (eg, sodium, T-type calcium) directly [39,52,60–62,66,69]. There is some evidence that levetiracetam may inhibit high voltage–activated neuronal calcium currents. Levetiracetam may also act by interfering with negative allosteric modulators of inhibitory GABA and glycine pathways in the brain [39,61,62,69]. It has recently been discovered that the binding site for levetiracetam in the brain is an integral membrane protein called synaptic vesicle protein 2A (SV2A); the interaction of levetiracetam with this protein appears to be associated with the drug's anticonvulsant effect [70]. Levetiracetam has demonstrated neuroprotective properties and may ameliorate seizure-induced brain damage [71,72]. Levetiracetam has also been reported to have an "antikindling" effect, which may diminish the likelihood of increasing seizure frequency over time [73,74]. Orally administered levetiracetam is approximately 100% bioavailable in dogs, with a serum $t_{1/2}$ of 3 to 4 hours (data on file at UCB Pharma, Smyrna, Georgia) [39,73,74]. Levetiracetam seems to exert an anticonvulsive effect that persists longer than its presence in the bloodstream would suggest [39,61]. In dogs, approximately 70% to 90% of the administered dose of levetiracetam is excreted unchanged in the urine; the remainder of the drug is hydrolyzed in the serum and other organs. There does not seem to be any appreciable hepatic metabolism of levetiracetam in human beings or dogs (data on file at UCB Pharma) [39,60–62,69,75]. The effective serum levetiracetam concentration in people is 5 to 45 μg/mL [53]. Because there is no clear relation between serum drug concentration and efficacy for levetiracetam and the drug has an extremely high margin of safety, routine therapeutic drug monitoring is not typically recommended for this drug in people [52,61,63,64]. However, although a therapeutic range has not yet been established for levetiracetam in either dogs or cats, human therapeutic ranges should serve as a reasonable population target until such information is available. Even without a range based on a sample population, monitoring is recommended to establish the therapeutic target for the individual patient. Monitoring should establish a baseline and then be repeated in the event that the patient becomes uncontrolled or the client becomes noncompliant. The author recommends an initial dosing schedule of 20 mg/kg of body weight administered every 8 hours based on pharmacokinetic data and clinical experience (data on file at UCB Pharma) [39,75]. This dose can be increased by 20-mg/kg increments until efficacy is achieved, side effects become apparent, or the drug becomes cost-prohibitive.

Long-term toxicity data for levetiracetam in dogs confirm that the drug is extremely safe. In one study, dogs were administered oral levetiracetam at doses up to 1200 mg/kg/d for 1 year. One of eight dogs receiving 300 mg/kg/d developed a stiff and unsteady gait. Other side effects (eg, salivation, vomiting) were confined to dogs receiving 1200 mg/kg/d. There were no treatment-related mortalities and no treatment-related histopathologic abnormalities (data on file at UCB Pharma). The author has used levetiracetam in dogs as an add-on therapy with favorable results. In a recent report, use of levetiracetam as an add-on drug in epileptic dogs was associated with a significant reduction (54%) in seizure frequency, with no apparent side effects [76]. Because of its paucity of side effects and lack of hepatic metabolism, levetiracetam is an attractive anticonvulsant choice for patients with hepatic dysfunction [77].

The author and colleagues are currently investigating the use of oral levetiracetam as an add-on anticonvulsant therapy for cats receiving PB [78]. Levetiracetam seems to be well tolerated in this species, usually with no apparent side effects. The $t_{1/2}$ of elimination is approximately 8 hours after oral administration. A dose of 20 mg/kg administered orally every 8 hours typically achieves a serum drug level within the therapeutic range reported for people. Two cats have experienced transient inappetence and lethargy that resolved without dose adjustment within 2 weeks. Although there is some degree of variability among cats, the mean reduction of seizure frequency in cats receiving levetiracetam as an add-on drug is approximately 60%. The author considers levetiracetam to be the preferred add-on anticonvulsant drug for cats receiving PB because of the lack of serious side effects and evidence of efficacy.

Zonisamide

Zonisamide is a sulfonamide-based anticonvulsant drug recently approved for human use; it has demonstrated efficacy in the treatment of focal and generalized seizures in people, with minimal side effects [39,79–87]. Suspected anticonvulsant mechanisms of action include blockage of T-type calcium and voltage-gated sodium channels in the brain, facilitation of dopaminergic and serotonergic neurotransmission in the central nervous system, scavenging free radical species, enhancing actions of GABA in the brain, inhibition of glutamate-mediated neuronal excitation in the brain, and inhibition of carbonic anhydrase activity [52,53,79–81,84,86–88]. Zonisamide is metabolized primarily by hepatic microsomal enzymes, and the $t_{1/2}$ in dogs is approximately 15 hours [39,89,90]. In people, it has been shown that the elimination $t_{1/2}$ of zonisamide is dramatically shorter in patients already receiving drugs that stimulate hepatic microsomal enzymes in comparison with patients who are not receiving such drugs [83,86,88,91]. A similar phenomenon seems to occur in dogs [39,88–92]. When used as an add-on therapy for dogs already receiving drugs requiring hepatic metabolism (eg, PB), the author recommends an initial oral zonisamide dose schedule of 10 mg/kg of body weight administered every 12 hours. This dose regimen has been shown to maintain canine serum zonisamide concentrations within the therapeutic range reported for people (10–40 μg/mL) when used as an add-on therapy [93]. For dogs not concurrently receiving drugs that induce hepatic microsomal enzymes, it is recommended to start zonisamide at a dosage of 5 mg/kg of body weight administered every 12 hours. The author generally checks trough serum zonisamide concentrations after approximately 1 week of zonisamide treatment. Zonisamide has a high margin of safety in dogs. In one study, minimal side effects occurred in Beagle dogs administered daily zonisamide doses up to 75 mg/kg of body weight per day for 1 year [94].

In one study, zonisamide was found to decrease seizure frequency by at least 50% in 7 of 12 dogs with refractory idiopathic epilepsy. In this responder group, the mean reduction in seizure frequency was 81.3%. In 6 of the 7 responder dogs, PB was able to be reduced by an average of 92.2%. Mild side effects (eg, transient sedation, ataxia, vomiting) occurred in 6 (50%) dogs; none of the side effects were considered severe enough to discontinue zonisamide therapy [93]. In a more recent study of refractory epileptic dogs, 9 of 11 dogs that received zonisamide were responders, with a median seizure reduction of 92.9%; transient sedation and ataxia occurred in six dogs [95].

Zonisamide has been shown to be effective as a sole anticonvulsant drug in people [96–98]. The author has used zonisamide as a sole anticonvulsant drug in a large number of dogs. These have been almost exclusively small-breed patients whose owners wished to avoid side effects associated with PB and Br use. Zonisamide seems to be effective as a sole anticonvulsant therapy, with few to no apparent side effects in dogs.

The author has treated two epileptic cats with zonisamide as an add-on to PB therapy. One cat became anorexic, necessitating drug discontinuation. The other cat experienced a substantial reduction in seizure frequency. This cat also had no side effects or blood work abnormalities attributable to zonisamide therapy after approximately 1 year of administration. Further data are needed regarding the use of zonisamide in cats before it can be recommended for use in this species.

THERAPY FOR CLUSTER SEIZURES AND STATUS EPILEPTICUS

Cluster seizures and status epilepticus hold the unfortunate role of being the most life-threatening and difficult to treat types of seizure activity in cats, dogs, and people. There are a number of definitions in the literature for cluster seizures and status epilepticus [1,3,31,99–105]. The author considers cluster seizures to include two or more discrete seizure events within a 24-hour period. A discrete seizure implies that the patient fully recovers before experiencing a subsequent seizure episode. Status epilepticus is continuous seizure activity lasting more than 5 minutes or recurrent seizures between which the patient does not fully recover. There is obvious overlap between these types of seizure activity, and cluster seizures may progress to status epilepticus in some patients. Unabated seizure activity can lead to severe consequences, such as hyperthermia, aspiration pneumonia, disseminated intravascular coagulation, and permanent brain injury [1,3,31,99–105]. It is vitally important in such severe cases to halt seizure activity, treat any seizure-associated problems (eg, brain edema), and provide attentive monitoring and nursing care. In the author's experience, many cases of cluster seizures, and most cases of status epilepticus, require measures that produce heavy sedation or anesthesia; these patients typically require tracheal intubation and close monitoring in an intensive care unit setting. The following discussion focuses specifically on drug options for emergency seizure control; more detailed information regarding the management of the cluster seizure and/or status epilepticus patient can be found in the listed references.

Intravenous diazepam (0.5–1.0 mg/kg) is the preferred initial choice to halt seizure activity because of its rapid onset of action and safety. Despite this, diazepam often results in temporary cessation of seizure activity or fails to halt seizure activity entirely. If seizure activity is repeatedly ceased with intravenous diazepam boluses, a diazepam intravenous CRI at a dose of 0.5 to 2.0 mg/kg/h may be successful [1]. If intravenous diazepam fails to halt seizures, another drug (eg, pentobarbital, phenobarbital) should be instituted. Other intravenous benzodiazepine drugs have been suggested for emergency treatment of seizures in dogs and cats, but clinical data regarding these drugs are lacking. These drugs include clonazepam, midazolam, and lorazepam [1–3,106]. Intravenous clonazepam was previously discussed and is not available in the United States at this time. A dose range of 0.05 to 0.2 mg/kg of body weight has been recommended for intravenous clonazepam in dogs [2,106]. Midazolam may be more effective and somewhat safer than equivalent doses of diazepam; midazolam has a rapid onset of action and a short elimination $t_{1/2}$ after intravenous or intramuscular administration. A recommended dose range for intravenously or intramuscularly administered midazolam for dogs and cats is 0.066 to 0.22 mg/kg of body weight [106–108]. Lorazepam has more potent activity at the benzodiazepine receptor than diazepam and lasts considerably longer than diazepam after intravenous administration. The use of intravenously administered lorazepam has become preferable to intravenously administered diazepam in managing human patients with status epilepticus [103–106]. An intravenous dose of 0.2 mg/kg of body weight has been shown to be well tolerated by dogs and achieves serum drug levels within the range considered therapeutic for people [106,109,110]. To the author's knowledge, there are no clinical studies addressing the clinical efficacy of lorazepam in dogs or any information regarding the use of this drug in cats. Administration of benzodiazepine drugs via the intrarectal and intranasal routes has been investigated in dogs. These routes of drug administration are advantageous when intravenous access is difficult to achieve. Owners of dogs that tend to experience cluster seizures or status epilepticus can administer these drugs at home during seizure activity. Potential disadvantages of intranasal administration of drugs versus intrarectal drug administration include technical factors (eg, drug loss attributable to swallowing or sneezing) and increased risk of an owner being inadvertently bitten by a pet during a seizure episode. Diazepam (0.5 mg/kg of body weight) and lorazepam (0.2 mg/kg of body weight) have been demonstrated to reach serum levels in dogs within the suspected therapeutic range within minutes after intranasal administration [110–112]. Similarly, intranasal administration of midazolam to dogs has been shown to achieve serum drug levels rapidly nearly three times that achieved after oral drug administration [113]. Diazepam has been shown to be well absorbed after intrarectal administration in dogs and effective as an at-home treatment of dogs with cluster seizures; the recommended dose range is 1 to 2 mg/kg of body weight, with the higher end of the range being used for dogs on chronic (>4 weeks) PB therapy [1–3,114,115]. Lorazepam does not seem to be absorbed well after intrarectal administration to dogs [106,109]. Midazolam is also suspected to be poorly absorbed after intrarectal administration; however, this is based on pharmacokinetic data from only one dog [108].

Intravenous barbiturate therapy is commonly used when intravenous benzodiazepine therapy fails to terminate seizure activity or if repeated dosing of intravenously administered benzodiazepine is necessary to control seizures.

Because of the potential for respiratory and cardiovascular depression with barbiturates, these drugs should be given to effect, with meticulous patient monitoring [1–3,31,103–105,112]. Pentobarbital is usually successful in abolishing motor manifestations of seizure activity within several minutes of intravenous administration but is not generally considered an anticonvulsant drug. The dose range for intravenous pentobarbital is 2 to 15 mg/kg of body weight. Compared with diazepam, it may require several minutes for pentobarbital to take effect [1,2,31,103–105,112]. If seizure activity is recurrent, an intravenous pentobarbital CRI can also be administered at a dose range of 0.5 to 4.0 mg/kg/h [1,2,31]. In addition to lacking anticonvulsant activity, pentobarbital is often associated with paddling activity during recovery; such activity may be confused with continued seizure activity [1]. Intravenously administered phenobarbital (2–6 mg/kg of body weight) requires approximately 15 to 20 minutes for clinical effect, so it is important not to give an overdose during this lag period. The serum level of PB increases by approximately 5 μg/mL per 3 mg/kg of body weight of intravenously administered drug. For patients not already receiving PB therapy, intermittent bolus injections (eg, 3–6 mg/kg of body weight) can be cautiously administered every 15 to 30 minutes to attain a serum PB level within the therapeutic range [1–3,106]. Alternatively, an IV CRI of PB (2–4 mg/kg/h) can be instituted [1]. When using barbiturates to control recurrent seizures, the author prefers using pentobarbital to terminate seizure activity, followed by a PB CRI.

Propofol is a phenolic injectable anesthetic agent that has been demonstrated to have GABA agonistic activity in the brain; propofol also decreases intracranial pressure (ICP) and brain metabolic activity. Propofol has the advantageous properties of being rapidly acting and quickly metabolized [2,105,107,112,116]. Propofol has proven to be useful in the treatment of cluster seizures and status epilepticus in human and small animal patients [1,2,31,103–105,107,112,116]. A bolus dose of 1 to 6 mg/kg should be administered slowly to effect. Because transient apnea is a commonly reported effect of bolus propofol administration, the clinician should be prepared to intubate the patient and assist with respirations. Apnea is not likely to occur if propofol is administered slowly and to effect [1,31,107,112,116]. Once seizure activity is halted, an intravenous propofol CRI can be initiated (0.1–0.6 mg/kg/min) [1,107,112]. In addition to its effects on respiratory activity, propofol has cardiovascular depressant effects. Careful monitoring is required when using propofol, similar to the situation with barbiturate use. Clonic motor activity, similar to that seen with pentobarbital use, can occur with propofol; this is most likely to take place when patients are waking up from propofol [107,112,116]. Transient seizure activity at the time of propofol induction and discontinuation has been reported in people [103,105]. The author has found propofol to be useful in the treatment of cluster seizures and status epilepticus in dogs and cats. Continuous infusion of propofol can be expensive when used in large-breed dogs, however.

Etomidate is an imidazole injectable anesthetic drug that has GABA-ergic activity in the brain and also decreases brain metabolic activity. Etomidate also may protect neurons from hypoxic damage and decrease ICP. It is rapidly acting after intravenous administration. The intravenous dose for etomidate when used as an induction agent is 1 to 3 mg/kg of body weight [2,112]. Although transient apnea may occur after injection of etomidate, this drug has minimal effects on the respiratory and cardiovascular systems [2,112]. The author has no clinical experience with the use of etomidate and is unaware of any studies investigating its use for treating seizure disorders in dogs or cats.

Fosphenytoin is the phosphate ester injectable prodrug form of phenytoin and is widely used in human medicine for the emergency treatment of seizure patients. After intravenous or intramuscular injection, fosphenytoin is rapidly converted to phenytoin (the active drug) by serum and tissue phosphatases. Unlike injectable phenytoin, fosphenytoin use is not associated with severe phlebitis and pain at the injection site. An intravenous dose range of approximately 10 to 20 mg/kg of body weight administered at a rate between 50 and 150 mg of phenytoin equivalents (PE) per minute is well tolerated in people and results in serum phenytoin levels within the therapeutic range (1–2 mg/L) within minutes [103–105,117]. Similar doses have been administered to dogs experimentally and achieve serum phenytoin drug levels within the therapeutic range reported for people [118,119]. A distinct advantage of fosphenytoin compared with other injectable anticonvulsant drugs is its relative lack of sedative effect. Although generally well tolerated, potential side effects of fosphenytoin use reported in people include hypotension, cardiac arrhythmias, nystagmus, ataxia, and somnolence [103–105,117]. To the author's knowledge, there are no clinical data regarding the use of fosphenytoin in dogs.

Intravenous levetiracetam has shown some promise as a treatment for experimental status epilepticus in a rat model. In this study, intravenous levetiracetam and diazepam seemed to potentiate each other's anticonvulsant effect [120]. Intravenous levetiracetam is well tolerated in dogs, even at high doses (eg, 400 mg/kg of body weight; data on file at UCB Pharma). In addition to overall safety compared with other injectable anticonvulsant drugs, levetiracetam does not cause sedation. The author is currently investigating the clinical use of intravenously administered levetiracetam in dogs with cluster seizures or status epilepticus. Although preliminary, results are encouraging.

INEFFECTIVE AND CONTRAINDICATED DRUGS

There are a number of older drugs that are generally ineffective in dogs, primarily because of their extremely short elimination $t_{1/2}$ in this species. These drugs are known or suspected to be toxic to cats as well. They include phenytoin, carbamazepine, valproic acid, and ethosuximide [1]. More recently introduced drugs that have been suggested for use in dogs include vigabatrin, lamotrigine, oxcarbazepine, tiagabine, and topiramate [39,121]. Although there is limited information regarding the use of these drugs in dogs, their short elimination $t_{1/2}$ in combination with their expense predicts that they may not be useful in managing canine seizure disorders. One study evaluating vigabatrin in refractory epileptic dogs found it to be of questionable efficacy; in addition,

2 of the 14 dogs receiving the drug developed hemolytic anemia [121]. Lamotrigine has an elimination $t_{1/2}$ of only 2 to 3 hours in dogs and undergoes significant hepatic metabolism to a potentially cardiotoxic compound. [39,45] Oxcarbazepine seems to induce its own hepatic metabolism in dogs, and has an elimination $t_{1/2}$ of only 1 hour after 8 days of repeated oral dosing [122]. Tiagabine has an elimination $t_{1/2}$ of approximately 2 hours in dogs and has been shown to cause marked sedation and visual impairment at relatively low doses [123]. The elimination $t_{1/2}$ of topiramate in dogs is only 2 to 4 hours [124]. Because of lack of toxicity data for cats, none of these aforementioned newer anticonvulsant drugs can be recommended for treating feline seizure disorders.

References

[1] Thomas WB. Seizures and narcolepsy. In: Dewey CW, editor. A practical guide to canine and feline neurology. Ames (IA): Iowa State Press (Blackwell Publishing); 2003. p. 193–212.

[2] Boothe DM. Anticonvulsants and other neurologic therapies in small animals. In: Boothe DM, editor. Small animal clinical pharmacology and therapeutics. Philadelphia: WB Saunders; 2001. p. 431–56.

[3] Podell M. Antiepileptic therapy. Clin Tech Small Anim Pract 1998;13(3):185–92.

[4] Marson AG, Kadir ZA, Hutton JL, et al. The new antiepileptic drugs: a systematic review of their efficacy and tolerability. Epilepsia 1997;38:859–80.

[5] Schwartz-Porsche D, Loscher W, Frey HH. Therapeutic efficacy of phenobarbital and primidone in canine epilepsy: a comparison. J Vet Pharmacol Ther 1985;8:113–9.

[6] Quesnel AD, Parent JM, McDonell W. Clinical management and outcome of cats with seizure disorders: 30 cases (1991–1993). J Am Vet Med Assoc 1997;210(1):72–7.

[7] Barnes HL, Chrisman CL, Mariani CL, et al. Clinical signs, underlying cause, and outcome in cats with seizures: 17 cases (1997–2002). J Am Vet Med Assoc 2004;225(11): 1723–6.

[8] Cochrane SM, Parent JM, Black WD, et al. Pharmacokinetics of phenobarbital in the cat following multiple oral administration. Can J Vet Res 1990;54:309–12.

[9] Hojo T, Ohno R, Shimodo M, et al. Enzyme and plasma protein induction by multiple oral administrations of phenobarbital at a therapeutic dosage regimen in dogs. J Vet Pharmacol Ther 2002;25:121–7.

[10] Levitski RE, Trepanier LA. Effect of timing of blood collection on serum phenobarbital concentrations in dogs with epilepsy. J Am Vet Med Assoc 2000;217(2):200–4.

[11] Dayrell-Hart B, Steinberg SA, Van Winkle TJ, et al. Hepatotoxicity of phenobarbital in dogs: 18 cases (1985–1989). J Am Vet Med Assoc 1991;199(8):1060–6.

[12] Muller PB, Taboada J, Hosgood G, et al. Effects of long-term phenobarbital treatment on the liver in dogs. J Vet Intern Med 2000;14:165–71.

[13] Jacobs G, Calvert C, Kaufman A. Neutropenia and thrombocytopenia in three dogs treated with anticonvulsants. J Am Vet Med Assoc 1998;212(5):681–4.

[14] Weiss DJ, Smith SA. A retrospective study if 19 cases of canine myelofibrosis. J Vet Intern Med 2002;16:174–8.

[15] Weiss DJ. Bone marrow necrosis in dogs: 34 cases (1996–2004). J Am Vet Med Assoc 2005;227(2):263–7.

[16] March PA, Hillier A, Weisbrode SE, et al. Superficial necrolytic dermatitis in 11 dogs with a history of phenobarbital administration (1995–2002). J Vet Intern Med 2004;18: 65–74.

[17] Ducoté JM, Coates JR, Dewey CW, et al. Suspected hypersensitivity to phenobarbital in a cat. J Feline Med Surg 1999;1:123–6.

[18] Gieger TL, Hosgood G, Taboada J, et al. Thyroid function and serum hepatic enzyme activity in dogs after phenobarbital administration. J Vet Intern Med 2000;14:277–81.
[19] Daminet S, Ferguson DC. Influence of drugs on thyroid function in dogs. J Vet Intern Med 2003;17:463–72.
[20] Muller PB, Wolfsheimer KJ, Taboada J, et al. Effects of long-term phenobarbital treatment on the thyroid and adrenal axis and adrenal function tests in dogs. J Vet Intern Med 2000;14:157–64.
[21] Dyer KR, Monroe WE, Forrester SD. Effects of short- and long-term administration of phenobarbital on endogenous ACTH concentration and results of ACTH stimulation tests in dogs. J Am Vet Med Assoc 1994;205:315–8.
[22] Foster SF, Church DB, Watson ADJ. Effect of phenobarbitone on the low-dose dexamethasone suppression test and the urinary corticoid:creatinine ratio in dogs. Aust Vet J 2000;78(1):19–22.
[23] Aitken MM, Hall E, Scott L, et al. Liver-related biochemical changes in the serum of dogs being treated with phenobarbitone. Vet Rec 2003;153:13–6.
[24] Gaskill CL, Hoffman WE, Cribb AE. Serum alkaline phosphatase isoenzyme profiles in phenobarbital-treated epileptic dogs. Vet Clin Pathol 2004;33:215–22.
[25] Gaskill CL, Miller LM, Mattoon JS, et al. Liver histopathology and liver and serum alanine aminotransferase and alkaline phosphatase activities in epileptic dogs receiving phenobarbital. Vet Pathol 2005;42:147–60.
[26] Trepanier LA. Use of bromide as an anticonvulsant for dogs with epilepsy. J Am Vet Med Assoc 1995;207(2):163–6.
[27] Pearce LK. Potassium bromide as an adjunct to phenobarbital for the management of uncontrolled seizures in dogs. Prog Vet Neurol 1990;1:95–101.
[28] Podell M, Fenner WR. Bromide therapy in refractory canine idiopathic epilepsy. J Vet Intern Med 1993;7:318–27.
[29] Boothe DM, Dewey C, Slater M. Comparison of phenobarbital and bromide as first choice anticonvulsant therapy in the canine epileptic. [abstract]. J Vet Intern Med 2002;16(3): 369.
[30] Dewey CW, Ducoté JM, Coates JR. Intrarectally administered potassium bromide loading in normal dogs. [abstract]. J Vet Intern Med 1999;13(3):238.
[31] Podell M. How do I treat status epilepticus. In: Proceedings of the 23rd Annual American College of Veterinary Internal Medicine Forum, Baltimore, MD; 2005. p. 366–8.
[32] Trepanier LA, Van Schoick A, Schwark WS, et al. Therapeutic serum drug concentrations in epileptic dogs treated with potassium bromide alone or in combination with other anticonvulsants: 122 cases (1992–1996). J Am Vet Med Assoc 1998;213(10):1449–53.
[33] Trepanier LA, Babish JG. Effect of dietary chloride content on the elimination of bromide by dogs. Res Vet Sci 1995;58:252–5.
[34] Gaskill CL, Cribb AE. Pancreatitis associated with potassium bromide/phenobarbital combination therapy in epileptic dogs. Can Vet J 2000;41:555–8.
[35] Boothe DM, George KL, Couch P. Disposition and clinical use of bromide in cats. J Am Vet Med Assoc 2002;221(8):1131–5.
[36] Wagner SO. Lower airway disease in cats on bromide therapy for seizures. [abstract]. J Vet Intern Med 2001;15(3):562.
[37] Center SA, Elston TH, Rowland PH. Fulminant hepatic failure associated with oral administration of diazepam in 11 cats. J Am Vet Med Assoc 1996;209:618–25.
[38] Hughes D, Moreau RE, Overall KL, et al. Acute hepatic necrosis and liver failure associated with benzodiazepine therapy in six cats, 1986–1995. J Vet Emerg Crit Care 1996;6(1): 13–20.
[39] Dewey CW, Barone G, Smith K, et al. Alternative anticonvulsant drugs for dogs with seizure disorders. Veterinary Medicine 2004;99(9):786–93.
[40] Forrester SD, Brown SA, Lees GE, et al. Disposition of clorazepate in dogs after single-and multiple-dose oral administration. Am J Vet Res 1990;51(12):2001–5.

[41] Forrester SD, Wilcke JR, Jacobson JD, et al. Effects of a 44-day administration of phenobarbital on disposition of clorazepate in dogs. Am J Vet Res 1993;54(7):1136–8.
[42] Brown SA, Forrester SD. Serum disposition of oral clorazepate from regular-release and sustained-delivery tablets in dogs. J Vet Pharmacol Ther 1991;14(4):426–9.
[43] Scherkl R, Kurudi D, Frey HH. Clorazepate in dogs: tolerance to the anticonvulsant effect and signs of physical dependence. Epilepsy Res 1989;3:144–50.
[44] Palmer KJ, McTavish D. Felbamate: a review of its pharmacodynamic and pharmacokinetic properties, and therapeutic efficacy in epilepsy. Drugs 1993;45(6):1041–65.
[45] Rho JM, Donevan SD, Rogawski MA. Mechanism of action of the anticonvulsant felbamate: opposing effects on N-methyl-D-aspartate and γ-aminobutyric acid$_A$ receptors. Ann Neurol 1994;35:229–34.
[46] Sisson A. Current experiences with anticonvulsants in dogs and cats. In: Proceedings of the 15th American College of Veterinary Internal Medicine Forum, Lake Buena Vista, FL. 1997. p. 596–8.
[47] Yang JT, Adusumalli VE, Wong KK, et al. Felbamate metabolism in the rat, rabbit, and dog. Drug Metab Dispos 1991;19(6):1126–34.
[48] Adusumalli VE, Gilchrist JR, Wichmann JK, et al. Pharmacokinetics of felbamate in pediatric and adult beagle dogs. Epilepsia 1992;33(5):955–60.
[49] Yang JT, Morris M, Wong KK, et al. Felbamate metabolism in pediatric and adult beagle dogs. Drug Metab Dispos 1992;20(1):84–8.
[50] McGee JH, Erikson DJ, Galbreath C, et al. Acute, subchronic, and chronic toxicity studies with felbamate, 2-phenyl-1,3-propanediol dicarbamate. Toxicol Sci 1998;45: 225–32.
[51] Dayrell-Hart B, Tiches D, Vite C, et al. Efficacy and safety of felbamate as an anticonvulsant in dogs with refractory seizures [abstract]. J Vet Intern Med 1996;10(3):174.
[52] Johannessen SI, Battino D, Berry DJ, et al. Therapeutic drug monitoring of the newer antiepileptic drugs. Ther Drug Monit 2003;25:347–63.
[53] Bazil CW. New antiepileptic drugs. Neurologist 2002;8(2):71–81.
[54] Ruehlmann D, Podell M, March P. Treatment of partial seizures and seizure-like activity with felbamate in six dogs. J Small Anim Pract 2001;42:403–8.
[55] Sills GJ. The mechanisms of action of gabapentin and pregabalin. Current Opinion in Pharmacology 2006;6:108–13.
[56] Radulovic LL, Turck D, Van Hodenberg A, et al. Disposition of gabapentin (Neurontin) in mice, rats, dogs, and monkeys. Drug Metab Dispos 1995;23(4):441–8.
[57] Vollmer KO, Von Hodenberg A, Kolle EU. Pharmacokinetics and metabolism of gabapentin in rat, dog and man. Drug Res 1986;36(1):830–9.
[58] Govendir M, Perkins M, Malik R. Improving seizure control in dogs with refractory epilepsy using gabapentin as an adjunctive agent. Aust Vet J 2005;83:602–8.
[59] Platt SR, Adams V, Garosi LS, et al. Gabapentin therapy for refractory idiopathic epilepsy in dogs. J Small Anim Pract 2006; in press.
[60] Leppik IE. The place of levetiracetam in the treatment of epilepsy. Epilepsia 2001;42(Suppl 4):44–5.
[61] Hovinga CA. Levetiracetam: a novel antiepileptic drug. Pharmacotherapy 2001;21(11): 1375–88.
[62] Shorvon SD, van Rijckevorsel K. A new antiepileptic drug [editorial]. J Neurol Neurosurg Psychiatry 2002;72:426–8.
[63] Krakow K, Walker M, Otoul C, et al. Long-term continuation of levetiracetam in patients with refractory epilepsy. Neurology 2001;56:1772–4.
[64] Morrell MJ, Leppik I, French J, et al. The KEEPER trial: levetiracetam adjunctive treatment of partial-onset seizures in an open-label community-based study. Epilepsy Res 2003;54: 153–61.
[65] Grosso S, Franzoni E, Coppola G, et al. Efficacy and safety of levetiracetam: and add-on trial in children with refractory epilepsy. Seizure 2005;14:248–53.

[66] Mohanraj R, Parker PG, Stephen LJ, et al. Levetiracetam in refractory epilepsy: a prospective observational study. Seizure 2005;14:23–7.
[67] Alsaadi TM, Shatzel A, Marquez AV, et al. Clinical experience of levetiracetam monotherapy for adults with epilepsy: 1-year follow-up study. Seizure 2005;14:139–42.
[68] French J, Arrigo C. Rapid onset of action of levetiracetam in refractory epilepsy patients. Epilepsia 2005;46(2):324–6.
[69] Strolin Benedetti M, Coupez R, Whomsley R, et al. Comparative pharmacokinetics and metabolism of levetiracetam, a new anti-epileptic agent, in mouse, rat, rabbit and dog. Xenobiotica 2004;34(3):281–300.
[70] Lynch BA, Lambeng N, Nocka K, et al. The synaptic vesicle protein SV2A is the binding site for the antiepileptic drug levetiracetam. Proc Natl Acad Sci 2004;101:9861–6.
[71] Hanon E, Klitgaard H. Neuroprotective properties of the novel antiepileptic drug levetiracetam in the rat middle cerebral artery occlusion model of focal cerebral ischemia. Seizure 2000;10:287–93.
[72] Rekling JC. Neuroprotective effects of anticonvulsants in rat hippocampal slice cultures exposed to oxygen/glucose deprivation. Neurosci Lett 2003;335:167–70.
[73] Loscher W, Honack D, Rundfeldt C. Antiepileptogenic effects of the novel anticonvulsant levetiracetam UCB (L059) in the kindling model of temporal lobe epilepsy. J Pharmacol Exp Ther 1998;284:474–9.
[74] Klitgaard H. Levetiracetam: the preclinical profile of a new class of antiepileptic drugs? Epilepsia 2001;42(Suppl 4):13–8.
[75] Isoherranen N, Yagen B, Soback S, et al. Pharmacokinetics of levetiracetam and its enantiomer (R)-α-ethyl-2-oxo-pyrrolidine acetamide in dogs. Epilepsia 2001;42(7):825–30.
[76] Steinberg M, Faissler D. Levetiracetam therapy for long-term idiopathic epileptic dogs [abstract]. J Vet Intern Med 2004;18(3):410.
[77] Glass GA, Stankiewicz J, Mithoefer A, et al. Levetiracetam for seizures after liver transplantation. Neurology 2005;64:1084–5.
[78] Dewey CW, Barone G, Boothe DM, et al. The use of oral levetiracetam as an add-on anticonvulsant drug in cats receiving phenobarbital [abstract]. J Vet Intern Med 2005;19(3):458.
[79] Oommen KJ, Mathews S. Zonisamide: a new antiepileptic drug. Clin Neuropharmacol 1999;22:192–200.
[80] Leppik IE. Zonisamide. Epilepsia 1999;40(Suppl 5):S23–9.
[81] Mori A, Noda Y, Packer L. The anticonvulsant zonisamide scavenges free radicals. Epilepsy Res 1998;30:153–8.
[82] Faught E, Ayala R, Montouris GG, et al. Randomized controlled trial of zonisamide for the treatment of refractory partial-onset seizures. Neurology 2001;57:1774–9.
[83] Leppik IE, Willmore LJ, Homan RW, et al. Efficacy and safety of zonisamide: results of a multicenter study. Epilepsy Res 1993;14:165–73.
[84] Marmarou A, Pellock JM. Zonisamide: physician and patient experiences. Epilepsy Res 2005;64:63–9.
[85] Yamauchi T, Aikawa H. Efficacy of zonisamide: our experience. Seizure 2004;13(Suppl):S41–8.
[86] Brodie MJ, Duncan R, Vespignani H, et al. Dose-dependent safety and efficacy of zonisamide: a randomized, double-blind, placebo-controlled study in patients with refractory partial seizures. Epilepsia 2005;46(1):31–41.
[87] Faught E. Review of United States and European clinical trials of zonisamide in the treatment of refractory partial-onset seizures. Seizure 2004;13(Suppl):S59–65.
[88] Leppik IE. Zonisamide: chemistry, mechanism of action, and pharmacokinetics. Seizure 2004;13(Suppl):S5–9.
[89] Matsumoto K, Miyazaki H, Fujii T, et al. Absorption, distribution, and excretion of 3-(sulfamoyl [^{14}C] methyl)-1,2-benzisoxazole (AD-810) in rats, dogs and monkeys and of AD-810 in men. Drug Res 1983;33:961–8.

[90] Boothe DM, Perkins J, Dewey C. Clinical pharmacokinetics and safety of the anticonvulsant zonisamide in healthy dogs following single and multiple dosing [abstract]. J Vet Intern Med 2005;19(3):421.
[91] Shinoda M, Akita M, Hasegawa M, et al. The necessity of adjusting the dosage of zonisamide when coadministered with other antiepileptic drugs. Biol Pharm Bull 1996;19:1090–2.
[92] Saito M, Orito K, Takikawa S, et al. Pharmacokinetics of zonisamide administered alone and in combination with phenobarbital in dogs [abstract]. J Vet Intern Med 2005;19(3): 421–2.
[93] Dewey CW, Guiliano R, Boothe DM, et al. Zonisamide therapy for refractory idiopathic epilepsy in dogs. J Am Anim Hosp Assoc 2004;40:285–91.
[94] Walker RM, DiFonzo CJ, Barsoum NJ, et al. Chronic toxicity of the anticonvulsant zonisamide in beagle dogs. Fund Appl Toxicol 1988;11:333–42.
[95] Von Klopman T, Simon D, Rambeck B, et al. Prospective study of zonisamide therapy for refractory idiopathic epilepsy in dogs. J Small Anim Pract 2006, in press.
[96] Newmark ME, Dubinsky S. Zonisamide monotherapy in a multi-group clinic. Seizure 2004;13:223–5.
[97] Seki T, Kumagai N, Maezawa M. Effects of zonisamide monotherapy in children with epilepsy. Seizure 2004;13(Suppl):S26–32.
[98] Wilfong AA. Zonisamide monotherapy for epilepsy in children and young adults. Pediatr Neurol 2005;32:77–80.
[99] Platt SR, McDonnell JJ. Status epilepticus: clinical features and pathophysiology. Compend Contin Educ Pract Vet 2000;22(7):660–9.
[100] Bateman SW, Parent JM. Clinical findings, treatment, and outcome of dogs with status epilepticus or cluster seizures: 156 cases (1990–1995). J Am Vet Med Assoc 1999; 215(10):1463–8.
[101] Platt SR, Haag M. Canine status epilepticus: a retrospective study of 50 cases. J Small Anim Pract 2002;43:151–3.
[102] Saito M, Munana KR, Sharp NJH, et al. Risk factors for development of status epilepticus in dogs with idiopathic epilepsy and effects of status epilepticus on outcome and survival time: 32 cases (1990–1996). J Am Vet Med Assoc 2001;219(5):618–23.
[103] Lowenstein DH, Alldredge BK. Status epilepticus. N Engl J Med 1998;338(14):970–6.
[104] Sirven JI, Waterhouse E. Management of status epilepticus. Am Fam Physician 2003; 68(3):469–76.
[105] Manno EM. New management strategies in the treatment of status epilepticus. Mayo Clin Proc 2003;78:508–18.
[106] Platt SR, McDonnell JJ. Status epilepticus: patient management and pharmacologic therapy. Compend Contin Educ Pract Vet 2000;22(8):722–9.
[107] Ilkiw JE. Other potentially useful new injectable anesthetic agents. Vet Clin North Am Small Anim Pract 1992;22(2):281–9.
[108] Court MH, Greenblatt DJ. Pharmacokinetics and preliminary observations of behavioral changes following administration of midazolam to dogs. J Vet Pharmacol Ther 1992; 15:343–50.
[109] Podell M, Wagner SO, Sams RA. Lorazepam concentrations in plasma following its intravenous and rectal administration in dogs. J Vet Pharmacol Ther 1998;21:158–60.
[110] Mariani CL, Clemmons RM, Lee-Ambrose L, et al. A comparison of intranasal and intravenous lorazepam in normal dogs [abstract]. J Vet Intern Med 2003;17(3):402.
[111] Platt SR, Randell SC, Scott KC, et al. Comparison of plasma benzodiazepine concentrations following intranasal and intravenous administration of diazepam to dogs. Am J Vet Res 2000;61(6):651–4.
[112] Platt SR, McDonnell JJ. Status epilepticus: managing refractory cases and treating out-of-hospital patients. Compend Contin Educ Pract Vet 2000;22(8):732–40.

[113] Lui CY, Amidon GL, Goldberg A. Intranasal absorption of flurazepam, midazolam, and triazolam. J Pharm Sci 1991;80(12):1125–9.
[114] Podell M. The use of diazepam per rectum at home for the acute management of cluster seizures in dogs. J Vet Intern Med 1995;9(2):68–74.
[115] Wagner SO, Sams RA, Podell M. Chronic phenobarbital therapy reduces plasma benzodiazepine concentrations after intravenous and rectal administration of diazepam in the dog. J Vet Pharmacol Ther 1998;21:335–41.
[116] Steffen F, Grasmueck S. Propofol for treatment of refractory seizures in dogs and a cat with intracranial disorders. J Small Anim Pract 2000;41:496–9.
[117] Fischer JH, Patel TV, Fischer PA. Fosphenytoin: clinical pharmacokinetics and comparative advantages in the acute treatment of seizures. Clin Pharmacokinet 2003;42(1):33–58.
[118] Varia SA, Stella VJ. Phenytoin prodrugs: in vivo evaluation of some water-soluble phenytoin prodrugs in dogs. J Pharm Sci 1984;73(8):1080–7.
[119] Smith RD, Brown BS, Maher RW, et al. Pharmacology of ACC-9653 (phenytoin prodrug). Epilepsia 1989;30(Suppl 2):S15–21.
[120] Mazarati AM, Baldwin R, Klitgaard H, et al. Anticonvulsant effects of levetiracetam and levetiracetam-diazepam combinations in experimental status epilepticus. Epilepsy Res 2004;58:167–74.
[121] Speciale J, Dayrell-Hart B, Steinberg SA. Clinical evaluation of γ-vinyl-γ-aminobutyric acid for control of epilepsy in dogs. J Am Vet Med Assoc 1991;198(6):995–1000.
[122] Schicht S, Wigger D, Frey HH. Pharmacokinetics of oxcarbazepine in the dog. J Vet Pharmacol Ther 1996;19:27–31.
[123] Reddy DS. Tiagabine: a potent antiepileptic drug with selective GABA uptake inhibitory effect. Indian J Pharmacol 1998;30:141–51.
[124] Streeter AJ, Stahle PL, Holland ML, et al. Pharmacokinetics and bioavailability of topiramate in the beagle dog. Drug Metab Dispos 1995;23(1):90–3.

Vet Clin Small Anim 36 (2006) 1129–1173

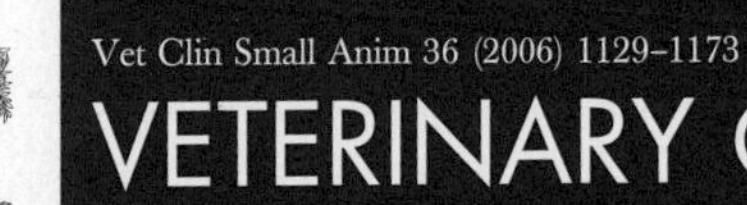

ELSEVIER
SAUNDERS
VETERINARY CLINICS
SMALL ANIMAL PRACTICE

Veterinary Compounding in Small Animals: A Clinical Pharmacologist's Perspective

Dawn Merton Boothe, DVM, PhD

Department of Anatomy, Physiology, and Pharmacology, 109 Greene Hall,
College of Veterinary Medicine, Auburn University, AL 36849, USA

The focus on individualized drug therapy as addressed by the paper on pharmacogenetics elsewhere in this issue is also manifested by the recent attention being drawn to compounding of animal drugs. Compounding of animal drugs has always been, and will continue to be, a vital aspect to the safe and effective delivery of drugs to veterinary patients. This reflects, in part, the sparsity of drugs approved by the US Food and Drug Administration (FDA) for use in animals compared to that in humans. The lack of commercially available drug formulations often leads the veterinarian to prescribe or dispense a product specifically designed and compounded for his or her patients' medical needs. Compounding has been defined by the National Association of Boards of Pharmacy (NABP; Model State Pharmacy Act) as the preparation, mixing, assembling, packaging, or labeling of a drug or device as the result of a practitioner's prescription drug order (or initiative) and based on the practitioner/patient/pharmacist relationship [1].

The last two descriptors, prescription driven and in the context of a veterinary client-patient relationship, are vitally important but often unrecognized or ignored descriptors of the definition. Indeed, in 1997, the US Supreme Court defined drug compounding as "a process by which a pharmacist or doctor combines, mixes, or alters ingredients to create a medication tailored to *the needs of an individual patient*" [2]. The issues surrounding compounding of animal drugs are complex, often confusing, at times apparently contradictory, and frustratingly dynamic. This manuscript is offered as a comprehensive review of compounding of animal drugs, with a specific focus on dogs and cats. A historical perspective is offered such that the role of compounding can be placed in the context of animal health care. A chronologic review of rules and regulations at the federal and state level includes a discussion of the basis for the regulations as well as very recent changes in the laws. Finally, those aspects of compounding that may place the health of a patient at risk, primarily because of

E-mail address: boothdm@auburn.edu

0195-5616/06/$ – see front matter
doi:10.1016/j.cvsm.2006.07.003

vetsmall.theclinics.com

therapeutic failure, are also addressed. The comprehensive nature of the manuscript is intended as a reference for veterinary practitioners interested in becoming familiar with the issues surrounding veterinary compounding. It is the author's hope that an appreciation of the risks and benefits of compounding in animals will lead the profession to take a more assertive role in the discussions and decisions regarding the compounding of animal drugs.

HISTORICAL PERSPECTIVE

Compounding is as old as drug use. Ultimately, it was compounding that led to the practice of pharmacy. Pharmacy is defined as the art and practice of preparing and preserving drugs and of compounding and dispensing medicine according to prescriptions of physicians. Pharmacy is practiced by an apothecary (one who prepares and sell drugs or compounds for medicinal purposes), who is commonly referred to as a pharmacist; the two terms are often used interchangeably. The earliest known record of apothecary dates back to 2600 BC in Babylon [3]. Among the best-known early compounders was the Italian physician, Galen (130–200 AD), whose principles of preparation and compounding directed drug formulations for another 1500 years. Although the first privately owned drug stores were established in Bagdad as early as the eighth century, it was not until the thirteenth century that pharmacy began to separate itself from medicine. It was only at this point that collections or stocks of drugs and accompanying books (pharmacopoeias) began to be generated. A major advent in the profession of pharmacy and the science of compounding was the development of drug standards. In the nineteenth century, the United States Pharmacopeia (USP) began its role in the provision of drug standards, thus ensuring strength and purity of drug materials. It maintains this often unrecognized yet critically important role today; its pharmacopeia (*United States Pharmacopeia/National Formulary* [USP/NF]) incorporates the legal standards recognized by the FDA [3–5].

Compounded products predominated into the twentieth century; as late as the 1930s and 1940s, 50% to 60% of human drugs were compounded by pharmacists [6]. However, in the late nineteenth century, the need for new therapeutically useful compounds led to the advent of pharmaceutic research and, shortly thereafter, pharmaceutic manufacturing. By the 1950s, advances in manufacturing technology led to the mass production of drugs, causing pharmacists to become largely dispensers rather than compounders of drugs. The 1980s and 1990s were accompanied by a resurgence in compounding in human medicine for a variety of reasons. Ongoing mergers between pharmaceutical companies have forced manufacturers to focus on more profitable drugs. According to the USP, more than 6500 previously approved drug products or drug combinations are no longer marketed, despite their recognized safety and efficacy [6]. Yet, the medical need for these discontinued products has not declined, and compounding has allowed their continued acquisition. Changes in the human health care system and the special needs of home health and hospice care patients have led to the generation of novel (many compounded) drug delivery systems. Orphan drugs (those used in a small percentage of patients) often require reformulation because they are unavailable in appropriate forms or strengths. A significant factor driving the increase in compounding in human medicine is the need to individualize drug therapy for special patient populations, such as geriatric and pediatric patients. As a result of these and other economic and health care–related issues, currently, more than 43,000 human drugs, or 1% of dispensed human drugs, are compounded each day by approximately 10% of human pharmacies [6].

The history of veterinary compounding has paralleled that of human compounding. Although hundreds of drugs are approved for animal use, limited availability of approved animal drugs has mandated the need for compounding of veterinary drugs more so than in human medicine. The current cost of approval of an animal drug is estimated at $15 to $20 million US, with a delay of 5 years.[1] The economic return of animal drug approval, not surprisingly, is low (generally less than $100 million[1]); subsequently, the financial incentive to pursue animal drug approval compared with human pharmaceutics is much less. Further, because of cost differences, rather than an approved veterinary drug, veterinarians often prescribe a human or human generic drug or (illegally) a compounded preparation that might be less expensive than the approved version. Unlike their human pharmaceutical counterparts, the financial basis of animal pharmaceutical companies generally is not large enough to allow simultaneous development of many animal drugs. As such, manufacturers of animal drugs (including generic animal drugs) pursue fewer animal drug approvals. A "catch 22" has resulted: fewer animal drugs lead to increased use of compounded or human approved drugs, decreasing the financial incentive for pursuit of animal drug approval.

Historically, compounding for animals generally has been implemented by veterinarians in private practice. However, within the last 5 years, compounding of animal drugs by pharmacists has dramatically increased. The current market has been estimated to be between $50 and $200 million US ($60–$80 million US [6][1]) compared with a market of $650 to $700 million US for the animal pharmaceutical industry; the estimates may be much lower than actual because of the lack of reporting by pharmacies that compound illegally. Whereas in the 1990s, few pharmacies offered compounding for animals, dozens exist now, with at least 14 pharmacies nationally advertising compounding exclusively for animals.[1] The increase in animal drug compounding is evidenced by advertisements (journal, television, and Internet); pharmacy exhibits at local, state, and national veterinary conventions; and current scientific literature (although limited). Indeed, to date, the *International Journal of Pharmaceutical Compounding* has devoted three issues [volumes 1(4) in 1997, 3(3) in 1999, and 5(2) in 2001] and more than 115 review or recipe articles to veterinary compounding since its inception in 1997.

[1] Data generated by Brakke Consultants, January 2004. Data provided courtesy of Wedgewood Pharmacy, 405 Heron Drive, Suite 200, Swedesboro, New Jersey 08085 1749.

The focus of pharmacists toward veterinary medicine reflects, in part, an improved standard of care for veterinary patients coupled with the lack of compounding training in veterinary curricula. However, a major factor is economically based. The advent of managed human health care, coupled with the decline in insurance reimbursement for human drugs (including recent changes in Medicare programs), has caused pharmacists to seek alternative markets [7]. Most veterinary compounding occurs for companion (nonfood) animals, in part, because of the restrictions placed by the FDA on compounding for food animals. The percentage of drugs prescribed in small animals that are dispensed as compounded products has been estimated to be 10%.[1]

The growth of veterinary compounding has been a healthy, and vital, adjuvant to the veterinary profession. The availability of compounding services enhances the veterinarian's ability to treat patients safely and effectively. Recipes that facilitate oral and otic drug delivery [8], identification of flavoring agents [9], and formulation of drugs unavailable in an approved preparation for any species (particularly for exotic or zoo animals) [10,11] are a few examples of the benefits. Safety can be enhanced by accuracy in dosing in extremely small patients. Compounding antidotes are available in anticipation of animal poisonings. Compounding allows access to drugs that are no longer available as pharmaceutical companies drop less economically beneficial drugs or in response to voluntary or federally mandated withdrawals (eg, cisapride, diethylstilbestrol). Compounding also can provide access to drugs temporarily unavailable (eg, cyclosporine). Finally, compounding offers improved compliance; under appropriate conditions, several drugs might be combined in a single dosage form for administration to a noncompliant patient. Among the more recent innovations in veterinary compounding is the advent of novel drug delivery methods that might allow more effective treatment, and safer administration, to fractious animals. However, by their nature, novel systems should be demonstrated to be safe and effective, but such demonstration rarely occurs for compounded products. Reformulation of any finished (eg, ready to administer) approved drug product into a compounded finished drug product alters the behavior of the finished version of the drug. Likewise, drugs compounded from a pure (bulk) substance do not necessarily behave as they do in an approved finished dosing form. Veterinarians should always question the quality, safety, and efficacy of the new (compounded) drug product.

The issues surrounding veterinary compounding are different than those surrounding human compounding. Unfortunately, animal caregivers, veterinarians, and pharmacists often are unaware of these differences. Accordingly, veterinarians should carefully consider the ethical, legal, and safety issues associated with use of compounded animal drugs. The first part of this article focuses on the regulation of veterinary compounding, including definitions, parties responsible for regulations, and the potential impact that regulation may have on provision of health care. The second part focuses on quality assurance as well as safety and efficacy considerations and includes a particular focus on transdermal drug delivery systems as an example of a novel drug delivery system being offered by compounding pharmacists.

RULES AND REGULATIONS FOR COMPOUNDING

The regulatory philosophy of the FDA toward veterinary and human drug compounding differs, potentially leading to confusion and misinterpretation of regulations. Failure of veterinarians or pharmacists to appreciate and address these differences can contribute to inappropriate compounding.

US Food and Drug Administration

The advent of pharmaceutic manufacturing in the early 1900s increased human exposure to drugs, and thus the risk of adverse drug events. In response to this increased risk, in 1908, Congress enacted the Federal Foods and Drug Act. This act provided for the formation of what eventually became the FDA; the act empowered the FDA to enforce its regulations [12]. Regulatory actions of the FDA are delineated in congressionally approved acts or their amendments. Thus, an act of Congress literally is necessary for the empowerment of the FDA with its regulatory actions. The regulations ("rules") established for implementation of the Food, Drugs, and Cosmetic Act (FDCA) and its subsequent amendments are published in codified form in the Code of Federal Regulations (CFR), which is available for public review. To facilitate understanding of the regulations by FDA staff and, to a lesser degree, industry and the public, the FDA may publish compliance policy guides (CPGs) for each set of regulations. The CPGs direct FDA regulatory actions. However, in contrast to an act or its regulations, which are legal documents, CPGs are not legally binding and are open to interpretation by the FDA. Indeed, the current CPG for compounding in animals (CPG 608.40) specifically states that the "guidance describes FDA's current thinking on what types of compounding might be subject to enforcement action." Because CPGs represent current interpretation of the laws by the FDA, they can be altered without public comment by the FDA (as happened for the most recent [2003] CPG for veterinary compounding) as it deems necessary to remain in compliance with the law. As a result, FDA regulatory guidelines are "moving targets" [13], contributing to difficulty in anticipating which activities might or might not be regulated by the FDA.

In the late 1930s, more than 100 persons died after being treated with sulfanilamide prepared in a toxic vehicle. The resultant public outcry was instrumental in the passage of the FDCA. With passage of the FDCA, as (manufactured) drugs increasingly were administered to people, the FDA focused its initial activities toward drug safety. However, because the law was intended to regulate the emerging pharmaceutical industry, and because compounding had, up to that time, proven vital to effective drug therapy, the act was not intended, nor was it interpreted by the FDA, to allow or prohibit the compounding of drugs [14]. In 1962, the FDCA was amended to include the assurance of drug efficacy in the mandated activities of the FDA. Again, compounding was not specifically addressed; further, animal drugs were not addressed. It was not until 1968, with passage of the Animal Drug Amendment, that animal drugs were distinguished from human drugs. This amendment of the FDCA provided for the formation of the Bureau of (later renamed the Center for) Veterinary Medicine (CVM) within the FDA. The mission of the CVM, as mandated by Congress, is assurance of animal and public health resulting from drug use in animals. Thus, although the regulatory activities of the CVM clearly focus on animal drug efficacy and safety, a major proportion of its actions address the impact of animal drug use on human health (eg, unsafe animal residues). Often, this mandated focus on public safety may lead to prioritization of issues related to food animal or public health over issues related to companion animal health.

Compounding of Human Drugs

Compounding of human drugs was not specifically addressed in the original FDCA or its 1962 amendment. Nevertheless, the FDA is empowered to regulate any drug (or any product intended to be used as a drug) and interprets a compounded drug to be an unapproved new drug (Neal Battalier, Office of Compliance, CVM, FDA, Rockville, Maryland, personal communication, 2005; Fred Richman, Office of Compliance, Center for Drug Evaluation and Research, FDA, Rockville, Maryland, personal communication, 2005). However, this interpretation is currently being challenged by selected representatives of the pharmaceutical industry (see later comment). As compounding increased toward the end of the twentieth century, FDA regulation of the human drug compounding was specifically addressed in 1997 with passage of the Food and Drug Administration Modernization Act (FDAMA). This act, which does not apply to veterinary medicine (compounding of animal drugs is addressed elsewhere in this article), included Section 503A, entitled "Pharmacy Compounding." Among other things, the FDAMA was intended to specifically legalize certain aspects of human compounding, including compounding from selected bulk substances (defined elsewhere in this article). However, to protect consumers, the act also attempted to provide the FDA with criteria by which inappropriate compounding could be identified and subsequently regulated. The intent of the FDAMA was "to ensure continued availability of compounded drug products as a component of individualized therapy, while limiting the scope of compounding so as to prevent manufacturing under the guise of compounding" [2].

These criteria included limiting the amount of drug product compounded in anticipation of need, and determining whether or not the compounding of the drug was individually patient driven. Additionally, because it was perceived by the FDA as an indication of manufacturing of inappropriate amounts of a compounded drug, the Pharmacy Compounding section of the FDAMA prohibited the advertisement of compounded products. However, this aspect of the law was subsequently challenged by the pharmacy profession, based on infringement of the second amendment (right of free speech). Ultimately, the US Supreme Court agreed that the restrictions on advertising did infringe on second amendment rights, and because the advertisement portions of the laws could not be easily separated from the remainder of the law, the entire Pharmacy Compounding section of the FDAMA was invalidated. The FDA is considering whether or not to pursue a revision of the Pharmacy Compounding section of the FDAMA and has rewritten its CPG for the FDAMA to remove restrictions in advertising (Fred Richman, Office of Compliance, Center for Drug Evaluation and Research, FDA Rockville, Maryland, personal communication, 2005). As this publication went to press, a recent ruling in the Federal District Court in Texas in response to a suit brought by pharmacists, found that "compounded drugs do not fall under the new drug definitions" and, as a result, are legal.

Compounding of Veterinary Drugs

In contrast to compounding of human drugs, federal regulation of veterinary compounded veterinary drugs is specifically and legally addressed by the Animal Medicinal Drug Use Clarification Act (AMDUCA) of 1994 [13,15]. As the animal counterpart to the FDAMA, it amends the FDCA. The major benefit of this act to the veterinary profession was legalization of the already common practice of extralabel drug use (ELDU) in animals [(Section 512 (a) (4)] as long as the conditions stipulated in the regulations are met. Regulations relevant to ELDU have been delineated for veterinarians by the American Veterinary Medical Association (AVMA) in a brochure [16] and a user-friendly algorithm (summarized in Box 1). Veterinary ELDU is legalized by the AMDUCA only for approved (human or animal) drugs and not for products that are intended for use as drugs but are not approved drugs (eg, herbs, botanicals, nutraceuticals). Such substances are perceived by the FDA to be (unapproved) drugs, and to fall under the FDA's regulatory jurisdiction. This includes novel ingredients, such as herbs and nutraceuticals, as well as products compounded outside the stipulations of the AMDUCA.

Compounding of animal drugs is specifically legalized by the AMDUCA (21 CFR Section 530). However, the compounding must be implemented in accordance with the relevant provisions of ELDU (see Box 1). As such, the AMDUCA stipulates that compounding must be performed by a licensed veterinarian or pharmacist (thus ensuring the rights of both professions to compound) in the context of a veterinary client-patient relationship and that no approved dosing form or concentration of the drug (human or animal) commercially exists for the treatment of the diagnosed condition.

The interpretation and implementation of compounding regulations of the AMDUCA are delineated in CPG 608.400: *Compounding of Drugs for Use in Animals*. The original CPG (written in 1996) for animal compounding regulations included the FDA's working definition of compounding as "any manipulation of a drug product to produce a dosage form drug other than that provided for by the labeled directions for use of the approved drug product." However, because CPGs are not legal documents, the inclusion of a definition was

Box 1: Conditions for veterinary compounding as stipulated by the Animal Medicinal Drug Use Clarification Act (AMDUCA)[a]

1. General stipulations of the AMDUCA for ELDU
   A. Use is by or on the order of a licensed veterinarian in the context of a valid veterinary client- patient relationship in the presence of a legitimate medical need.
   B. Advertising and promotion are not permitted.
   C. Records must be maintained for 2 years (or longer if mandated by the state or federal government) regarding ELDU and should include the following:
      i. Name of drug and active ingredients
      ii. Condition, species, and number of animals treated
      iii. Dose and duration of treatment (for food animals, specific information pertaining to drug residues)
   D. The label should bear the following:
      i. Name and address of the prescribing veterinarian or name and address of the prescribing veterinarian and name and address of the dispensing pharmacy
      ii. Name of the drug or each active ingredient
      iii. Directions for use, including animal/group identification, dosing regimen (including route), and duration of therapy
      iv. Cautionary statements (and for food animal, pertinent residue information)
2. Specific stipulations of the AMDUCA for ELDU from compounded drugs:
   A. No marketed approved drug (human or animal) exists for the needed dosing regimen (for food animals, compounding from human drugs is not allowed if an approved animal drug is available).
   B. Compounding is performed by a licensed pharmacist or veterinarian in the scope of the professional practice.
   C. Adequate procedures and processes are followed that ensure the safety and efficacy of the compounded product.
   D. The scale of compounding is commensurate with the established need for the compounded product.
   E. All relevant state laws relating to compounding of drugs for use in animals are followed.

[a]The AMDUCA is a legal document; CPGs are guidelines but are not legally binding.

considered by the FDA to be misleading; as such, the definition is not included in the current version of the CPG. Rather, the updated CPG describes those activities not considered to be compounding. These include mixing, reconstituting, or other acts (on the drug) that are performed in accordance with the approved labeling provided by the manufacturer. Thus, any modification in the finished dosing form of the approved drug that is not specifically delineated on the drug label (which includes its accompanying package inserts) is considered as compounding. This includes modifications as simple as dilution beyond that stipulated on the label, crushing a tablet to be prepared in syrup, or the combination of two or more finished drug products in the same preparation. The FDA considers any compounded product (human or animal) to be a new finished (ie, ready for administration) drug and, because it undergoes no federally mandated approval process, an unapproved drug. As such, any compounded animal product, whether appropriate or not, is perceived by the FDA to fall under their perview. As with human compounded drugs, this viewpoint is being challenged by the pharmacy profession (see later discussion). The FDA assumes that public and animal health potentially are put at risk if compounded drugs are administered to veterinary patients, because the drugs are not accompanied by "adequate and well-controlled safety and effectiveness data," particularly if not compounded in "adherence with pharmaceutical chemistry and current good manufacturing practices" (CPG Section 608.400). The FDA anticipates that compounded products may cause adverse reactions or contain potentially harmful excipients and that the unscientific assignment of withdrawal times to compounded food animal products may lead to potentially harmful tissue residues. Accordingly, the laws (eg, the AMDUCA), regulations, and CPGs that address compounding of animal drugs include a strong focus on protection of human (public health) safety. The original CPG also included directions as to how compounding should be performed, but these are also absent in the updated CPG because regulating compounding to such an extent is outside the authority of a federal agency. It is the intent of the FDA to defer to state authorities for such regulations.

Several drug forms are used as a source for compounded animal drugs. Legal sources (according to the FDA) are limited to FDA-approved finished forms of animal or human drugs; the FDA makes no distinction as to which (animal versus human) is the preferred source in companion animals (Fig. 1). Because no other source is legalized, all other drug sources are considered by the FDA to be illegal, including non–FDA-approved finished drug products obtained outside the United States and bulk substances. A bulk drug substance is legally defined [21 CFR 207.3(a)(4)] for human and animals as "any substance that is represented for use in a drug and that, when used in the manufacturing, processing or packaging of a drug, becomes an active ingredient or a finished dosage form of the drug." In laymen's terms, any drug or drug preparation ingredient not prepared in a finished dosage form is considered to be a bulk substance. Whereas AMDUCA regulations specifically state that ELDU of drugs compounded from an approved animal or human drug is permitted (21 CFR Section 530), they further state that "nothing (in [Part 530]) shall be construed as permitting compounding from bulk drugs." This statement emphasizes that the law and its regulations do not address compounding from bulk drugs (ie, compounding from drugs is not legalized and thus, according to the FDA, is illegal). This exclusionary statement was included in the law, in part, because compounding from bulk substances is perceived by the FDA

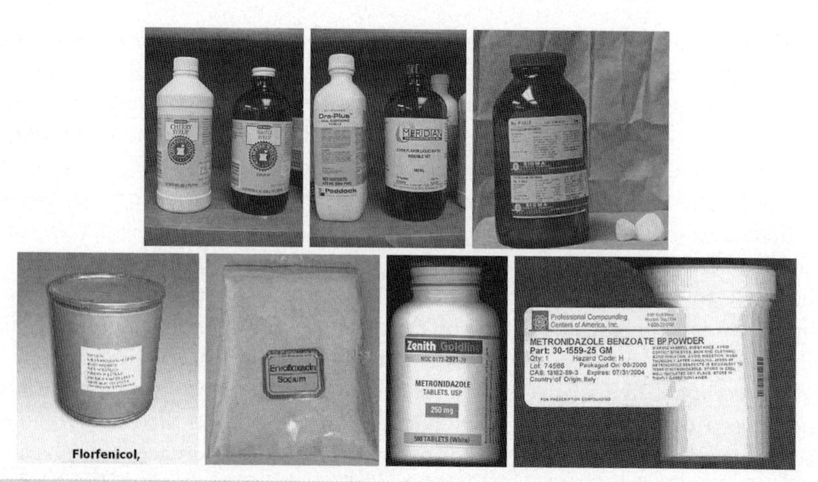

Fig. 1. Example of materials used for compounding (from *top left, clockwise*). Simple syrups are used to sweeten solutions. Bromide (potassium shown) is an example of a compound that is not available in any approved form in the United States. This particular version was purchased from a chemical company as the medicinal grade. Metronidazole hydrochloride is available in trade and generic (shown) preparations, but the benzoate form is only available as the pure substrate. The products to the lower left are bulk antimicrobials available on-line through Asian retailers; the purity and potency of these products should particularly be suspect. Each of the bulk drug substances shown should be accompanied by a valid certificate of analysis.

to place human beings at an increased risk to inappropriate drug residues. It is this statement in particular, and the CPG addressing this regulatory statement, that is the focus of challenge by the pharmacy profession as it seeks congressional action to change the FDA's interpretation of compounding from bulk substances in animals.

Confusion has surrounded the issue of compounding of animal drugs; this reflects, in part, the wording of the law. However, interpreting what is legal and what is illegal was complicated by the original CPG for the compounding aspects of the AMDUCA. These were written (in 1996) before, and in anticipation of, the regulations themselves. Consequently, the original (1996) CPG, which represented "current thinking" of the FDA at the time AMDUCA was passed, did not necessarily represent the final regulations of the law. Despite the fact that the AMDUCA specifically indicates that compounding from bulk substances is not addressed (and thus not allowed), the 1996 CPG implied a prioritization of FDA CVM regulatory action toward compounding from bulk substances. The CPG indicated that normally, regulatory action would not be pursued for compounding from bulk substances in small animals if an approved finished version of the bulk substance existed. This contradictory guideline was misinterpreted to mean that compounding from bulk substances was legal, leading to two negative sequelae. First, compounders abused (intentionally or not) the "tolerant" approach of the FDA toward compounding from bulk substances in nonfood animals; abuses ranged from compounding for food animals to compounding for nonfood animals but outside the stipulations of the AMDUCA. Further, the original CPG compromised the FDA's ability to regulate inappropriate compounding: the perception of tolerance complicated the FDA's ability to prove abuse. As such, in 2003, the CPGs for compounding regulations of the AMDUCA were updated to remove any implied prioritization of regulatory action or an attitude of toleration toward compounding from bulk substances, thus bringing the FDA into compliance with the law. As mandated by the FDA, the updated CPG for compounding of veterinary drugs also is in harmony with those written for the FDAMA, the human counterpart to the AMDUCA (CFR 503A).

The FDA specifically states in its 2003 CPG for animal drug compounding that the updated CPG do not apply to compounding of products if an approved animal or human drug is used as the source as long as such compounding adheres to conditions stipulated by the AMDUCA (because such action is legal, regulation is not indicated and no CPG is needed). Rather, the updated CPG focuses on the compounding of unapproved new animal drugs (those compounded outside the AMDUCA) "in a manner that is clearly outside the bounds of traditional pharmacy practice." In contrast to the 1996 CPG, the 2003 CPG specifically states that the AMDUCA does not permit veterinarians to compound unapproved finished drug products from bulk drug substances unless the finished drug is not a new animal drug. Because any compounded animal drug has been perceived by the FDA as a new (yet unapproved) animal drug, no circumstances exist in which compounding from bulk substances is allowed (except for bulk substances delineated in Appendix A of the CPG). It is this aspect of the law that has caused many distributors or suppliers of bulk drug distributors to decline their sale to veterinarians or pharmacists because of their concern over regulatory actions by the FDA. However, because the Federal District Court in Texas has recently indicated that a compounded drug is not a new (animal) drug, it is likely that sales will increase again. The increased flexibility afforded to compounders with this ruling, however, will be accompanied by an increased risk of inappropriate compounding.

Although the percentage of drugs prescribed or dispensed by veterinarians represented by compounded products is not known, in one study of 92 veterinarians,[1] up to 4% of small animal practices used compounded products, with one third of respondents noting that only approximately 1% of their drug products are compounded. The most common (92%) reason why respondents treated with a compounded drug was lack of availability of the desired product: the dose size or formulation is not available, the product requires flavoring to improve animal compliance, or the compounded product is less expensive (with the latter reason being inappropriate). Oral products are the most popular compounded product used by veterinarians, although 50% of responding veterinarians reported that transdermal gels were the first or second most commonly used product.

Bulk substances clearly are important to the provision of drugs in small animals. Of the top products compounded for small animal use in 1999, the first

6 are more than likely compounded from bulk substances, and as such, currently are illegal (Table 1)[17][1] even though, for some of them, approved versions of the drug exist. Interestingly, cyclosporine consistently is in the list of the top 10 products compounded for small animal use and has risen recently to being first in the list, despite the existence of animal-approved versions for oral and ophthalmic use. Cyclosporine is an example of a drug that might be compounded from the veterinary-approved product, the human-approved product, or a bulk substance. Of these, unless the approved versions contain ingredients that preclude compounding of the desired formulation, compounding is legal from the FDA's perspective only from the veterinary- or human-approved product.

Despite the changes in the 2003 CPG, the FDA has indicated verbally that its intent with the new CPG is not to alter regulatory priorities but, rather, to facilitate regulatory abilities. Regulatory action by the FDA is likely to focus, according to the CPG, on "compounding that is intended to circumvent the drug approval process and provide for the mass marketing of products that

Table 1
Top 10 products compounded for small animals, 1999, 2003, and 2004

Rank	1999[a]	2003 status[b]	[c]
1	Potassium bromide: capsules	Cyclosporine: drops; ointment during commercial ophthalmic product backorder	Cyclosporine (70%)
2	Metronidazole: suspension	Methimazole: flavored suspension, chewable treats, transdermal gels	Methimazole (67%)
3	Methimazole: oral liquid	Diethylstilbestrol oral capsules, chew treats	Diethylstilbestrol (32%)
4	Diethylstilbestrol capsules		Cisapride (30%)
5	Potassium bromide solution	Bromide: flavored suspension, chew treats	Bromide, metronidazole (28%)
6	Cyclosporine ophthalmic	Metronidazole chewable treats, usually as the less bitter metronidazole benzoate	Prednisone, enrofloxacin (14%)
7	Prednisone oral liquid		Phenylpropanolamine (12%)
8	Amitriptyline oral liquid		Amitriptyline (7%)
9	Chloramphenical: oral suspension		
10	PZI		
11	Cisapride		

Abbreviation: PZI, protamine zinc insulin.

[a]Based on 1999 publication (anonymous).

[b]Number in parenthesis refers to the status in 2003, when prepared as cited.

[c]2004 Data from Brakke report (number in parenthesis refers to percentage of 93 respondents who prescribe of dispense the product).

have been produced with little or no quality control or manufacturing standards to ensure the purity, potency and stability of the product." The implied prioritization or tolerance to compounding from bulk substances of the 1996 CPG has been replaced in the updated 2003 CPG with a delineation of 13 compounding actions that are to be considered for regulatory action by the CVM. This list is not inclusive and can be modified as needed by the CVM to remain in compliance with the law and to protect public safety. The following 13 actions are not necessarily listed in order of regulatory priority. In general, violations that may result in harm to public health (eg, involves compounding for food animals) are most likely to be regulated, followed by compounding that may harm animal health (Neal Battalier, Office of Compliance, CVM, FDA, Rockville, Maryland, personal communication, 2005). Regulatory action toward veterinary compounding for small animals is more likely to occur for the following reasons:

1. The health of the animal being treated with the compounded drug is not threatened, and suffering or death is not likely to result from failure to treat with the compounded product.
2. Compounding is done in anticipation of prescriptions, unless in limited amounts as indicated by a prescription issued in the confines of a veterinary client-patient relationship.
3. Compounding is performed using drugs prohibited for ELDU in food-producing or non–food-producing animals (currently, no drugs are prohibited for use in non–food-producing animals, but this clause allows for action should such drugs exist).
4. Compounding occurs from drugs with a restricted distribution system (drugs whose use is restricted by the FDA, such as thalidomide).
5. Compounding occurs from drugs that are not approved (this includes human or animal drugs in their manufactured finished dosing form and does not include bulk drugs) unless the product is specifically addressed for regulatory discretion by the FDA in Appendix A.
6. Compounding involves the use of commercial-scale manufacturing equipment (implying the manufacture of large amounts of drug products in anticipation of need, and thus not patient driven).
7. Compounding occurs for third parties with subsequent resell to individual patients (indicating that resale by a veterinarian to a client of a product compounded by a pharmacist is subject to regulatory action), or compounded products are offered at wholesale with intent to resale (the product is then considered an unapproved, manufactured drug). Few veterinarians or pharmacists realize that resale of compounded products is illegal. However, some State Boards of Pharmacy allow "for office use" products, which are intended for short-term dispensing to animals (clients) when prescription availability is precluded (eg, weekends or evenings). This is not to be confused with veterinary purchase of a large quantity of a compounded product, with the intent to dispense the product as a manufactured, approved product might be dispensed. Even if a manufactured version of the drug in need is not commercially available, a large quantity of the drug should not be compounded (manufactured) and

subsequently purchased, with the intent of re-selling the product to a client as part of routine dispensing.

8. Compounding is not in compliance with applicable state pharmacy laws.
9. Compounding results in piracy; that is, the compounded product mimics an FDA-approved (human or animal) product that is commercially available in a finished dosing form and appropriate for treating the patient. Importantly, this guideline indicates that cost is not a justifiable reason for use of a compounded product that replaces a more costly commercial product. The FDA perceives that compounded pirated products are more likely to be mislabeled compared with the commercial product because of the lack of approval. Unfortunately, piracy of commercially available pharmaceutic animal products is prolific (particularly equine products) and has a negative impact on the availability of approved animal drugs, including generics. Such compounding serves as a marked financial disincentive for pharmaceutical manufacturers to pursue approval of animal drugs.
10. Regulatory action of the FDA toward animal drug compounding also is more likely if the compounded label does not contain sufficient information as delineated in the AMDUCA regulations (including withdrawal times, name and address of the prescribing veterinarian, name of the active ingredients, directions for use, cautionary statements, and veterinary-specified withdrawal time; see Box 1).

The remaining three guides relate to food animals, including the use of human drugs, avoidance of drug residues, and scientific establishment of withdrawal times. Veterinarians should avoid as much as possible prescribing through those pharmacies whose practices in compounding clearly are in violation of the law. Note that the Federal Court's recent rulings regarding compounding of animal drugs includes a stipulation that those items (eg, portions of item 5) in the CPG that are in conflict with the ruling will be disallowed.

The CPG for the FDAMA state that compounding of human drugs from bulk substances is tolerated as long as an approved finished version of the drug exists. Pharmacists may not recognize (or agree) with the FDA's different regulatory stance when compounding animal drugs from bulk. Further, compounding from bulk may be easier for some products than compounding from a finished dosing form; and for some drugs, a finished dosing form does not exist. Thus, many animal drugs are compounded from bulk substances.

Despite the fact that the FDA does not intend to alter its regulatory stance toward compounding in small animals (including compounding from bulk substances), the 2003 CPG has had a negative impact on the provision of health care for some companion animal patients. The pharmacy profession has been particularly affected because of its inability to acquire some bulk substances in a timely fashion. Providers of bulk substances (eg, chemical companies) increasingly are removing veterinary-only chemicals from their catalogs. Others simply refuse to sell chemicals if medicinal use in animals is suspected. Further, because of the change in the CPG, the *Journal of the American Veterinary Medical Association* has declined publication of scientific articles that report results of studies using drugs compounded from bulk substances, even if such studies document failed delivery, for fear of implying their support of illegal activity. More disconcerting is the reaction of carriers of professional liability insurance, who recognize that compounding from bulk substances is illegal. Claims that involve compounded products are likely to be reviewed for coverage eligibility on a case-by-case basis in the context of current standard of care.

Not surprisingly, the 2003 CPG has elicited a significant response from the pharmacy profession. The International Academy of Compounding Pharmacists (IACP) has been particularly active in contesting the new CPG [2]. The IACP maintains that the right of pharmacists to compound is being violated (the basis for this argument is not clear), and the IACP is asking veterinarians to solicit the FDA to change the 2003 CPG [18]. However, the veterinary profession should closely examine the wisdom of supporting this action. The 2003 CPG do not infringe on the right of pharmacists or veterinarians to compound but, rather, provides restrictions, particularly as it pertains to compounding from bulk substances. Specifically, the current CPG undoes the previous "stance of tolerance" that the FDA took toward compounding from bulk substances in companion animals, because the stance led to the perception that compounding from bulk was allowed. The CPG, in essence, established different standards for food and companion animals. It is the interpretation by the FDA of AMDUCA as it relates to compounding from bulk substances that has led to the challenges in the most recent CPG by the IACP. Thus far, the challenges have been successful. As this publication went to press, a final ruling from the Federal District Court in Texas reaffirmed that, like human drugs, compounded animal drugs are not "new animal drugs" and accordingly, do not fall under FDA jurisdiction. This in essence precludes the FDA from oversight of compounded products, limiting their ability to curtail abusing compounding pharmacies that are actually manufacturing drugs. The ruling indicates that compounding from legal bulk substances will be allowed for non-food animals, as long as the compounding pharmacy is compliant. Although seemingly a resolution to the conundrum facing compounding pharmacists (balancing the need to compound quality products with the need to follow CPG), this ruling leaves several questions that may lead to confusion and facilitate abuse. Notably, "food-animals", "legal" bulk-substances and "compliant" are terms used, but not defined. Whether or not the FDA will appeal the decision is not yet clear, but this ruling may open the flood gates for abuse, whether intended or not. Reasons for restricting the use of bulk substances for compounded animal products are valid. These include protection of the public from inappropriate exposure to drugs, protection of the veterinary patient from therapeutic failure, and protection of pharmaceutical manufacturers from pirated products. For example, in the early 2000s, enrofloxacin injection was offered for purchase by a compounding pharmacy (Gatz Ridell, American Association of Bovine Practitioners, personal communication, 2003) (Fig. 2). The nature of the product (injectable preparation) indicates it was manufactured from a bulk drug substance. Because the active drug ingredient,

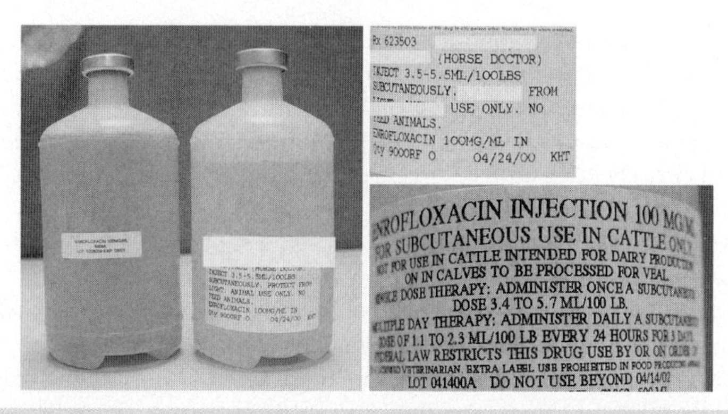

Fig. 2. Label from a compounded enrofloxacin product. This product clearly is in violation of the AMDUCA because, as an unapproved product, its use constitutes extralabel use of enrofloxacin in food animals. Note that the label contains the appropriate warnings regarding the use of enrofloxacin in food animals, including the statement, "extra-label use prohibited in food producing animals." This suggests that the maker of the product does not understand the concept of extra-label drug use. This product has been compounded from a bulk substance. The product was for sale while the original holder of the patent for the active drug ingredient still retained the patent for the active ingredient, indicating that the bulk substance was imported from a foreign source and thus, was probably illegal and renders the quality of the product suspect. Further, because a similar finished dosing form is available commercially, this product represents piracy and its use is a major disincentive for manufacturers of approved dosing forms to pursue drug approval. Other points for consideration include the following. Unlike some compounded products, the appearance of the label of this product indicates that the source is not a manufacturer, and thus, it is not an approved product. The presence of lot numbers and expiration dates (as seen on this label) contributes to the perception that a validation process and quality assurance program supports the product, which is unlikely for this product. Finally, the volume (500 mL) suggests that this is a multiple-animal use vial, a violation of the stipulation that compounding be implemented for individual patients.

enrofloxacin, was still under patent at the time the product was made, the bulk drug substance was probably purchased from a foreign site and probably was not inspected by the FDA. Quality of the active drug ingredient and the presence of potential contaminants would be a concern. Further, this product represented a violation of the AMDUCA and its regulations from several standpoints. The most disconcerting is that fluorinated quinolones are among the drug classes whose extralabel use in food animals is specifically prohibited. Because enrofloxacin is compounded from bulk and is intended for use in food animals represents the second violation. Third, because it mimics an approved version commercially available in the United States, it is a pirated product. Purchase of this product by veterinarians is a major disincentive for a drug company to pursue approval of an animal drug. Interestingly, the label for the product noted that "extra-label use of enrofloxacin in food-producing animals is prohibited," indicating that the "compounder" of this product did not understand the laws regulating animal drugs including, did not recognize that the use of this product constituted extra-label drug use. Limitations in compounding of bulk substances for small animals also may be prudent because abuses will occur. For example, a nationally-recognized compounding pharmacy that offers services for veterinary patients appears to have crossed the boundary from compounding to manufacturing, thus violating the intent of AMDUCA by manufacturing rather than compounding, animal products. Its DEA license was recently revoked by the Drug Enforcement Agency (DEA) for manufacturing rather than compounding scheduled products [19]. However, its activities are not limited to scheduled products. Exhibits offered by this pharmacy on its web site suggest compounding of its products represents manufacturing, with the source of drugs being bulk substances. Indeed, at one of the most recent national veterinary continuing education meetings attended by the author, a nationally recognized veterinary distributor exhibited products compounded by this pharmacy. Among the products was trilostane (see article on drugs used in the treatment of endocrine diseases elsewhere in this issue). Various sizes and concentrations of multiple-dose tablets were exhibited, each bearing labels similar to those of approved finished dosing forms. When queried regarding the legality of distributing a compounded product, the exhibitor indicated that the distribution was provided as "a service" to the profession. Several aspects of the intent of AMDUCA are being violated with this product. First, these products have undergone no approval despite the "finished" appearance given to this and other products compounded by this pharmacy. Lot numbers may indicate the products really have been manufactured, but if so, the rigorous quality assurance program implied by the lot number will not have been followed. Further, the basis for the expiration date should be suspect. Availability through a distributor facilitates the perception that the product is approved and is further evidence that the product is indeed manufactured. Second, although approved in the United Kingdom, trilostane is not available in the United States in any approved dosing form for any species. Yet, AMDUCA regulations state that compounding is allowed (only) from an approved drug (human or animal). The manufacturer of an approved form of the drug in the UK does not supply the drug for compounding in the US. As such, the source and quality of the drug substance used for this preparation should be of concern. Contributing to this concern is the findings by the UK manufacturer that several samples of the US compounded trilostane products have contained less than 90% of the labeled content. Third, successful promotion of this compounded product such that veterinary use becomes widespread may serve as a major disincentive to approval of this product for animal use in the US. Marketing analysis will have to take into account potential competition with the compounded product. Failure of a company to pursue approval results in not only the lack of availability of an approved version of the drug for animals, but also the loss of scientific studies that would establish the safety, efficacy, and appropriate dosing regimens. This same pharmacy has recently mailed postcards to veterinarians indicating the availability of pimobendan, another drug not approved in the United States. This compounded product also is available from the pharmacy in various sizes and drug concentrations, including its most "common" size of 100-count capsules. The product has even been "introduced" by *DVM* magazine. However, the importation of this product, like trilostane, is not legal. A mechanism does exist whereby permission can be granted by the FDA to import into the US a limited amount of a drug approved for use in another country [20]. This is the only FDA-sanctioned mechanism by which pimobendan or trilostane can be obtained. An argument might be made that non-prescription driven purchase of bulk-compounded pharmaceuticals by veterinarians is legitimate if the products are intended for office stock of inhospital use products (ie, the products will not be dispensed).

These and other episodes probably represent only a small number of the abuses that occur regarding compounding. Disconcertingly, the recent federal ruling also indicated that pharmacies are not required to submit to FDA inspection of their records unless the FDA can first demonstrate that the pharmacy is not compliant with applicable state laws, and does not operate as a retail pharmacy. The FDA may have a difficult time demonstrating the lack of compliance if it does not have access to the pharmacy records. Thus, the ability of the FDA to regulate compounded animal drugs at any level has been markedly curtailed. Limitations in state oversight are addressed below. As long as compounding from bulk is legal, unless the pharmacy profession successfully self-regulates and the veterinary profession self-educates, abuses are going to continue to put veterinarians, their patients, and the food-animal-product consuming public in harms way. Fortunately, the pharmacy profession is taking an increasingly active role in educating its members regarding the rules and regulations as they pertain to compounding for animals, and in discouraging inappropriate compounding (Gigi Davison, North Carolina State University, personal communication, 2006).

The CVM recognizes that medical conditions may exist in which a drug compounded from bulk substance may be necessary. Currently, mechanisms do exist whereby written evidence of FDA tolerance (regulatory discretion) to compounding from bulk substances can be obtained. For example, of the list of compounding actions likely to draw FDA regulation, item 5 refers to Appendix A of the CPG. This appendix is a list of less than 15 bulk drug substances that might be used for compounding of poison antidotes, for food animals. In such cases, the CPG indicates, assuming all other AMDUCA stipulations are appropriately met, that the CVM follows regulatory discretion, that is, ordinarily does not object to the compounding, even if done in anticipation of need. Because this appendix is in the CPG (and not the regulations), the list does not legalize compounding from these bulk substances. Further, the absence from Appendix A of a product critical to animal health does not necessarily imply that the CVM is going to regulate compounding from that bulk substance. However, the CVM may be recalcitrant to expand the list to include other medically necessary substances because of concern as to "where to draw the line" and the risk of abuse. In addition to Appendix A, the CVM may, depending on the circumstances, offer regulatory discretion for other medicines for individual patients. Potassium bromide, for example, is an important antiepileptic for dogs that is not available in an approved form and can only be compounded from bulk. Chemical companies may refuse to sell bulk bromide to a veterinarian. However, written documentation from the Division of Compliance (240 276 9200) stating that the CVM does not object to a specific use of a product may be sufficient for the company to allow the sale.

Unfortunately, this approach to regulatory discretion must be sought for each patient; as such, it is unlikely to be pursued in all instances of need. Further, the CVM is unlikely to have the resources necessary to address all legitimate requests. Among the most effective mechanisms for increasing availability of medically necessary drugs compounded from bulk in companion animals might be the generation of a second set of CPGs that focus on nonfood animals. This, in essence, may have been accomplished with the recent federal ruling. A major disadvantage of the legal use of bulk substances is the inability to confirm the quality of the products, thus putting animals at risk (see the second part of this series). Finally, imported materials might be used in acts of terrorism, and neither the FDA nor Congress is likely to become more lenient in regulations related to bioterrorism.

Despite current CPG which indicate conditions under which the FDA is likely to regulate compounded animal drugs, the FDA does not regulate all compounding that is or seems to be in violation of the law. However, resources of the CVM often must prioritize illegal activities that place human health at a risk, giving the appearance of tolerating (but, in fact, neither ignoring nor condoning) activities that clearly are not legal. The lack of apparent activity also may reflect the legal environment under which the FDA must regulate: often, regulatory action is planned or ongoing, but the activities cannot be publicized because of legal considerations. Finally, some aspects of compounding are outside the regulatory jurisdiction of the FDA. In its compounding CPG, the FDA notes its intent to defer to state authorities (eg, State Boards of Pharmacy) regarding day-to-day regulation of compounding and to coordinate regulatory efforts with individual states.

The DEA also plays a role in regulation if the drug in question falls under the jurisdiction of the DEA. For example, a nationally recognized Internet-based pharmacy that compounds for human and veterinary medicine (previously mentioned) has recently had its DEA licensed revoked. In the *Federal Register* describing this process [2], the owner of the pharmacy admitted that more than 80% of its sales were made directly to a physician or veterinarian rather than to an individual patient. Examples cited included individual sales of injectable stanozolol and boldenone undecylenate (to veterinarians) as well as injectable diazepam (to a physician). Other sales included testosterone, buprenorphine, and phenylpropanolamine. Discrepancies in records, inability to account for all substances, volume of drugs being manufactured, and direct sales to veterinarians and physicians are some of the violations cited by the DEA as justification for revocation of the license. Although the loss of the DEA license should not affect compounding of other products by this pharmacy, several of these violations are also violations of the intent of the FDAMA and AMDUCA.

State Regulations

In addition to federal laws (eg, the AMDUCA), all actions related to pharmacy, including compounding, are regulated by State Boards of Pharmacy. However, individual states vary in the applicability of these laws to compounding veterinarians. Not all states recognize a veterinarian's right to compound. Selected states have specific regulations for veterinary compounding; in their absence, human compounding regulations may apply. However, a conundrum in the regulation of compounding for animals exists in many states. State Boards of Pharmacy often defer to State Boards of Veterinary Medicine on issues regarding compounding in animals. Yet, State Boards of Veterinary Medicine are likely to indicate that the issues are not in their jurisdiction and defer back to the State Board of Pharmacy (Gigi Davidson, North Carolina State University, personal communication, 2006). The Food and Drug Administration has no regulatory role in the act of compounding, and appears to be loosing its ability to regulate–when desired–the compounded product. Thus, compounded animal products may not be regulated at any level. In light of the changes in human and animal compounding CPGs, some State Boards of Pharmacy are re-examining their rules and regulations regarding compounding. The NABP [21]) is a nonregulatory organization that attempts to provide standards and conformity for individual State Boards of Pharmacy. Currently, this association is generating standard regulatory guidelines (within a Model Practice Act) regarding many aspects of pharmacy practice, including compounding, which might be implemented among the states. Because the NABP has recognized the increase in veterinary drug compounding, it has begun to address problems and concerns of the veterinary profession, such as compounding by pharmacists who are unaware of differences in regulatory philosophy or "rogue" pharmacists who are indifferent to the regulations. The NABP web site provides a link to each state Board of Pharmacy, which, in turn, generally provides information regarding the state regulations as well as a venue through which queries or complaints regarding inappropriate pharmacy activity can be made. Veterinarians who dispense or prescribe compounded drugs should become aware of the relevant state laws; the AVMA web site may be a venue where recently approved or currently considered bills can be reviewed [22].

Role of the Veterinary Pharmacist

Pharmacists are the only health care professionals formally trained in the art and science of pharmaceutic compounding. However, the extent of formal training among the schools or colleges of pharmacy ranges from limited to nonexistent, however.

The extant of training in the art and science of compounding is variable among pharmacy schools, ranging from limited to absent. Even less training is provided in veterinary schools. Yet, the right to compound drugs guaranteed to veterinarians by AMDUCA reflects, in part, the recognition that no other allied health profession sufficiently addresses the interests of animal health and well-being. Pharmacy training largely focuses on the provision of human, not animal, health care as is reflected in the oath that pharmacists take upon graduation. Pharmacists may approach compounding for animals with a standard of care lower than that followed for human drugs. The pharmacists' expertise is detrimentally impacted without training in species differences in physiology, pharmacology, or disease pathophysiology. Differences in drug absorption, drug interactions or adverse drug events will be underestimated. Selected pharmacists may pursue post-graduate education in animal-related issues, but training generally is designed by pharmacists, not veterinarians. The approach to provision of animal care by pharmacists may also be negatively impacted by the perceived position of animals. For example, the property status of animals may overwhelm their patient status, leading pharmacists to take liberties in drug substitution or prepations that would not be taken for a human patient (Katrina Mealey, Washington State University, personal communication, 2001). Consider, for example: if transdermal PLO gels are as effective for systemic drug delivery in animals as suggested by their promotion, then why is this method of drug delivery not a popular method for administration of drugs to humans, and particularly, children? Veterinary compounding offers a financial incentive that is likely to ensure continued growth of this profession and, with that growth, potential increases in inappropriate pharmacy practices.

Despite the current voids in veterinary pharmacy education, the veterinary profession serves to benefit from a focus on improved provision of veterinary health care by pharmacists. At least two organizations have been established to facilitate expertise in veterinary pharmacy: the Society of Veterinary Hospital Pharmacists (SVHP), and the American College of Veterinary Pharmacists (ACVP). Both are striving to improve the education of pharmacists in special needs and to address concerns of the veterinary profession regarding the dispensing (including compounding) of animal drugs. The former has established an experience- and examination-based certification program for academic veterinary pharmacists comparable to that of the American Board of Veterinary Practitioners (successful candidates are "diplomates" of the International Academy of Veterinary Pharmacists). The program is based on experience, coursework, and examination, leading to diplomate status in the International Academy of Veterinary Pharmacists. Despite the inclusion of "college" in its title, the ACVP is not a college recognized by and has no formal affiliation with the AVMA. Rather, its organization is an offshoot of the American Academy of Apothecaries. The ACVP also is developing a program similar to that of the SVHP, but will be inclusive of all interested pharmacists. Further, the NABP and the Association of Veterinary State Boards have developed a verification program for Internet pharmacies. The Verification of Internet Pharmacy Program (VIPP) has been implemented for human pharmacies; those that pass this voluntary screening process would be provided a "seal of approval" indicating that the pharmacy has met state and federal regulatory requirements.

The presence of the seal should increase consumer confidence in the appropriateness of practices by the approved pharmacy. The success of this program is dependent on volunteer participation by pharmacists, which, in turn, depends on physicians (or veterinarians) being willing to encourage client use of approved pharmacists. A second validation program has also been recently implemented. The Professional Compounding Accreditation Board [23] offers a validation program and an indicator seal that can be used by pharmacists completing certification. However, the certification process is not particularly robust, and care should be taken in assuming that a "seal" is associated with a stringent process. Finally, the IACP has taken a proactive attitude in resolving at least some of the issues that put users of compounded products at risk. It has offered labeling guidelines for products compounded for human use. The AVMA is in dialog with the IACP to ascertain why these guidelines should not also apply to compounded animal drugs (Elizabeth Curry Galvin, Director of Scientific Activities Division, AVMA, personal communication, 2006). Until evidence of competence in the compounding of animal drugs is easily appreciated of a pharmacy, veterinarians should seek a pharmacist who is aware of and follows the regulations for veterinary compounding (see Box 1).

Veterinary Compounder

As the need for compounded products increases, veterinarians are likely to offer compounding through their practice. Indeed, veterinarians are specifically targeted with advertisements for compounding materials (eg, flavoring) and equipment. State rules and regulations that have an impact on compounding should be and, for many states, must be adhered to by veterinary compounders. The veterinarian is no less expected to adhere to proper pharmacy practices than is the pharmacist (Box 2). However, compounding represents a major void in the education of the veterinarian. In the author's experience, many veterinary students resist laboratories that introduce them to calculations and even the basic concepts in the art and science of compounding. If veterinarians are to maintain their right to compound, the profession must correct this deficiency and become more proactive in the proper education of compounding of drug products. The recent trend of law schools to offer individual courses or minor courses of studies that specialize in veterinary medicine should cause the profession to take pause and strongly consider its role in the liability of dispensing and prescribing drugs. The AVMA Professional Liability Insurance Trust has been addressing the role of compounding in veterinary medicine.[1] Some compounding is legal, and some is illegal; the line between the two is not distinct. Thus, each liability case that involves compounding is likely to be considered individually, and the current standard of care is likely to be the basis for decision making surrounding litigation. A pharmacist can not dispense any prescription drug, whether as a manufactured finished, dosing form or a reformulated or compounded product, without a prescription. The prescription becomes the legal document which orders the medication. In the event that the product proves ineffective or unsafe,

Box 2: Criteria of a desirable compounding pharmacy or pharmacist

1. Is legitimate, based on the following:
   A. Appropriate licensure or registration in all applicable states
   B. Conformation to relevant laws in all appropriate states
2. Maintains and enforces policies and procedures that ensure the following:
   A. Integrity, legitimacy, and authenticity of the prescription drug order, including a valid veterinary client patient relationship
   B. Compliance with applicable generic substitution statues and regulations
   C. Compliance with all appropriate state (including Pharmacy and DEA) and federal (including the AMDUCA and its CPG and DEA) laws
   D. Reasonable verification of patient/client/prescriber identity
   E. Patient/client confidentiality
   F. Interactive, meaningful, and appropriately educated consultation with the client/pet owner regarding the following:
      i. Use of the drug
      ii. Recalls of any drugs (in a timely fashion)
      iii. Disposal or return of unused or damaged drugs
   G. User-friendly mechanism for the receipt and subsequent report to appropriate medical bodies of the following:
      i. Medication errors
      ii. Adverse drug events
      iii. Delay in receipt of prescription
   H. Prospective drug use review before dispensing of a medication to a patient
3. Maintains and implements policies that ensure adherence to state and national quality assurance/quality improvement
4. Maintains legible and reasonably retrievable records of the following:
   A. Source of compounded ingredients
   B. Ingredients, active and inactive
   C. Formulas
   D. Assurance of quality of raw ingredients
   E. Adverse events, including product failure
5. Implements procedures that minimize risk to human beings of exposure to harmful ingredients attributable directly or indirectly (including through the food supply)
6. Maintains and implements policies that ensure neither prescription, over- the-counter, nor ethical animal products are diverted from veterinarians to pharmacies with the intent to circumvent sales policies of manufacturers of animal products
7. Bases compounding protocols on guidelines provided in the USP general chapter (1075) on good compounding practices, the *USP Pharmacist's Pharmacopeia*, and *Remington: The Science and Practice of Pharmacy*
8. Is aware of and adheres to the criteria for appropriate compounding in animals as delineated in the AMDUCA and its regulations (CFR 21 CFR Section 530) and the most recent CPG (608:400)

the ultimate determinant of liability, whether pharmacist, veterinarian, or both, will be determined on a case-by-case basis. Among the issues to be considered will be whether or not the use of the product reflects the current standard of care. The pharmacists' responsibility lies in the preparation and dispensing of the product. Pharmacists will point out that it is not their responsibility to assure safety or efficacy of a compounded product. This responsibility lies with the prescribing clinician. However, this division of responsibility is true only to a point. Clearly, it is in the best interest of the patient–veterinary or human–for pharmacists and clinicians to approach the provision of health care as a partnership, both taking an equal role in the likelihood of therapeutic success–or failure–of any compounded preparation prescribed or dispensed for a patient. Whereas a veterinarian might not be susceptible to criminal charges when prescribing an inappropriately compounded product, civil liability may drive the profession to be more responsible in regard to the prescription of a safe and effective compound.

Thus far, this article has focused on the rules and regulations that guide the compounding of animal drugs. However, a major consideration regarding compounded products is their formulation and the impact that it has on changes in the disposition of the drug. Compared with their manufactured counterparts, compounded drug products are more likely to cause adverse drug events. The second part of this article addresses the practice of compounding by veterinarians and pharmacists, with a particular emphasis on the potential for adverse drug events. The most likely adverse drug events involve pharmaceutic inactivation of the compounded drug during its preparation and variability in drug absorption, either of which can lead to adverse events.

GENERATING CONFIDENCE IN COMPOUNDED PRODUCTS

The promotion of compounded products through advertisements and exhibits often is misinterpreted by veterinarians (and their clients) as evidence of safety and efficacy of those products.

The Federal Court has recently (June 2006) ruled that pharmacists may continue to compound customized drugs for individual patients and that the compounded product does not constitute a new drug, thus rejecting the FDA's stance on compounded drugs being new unapproved drugs, and thus under FDA jurisdiction. Hailed as a victory, pharmacists noted in response to the ruling that "doctors can write customized prescriptions with the confidence that those drugs will be dispensed according to their exact directions." Ignoring the optimistic observation that "exact directions" are going to be provided (let alone followed for veterinary patients), what is not pointed out in the remarks is what is lost with the possible removal of FDA oversight of compounded products: confidence in the product itself. This ruling has recently been applied to veterinary compounded drugs; however, further appeals are likely to be pursued. The courts are also expected to address the legality of compounding from bulk substances in non-food–producing animals and the FDA's ability to inspect pharmacies. Rather than react to these considerations as an infringement of government on individual rights, the veterinary profession might prudently consider the advantages of federal oversight (rather than state oversight) on compounding and look for compromises that protect the patient without precluding access to necessary medicaments.

For manufactured drugs, the FDA drug approval process involves scientific validation of not only the safety and efficacy of a drug but the methods of its manufacture. Approved manufactured products have been scrutinized with regard to quality control in drug content, stability, and strength as well as accuracy in labeled contents (generally within ±10%–20%) between and within lots. Expiration dates are based on stability and other relevant studies under appropriate environmental conditions; all data are inspected by the FDA. Labeling requirements ensure tracking of products through the marketing process. Labels are reviewed for accuracy and adequacy, meaning that sufficient information is provided so that clinicians can make informed decisions regarding the use and safety of the product (including storage conditions and shelf life).

Drugs approved by the FDA undergo rigorous scientific testing to ensure drug quality, safety and efficacy. Predefined toxicity studies in the target species are mandated at specified doses and durations in order to provide reasonable assurance of safety. Pharmacokinetic data generally are required to determine elimination rates necessary for the design of appropriate dosing regimens. Data also include bioavailability and bioequivalency studies for nonintravenous preparations and generic preparations respectively. Controlled clinical trials are required to ensure both safety and efficacy. In all cases, studies are based on the manufactured finished dosing form in the approved species. As such, data generated during the approval process can not be directly extrapolated to compounded products. Finally, and equally important, postmarket surveillance programs are required of manufacturers of approved products for the report of adverse events, including therapeutic failure. Manufacturers are mandated to report adverse events to the FDA, which, in turn, reports the information back to the public (veterinarians and clients).

Similar mechanisms of assurance simply do not exist in any fashion for compounded products. Although the FDA perceives a compounded drug to be a new animal drug (a perception recently disallowed by the Federal Court), it does not approve compounded products. Further, no funding agency is mandated to provide data that ensures the quality or accuracy of preparation or the efficacy and safety of compounded products. Indeed, no funding agency is easily identifiable that should have a vested interest in providing such information. Manufacturers of the drug from which compounding is done are unlikely to be willing to fund studies if doing so is likely to result in competition for their products (as would occur if bulk or generic substances are used). Further, such support may imply to the FDA manufacturer sponsorship of an unapproved drug product, sponsorship that is forbidden by the FDA. Finally, manufacturers that fund studies demonstrating the ineffectiveness of compounded products might be perceived as being financially motivated (by disproving the efficacy of a competing product), a public perception that many companies would like to avoid. The pharmacy profession conceivably should be willing to fund such studies because it has the greatest financial incentive to do so. As long as physicians and veterinarians embrace compounded products in the belief that they are properly prepared and, if properly prepared, are therefore efficacious and safe, however, the motivation for pharmacists to participate in (let alone fund) studies that validate compounded products is lacking. The FDA cannot be counted on to be a "watch dog" for all compounded products because it does not have the resources to police the large number of pharmacies currently offering compounded products. Further, pharmacies (including State Boards) are protective of their rights as pharmacists; legal resistance by pharmacists toward regulation further stresses FDA time and financial resources, limiting the FDA's ability to regulate activity. Finally, even if the FDA should be successful in implementing regulatory action, the punitive actions available to the FDA, unfortunately, often have a minimal impact on the offending pharmacy. Pharmacies (generally the most abusive) that are successfully regulated ("closed down") may appear in another state, under another name, but often with the same inappropriate compounding activities. State Board action may likewise be successful, but such action may simply force the pharmacy to another state. The advent of Internet pharmacies further complicates regulatory action.

The risks associated with the approved finished dosing form of a drug also are of concern in the compounded product. Compounded products are associated with additional risks, however, simply because they are compounded, with therapeutic failure attributable to failed drug delivery perhaps being the most likely adverse effect. Adverse events associated with compounded products may occur at the pharmaceutic phase (during preparation) or because an inappropriate method of delivery has been compounded at the pharmacokinetic phase (changes in drug absorption).

PHARMACEUTICS OF COMPOUNDING: ROLE OF QUALITY ASSURANCE

Failure at the pharmaceutic phase of drug preparation might occur for many reasons, beginning with the selection of ingredient sources, through implementation of the compounding recipe (protocol), to storage of the finished compounded product.

Ingredient Source

The use of an approved finished dosing form of a drug for compounding offers a major advantage to use of a bulk substance. Whereas the bulk substance used in the approved version of a drug has passed stringent tests of analysis regarding drug ingredients and presence of contaminants, the bulk substance used in compounded products is not necessarily associated with a similar guarantee and the burden of purity and accuracy lies with the pharmacist. All products, active ingredients, or excipients (eg, fillers, preservatives), domestic or foreign, should meet USP or equivalent standards or should be purchased after FDA inspection. The activities of the USP are integral to the protection and promotion of health as it relates to pharmaceutic products. Founded in 1820, this nonregulatory organization establishes standards for medicines and products of other health care technologies (including new drug delivery systems). Its original mission of the standardization of medicinal compounds among the states remains a core activity [4]. Today, the USP generates standards for close to 4000 prescriptions and nonprescription drugs or other health care products; the standards are published annually in the USP and the USP/NF publications, which are officially recognized by the FDCA.

For products that do not meet USP or similar standards, FDA inspection of the product should be expected. However, the pharmacist should be specifically queried about the product itself, not the manufacturer or the site of production. A bulk product may be obtained from a site that is FDA inspected, but this does not assure that the specific product has been inspected. Although the FDA must inspect bulk substances to be used in finished dosage forms, but is under no mandate to inspect bulk substances to be used in compounded products. Thus, chances of FDA inspection of a bulk substance used in compounding are slight. All bulk products used in compounding should be accompanied by a certificate of analysis that delineates the purity of the product, thus ensuring that the proper amount of drug is present (ie, the product is correctly labeled in regard to drug content) and that no potentially damaging contaminants (including degradative products, metals, and microbial contaminants) are present. Pharmacists should maintain evidence of the source of ingredients as well as the certificate of analysis of each. The need for validation of substance source is paramount, because bulk substances are increasingly being acquired from noninspected foreign (particularly Asian) sources at a price much lower than their domestic counterparts. Drugs that are still under US patents are often obtained in this manner. For example, the approved pharmaceutic ingredient (API) for enrofloxacin has been held by Bayer Animal Health, which has maintained patent rights and does not sell bulk substance to compounders (Neal Battalier, Office of Compliance, CVM, FDA, Rockville, Maryland, personal communication, 2005). As such, pharmacies that compounded enrofloxacin from bulk substances (eg, transdermal gels) before the patent expiration last year were likely to be obtaining the bulk drug from a foreign non–FDA-inspected source. The need for documentation of the source of bulk ingredients cannot be overemphasized, particularly if the FDA is ultimately directed by Congress to tolerate compounding from bulk substances.

Substitutions of drugs to be used for compounding should be made cautiously and never by the pharmacist independent of the veterinarian. The salt form of the drug might affect drug delivery not only because of differences in stability, pH, and bioavailability but because the active drug content may differ. Metronidazole benzoate, the more palatable salt preferred for treatment in cats, contains less active drug than the less palatable metronidazole hydrochloride; the dose of the benzoate salt should be increased by 1.6 (ie, 16 mg/kg rather than 10 mg/kg).

Bromide offers another example: the sodium (molecular weight [MW] = 23) salt bromide (MW = 79) at a dose of 1 g contains more bromide (774 mg) than the potassium (MW = 35) salt (692 mg). Failure to adjust to the amount of active drug in a salt form might lead to adverse events [24].

Mathematical Errors

Mathematical errors are probably the most common reason for pharmaceutic compounding errors as well as, potentially, the most lethal. Mistakes during the preparation of a compounded product are particularly egregious because they can lead to marked under- or overdosing; however, with proper care, such mistakes are avoidable. Their potential emphasizes the importance of basing all compounding on written protocols and recording unique actions taken during compounding each prescription. Compounding is predisposed to mathematic mistakes, because, by its nature (eg, prescription driven, small volumes), much of the equipment and technology that facilitates accuracy and precision of finished dosing forms is not (and should not be) used. The author has experienced the impact of mathematic errors in compounding during a clinical trial based on compounded products. Five previously well-controlled dogs with epilepsy receiving phenobarbital from the same lot of a compounded product experienced breakthrough seizures, all within the same month. Serum phenobarbital concentrations in each of the seizuring patients had decreased by 50%; phenobarbital content measured in random samples from the common source lot was also found to be less than 50% of the labeled content. Eventually, that pharmacy was closed after FDA regulatory action, only to reopen in another state. Unfortunately, therapeutic failure often is difficult to identify, particularly if clinical signs of response are not discreet. In this instance, the mistake was identified only because the same clinician was handling the patients, the clinical signs of therapeutic failure were obvious, and monitoring documented low drug concentrations.

Preparation and Storage Failure: Product Integrity

The more sophisticated a compounded preparation, the more likely it is that adverse events are going to occur because of diminished or excessive drug delivery. The preparation and storage of a pharmaceutic product may be associated with adverse events attributable to factors including, but not limited to, drug interactions (between drugs in the same preparation), stability (affected by excipients, diluents, concentration, and storage conditions), product pH, osmolality, osmolarity, and microbial growth. The multimillion dollar cost of FDA drug approval includes analysis that ensures stability of the approved product in its final dosage form under the storage conditions delineated on the label. Factors that lead to instability are relevant both to finished dosing forms and compounded products; however, studies that establish stability are relevant only to the product being tested and cannot be extrapolated to others. Unfortunately, compounded products generally are not subject to the same studies that establish or document stability under recommended or used conditions of preparation, storage, and use. Indeed, the basis for recommended storage conditions of compounded products is not clear, since they generally are not based on scientific studies.

Chemical reactions (eg, oxidation, reduction, hydrolysis) are facilitated by environmental changes in humidity, light, pH, presence of oxidizing trace metals, and temperature [25,26]. Excipients may enhance instability because of changes in pH or the presence of disintegrating agents. Degradation products (drugs or excipients) can cause adverse events. In general, although the use of approved finished dosing forms is preferred because of purity and accuracy, bulk substances are often preferred for compounded products, because excipients that are critical to the finished dosing form increase the risk of instability in a compounded product.

Product pH

The importance of pH in a drug preparation cannot be overemphasized. Often, the specific salt of a drug is selected because of its ability to remain stable. Simple syrups (which tend to be acidic) can alter drug pH, and thus ionization (diffusibility) or stability. Even preservatives should be added cautiously. Not only can their addition alter drug pH and stability, but adverse reactions to the preservative may occur. Combinations of drugs increase the risk of drug interactions, in part, because of the impact on the pH of the preparation. For example, weak acids and weak bases are likely to inactivate one another chemically.

Omeprazole offers a good example of the influence of compounding on formulation pH and drug efficacy. An equine preparation of omeprazole that mimics the commercial product but at a markedly reduced cost is available (illegally) through compounding pharmacies. The manufacturer of the commercial product demonstrated that of 10 compounded products tested, none contained close to 100% of the labeled omeprazole concentration (Fig. 3). The percentage of actual drug compared with labeled content was markedly variable; only 2 products contained within 50% of the labeled content, whereas

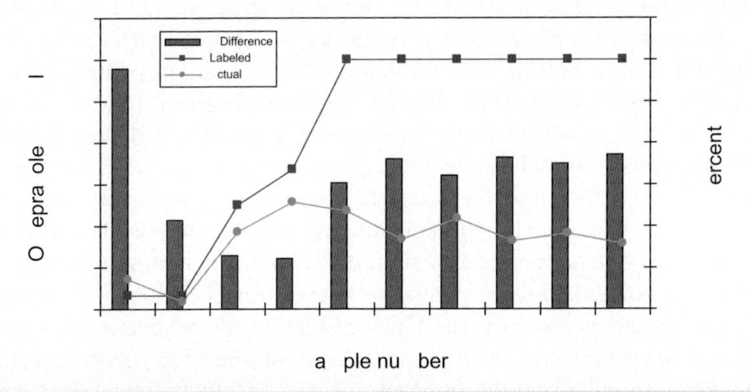

Fig. 3. Percentage difference (*bar*) between labeled and actual content of omeprazole in 10 compounded paste products that mimic the commercial preparation (*Data courtesy of* Frank Hurtig, DVM, Eagle, ID.)

6 contained less than 30% of the label claim. It is not surprising that a clinical trial of the two products in Thoroughbred race horses found the compounded product to be ineffective, whereas the commercial product was effective in controlling gastric ulcers in horses [27]. The content and preparation of compounded products may have played a role in the lack of efficacy. The pH of the compounded omeprazole paste intended for use in horses was substantially lower at 3.4 compared with the manufactured product at 8.4. As a weak-based drug, omeprazole is essentially ionized at a pH of 3.4, and is thus poorly diffusible.

Drug Interactions

The combination of two or more drugs in the same preparation to render therapy more convenient should be done cautiously. The more drugs mixed together in a single preparation, the greater is the risk of chemical drug interactions. Interactions are not limited to drugs but may occur between the drugs or excipients. For example, only 54% of a fluorinated quinolone (orbifloxacin) was found to be present when prepared in one product as a vehicle compared with simpler syrups [28]. Because it is the veterinarian who is ultimately responsible for a prescribed product, and because a pharmacist compounds that which is requested, veterinarians must assume the responsibility of ensuring that no combination product is to be used unless evidence exists supporting the lack of drug interactions.

Particle Size

The physical attributes of a compounded product can have an impact on therapeutic success. The presence of macroscopic or microscopic precipitates indicates undissolved, and thus nondiffusible, ineffective drug and should be cause for avoiding use of the product. Sedimentation of undissolved particles may result in caking at the bottom of the drug receptacle; difficulty in shaking or rapid sedimentation after shaking can result in erratic and unpredictable doses. Crushing of any oral tablet may result in unequal particle sizes in the preparation, which, in turn, yields different surface areas and different rates of absorption. Although vigorous shaking might randomly distribute the different-sized particles equally in the syrup, sedimentation of the particles (at different rates) is likely to occur before the dose can be accurately removed. Consistency between doses is lost, and for drugs characterized by a narrow therapeutic window, toxicity may occur. Manipulating the suspension (visible particles) so that it becomes a solution probably should be avoided. Filtering visible particles with the intent of removing excipients and fillers is also likely to remove drug that is retained in the filtered particles. Fine crushing of the product so that it is no longer a suspension increases the concentration of soluble excipient; chemicals, including those added to the finished dosing form to facilitate degradation, can cause drug instability. Finally, although methods intended to assure drugs are dissolved, and thus more likely to passively diffuse, the drugs simultaneously become more susceptible to degradation than are drugs in suspension [29].

Oral Products

Dispersing a tablet in a flavoring solution is preferred to simply crushing tablets or adding the contents of a capsule to food or water so that the amount administered is not certain [30,31]. Crushing an oral tablet for preparation in a syrup may lead to unequal distribution of dissolved drug in the finished preparation, and mixing the drug so that it is equally distributed throughout the preparation may not be possible. Repackaging oral tablets or capsules into smaller dosing units may also affect drug efficacy. Diluents, such as starch and dextrose, might impede oral absorption. Preparation of an oral formulation from an injectable solution to enhance accuracy of dosing is more likely to be appropriate if the drug salt is the same in both preparations. Compared with an approved oral preparation, however, absorption is more rapid (and peak concentrations higher) if an injectable solution is used to formulate the oral preparation [8]. Preparation of oral drugs from injectable drugs for which no oral form exists must be done much more cautiously, because the lack of an oral preparation may reflect the inability to make an effective oral product (see section on pharmacokinetic changes). The addition of flavoring agents to oral products may increase drug instability because of changes in pH or the increased risk of microbial growth (ie, with syrups).

Injectable Products

Administration of injectable products is inherently associated with a higher level of risks compared with administration of topical or oral products because of more rapid drug delivery, the risks associated with administration of suspensions rather than solutions, the potential impact of impurities (including endotoxin), and the need for sterility. Actions taken to ensure sterility and removal of impurities may cause drug degradation. Endotoxin (which is essentially ubiquitous in the environment) is difficult to remove. Without testing, its absence is impossible to document; yet, its presence can be lethal. The USP has generated guidelines and state laws generally delineate regulations specifically for the compounding of injectable products. Veterinarians should be reluctant to prescribe compounded injections, and when doing so, they must be confident that the compounding pharmacist follows these criteria.

Topical Products

Although administration of topical products generally is associated with fewer risks compared with administration of systemic products (the exception would be ophthalmic products, which also should be sterile), compounding the proper product can be challenging. The USP has promulgated guidelines for the compounding of topical ingredients [5,31]. Those factors previously discussed pertain to topical products. Because only dissolved drug can move into the skin, additional guidelines are designed to ensure drug dissolution. For example, solid ingredients should be reduced to the smallest reasonable particle size, and the active ingredient should then be added to other substances necessary to dissolve the drug to achieve a uniform liquid or solid dispersion. Uniformity of dispersion should be demonstrated by spreading a thin film of the finished formulation on a flat transparent surface. Visual examination of a compounded product should be implemented to identify obvious problems with dissolution, for example. Care must be taken to ensure that ingredients are not caustic, irritating, or allergenic Vehicle selection can be impressively difficult: undissolved drug cannot pass into the skin, and drug that has too great an affinity for the vehicle remains in the vehicle.

Toxicity

In addition to excipients and contaminants, ingredient products intentionally included in a compounded product may become problematic. Benzoic acid (alcohol or benzoate) is a preservative commonly added to oral and parenteral drugs at concentrations of 5% or higher. Pharmacists may not be aware that the glucuronide deficiency of cats predisposes them to toxicity with products containing benzoic acid [32]. A single 450-mg/kg dose can be lethal, and 200 mg/kg/d cannot be tolerated with multiple dosing. A product containing 5% benzoic acid contains 5 g/dL or 50 mg/mL (50 mg/g for nonsolutions), limiting a single dose to 9 mL/kg or a daily dose to 4 mL (4 g). Drugs also can be prepared as benzoate salts. Despite their sensitivity to benzoates, cats can tolerate metronidazole benzoate salt safely: 40% of the preparation is benzoate, and a dose of 20 mg/kg delivers metronidazole at a rate of 12 mg/kg and benzoate at a rate of 8 mg/kg [24].

Finally, improper facilities management can contribute to adverse drug events associated with a compounded product. Failure to adhere to strict cleansing procedures may result in contamination of compounded drugs with drugs from previous compounding procedures or cleansing agents.

Documentation of Adverse Events Caused by Compounded Products

Unfortunately, few published reports exist that delineate adverse events resulting from inappropriate compounding. Several human studies have demonstrated frequent errors with two of the most commonly compounded products: intravenous admixtures [33] and products prepared for parenteral nutrition [34]. The *Kansas City Star* generated national interest in an investigative article that focused on compounding mistakes (Donna McGuire and Mark Morris, personal communication, 2002). Specific instances of morbidity and mortality resulted from microbial contamination of presumed sterile products, with miscalculation leading to over- and underdosing of drugs and inadvertent inclusion of toxic compounds. The report also cited an unpublished study by the FDA that found 34% of 29 tested products did not meet FDA standards, primarily because the products contained less drug than the labeled content. Yet, despite these indications of frequent problems, the FDA receives few reports regarding adverse events related to compounded products, in part, because there is no mandated adverse event reporting for these products. Similar or worse problems occur with veterinary compounding; however, unless reported, their occurrence is lost to the profession. The author's experience with failure of compounded phenobarbital was previously described. Potassium bromide offers another example. It is relatively easy to formulate as a liquid. Purchased as a pure (crystalline) preparation, it is added to water with or without a flavoring agent. As a salt, it is stable, and the concentration of the final preparation is sufficiently high that microbial growth is unlikely. Yet, the author has documented several cases of seizures in previously well-controlled epileptic animals. Decreased serum bromide concentrations, despite no change in dose or diet, were ultimately associated in each case with mislabeled solutions compounded by pharmacists or veterinarians. Other instances of inappropriate veterinary compounding are becoming evident, although most have been reported for equine products. Mislabeled compounded omeprazole paste was previously discussed. A veterinary equine ivermectin product that mimics a commercial preparation approved for use in horses was found to be within 90% of the labeled content in only 2 of 11 products (although all products were within at least 70% of the label claim); the reasons for mislabeling were not identified. A different study compared compounded products with FDA-approved versions of several drugs. The content and purity of compounded preparations varied from the FDA-approved versions. Drug studied and the percentage of accuracy in labeled content included ketoprofen (1 product contained only 50% of the labeled content, whereas 12 of 13 products contained close to 100%), amikacin (percentage of the labeled content ranged from 59% to 140%, whereas that of none of the products was within 10%), and boldenone (all within 15% of labeled content, but 2 of 5 products contained up to 5% impurities) [35].

Recommendations for Compounded Products

"Keep it simple" is a prudent approach to compounding. Actions that minimally change a product, such as diluting a solution or adding a flavoring agent, are less likely to have a negative impact on drug action than more complex actions. Even so, changes in drug stability, pH, or drug-vehicle interactions may have a negative impact on the drug.

Compounders have at their disposal several texts that provide guidance regarding stability of drugs when mixed with various ingredients, including other drugs. These include *Remington's Practice and Science of Pharmacy* (previously *Pharmaceutical Sciences*) [36], which provides guidance regarding the stability and optimal vehicle conditions for (human) drugs (bulk and finished). *Trissel's Handbook on Injectable Drugs* [37,38] and *King's Guide to Parenteral Admixtures* [39] delineate chemical drug incompatibilities among drugs in solution, and other similar texts are available [39–42]. Formularies of the USP [5,31] not only provide standards but general chapters on pertinent pharmaceutics, including compounding practices. The USP has contributed to the validation of pharmacy compounding through chapters in the USP/NF [general chapters 795, 1206, and (1075), with the latter pertaining to good compounding practices]. More recently, USP has published the *Pharmacists' Pharmacopeia* which contains relevant chapters in one text. In response to the dramatic upswing in compounding that has taken place in human and veterinary medicine, the chapters currently are under revision, and monographs are currently being generated to guide compounding of veterinary products, with bromide being the first. Reputable compounding pharmacies should be expected to have a copy of this pharmacopeia. Content also is relevant to compounding veterinarians. A reputable compounding pharmacist should include copies of these or similar texts in his or her compounding library. Veterinary compounders might also contact a pharmacist or the technical services 800 telephone number of the drug manufacturer for the product being used.

All compounded products should be labeled with a beyond-use date (with expiration dates being reserved for approved products). In general, compounded preparations are intended for immediate rather than long-term use, and lengthy expiration dates typical of approved products are not necessary for compounded products [26]. As such, beyond-use dates tend to be short. Lengthier dates should be based on scientific studies, although these are seldom available. Manufacturers and published resources may provide some data; however, the data are applicable only as long as the conditions (including ingredients [active drug or excipients], pH, and range of drug concentrations) are the same. The USP offers some guidelines when no information is available. For example, for solid dosing forms, the date should not be more than 25% of the time remaining for the expiration date of an approved drug used for compounding or for 6 months, whichever is less. For water-containing products, the date should be 14 days or less unless scientific evidence exists to the contrary. In general, compounded products should be stored in cool (often refrigerated, but exceptions occur) temperatures protected from light [5,30].

Materials and equipment [43] to be used in compounding increasingly are being promoted directly to veterinarians and pharmacists, including flavoring systems, chew tablets, and other methods of drug delivery. "Recipes" often are provided. No approval process exists for these products, and promotion should not be interpreted as assurance of efficacy. For example, a flavoring system that has been used for compounding of pediatric medicaments for a decade is being marketed to veterinary hospitals and veterinary compounding pharmacists. The system includes 20 different flavors appealing to animals as well as a formulary of approximately 300 recipes. The recipes are not based on scientific studies, nor are they limited to drugs whose stability has been documented in the flavoring systems.

The potential pitfalls of compounding can be reduced and the attributes supported through several actions (see Box 1). A veterinarian who selects compounded products for therapeutic intervention should consider visiting the facilities of the pharmacy being recommended to the client. The pharmacist responsible for compounding should be queried regarding training in veterinarian medicine and specific qualifications regarding compounding (see Box 1). Personnel and facilities of the pharmacy should be dedicated to compounding.

Although State Pharmacy Model Practice Acts direct pharmacists to follow activities intended to facilitate quality assurance, these directives focus on record keeping, evaluation of equipment, and tracking of materials and do not guarantee accuracy. A well-designed and well-implemented quality control program would include verification of the accuracy of selected compounded products by measuring actual drug content. This would be particularly important for drugs characterized by a low therapeutic index or drugs that tend to be unstable. However, measuring drug content is costly. Quality assurance should be implemented only by laboratories that follow good laboratory practices, and expecting all compounding activities to be verified through drug analysis is unreasonable. Nevertheless, expecting a compounding pharmacy to follow a well-designed quality assurance program is not only reasonable but paramount. Quality assurance in compounded products is partially but not adequately addressed by state pharmacy laws. Most state laws, in concert with the NABP, direct the pharmacist to implement good compounding practices intended to ensure that a compounded product is made appropriately and is free of potentially harmful contaminants. The compounding veterinarian should (and, in many states, is mandated to) follow those state laws (veterinary medical or pharmacy) that delineate any applicable requirements for quality assurance. Prescribing veterinarians should likewise assure themselves that the dispensing pharmacy is adhering to state laws. Pharmacies also should adhere to standards delineated by the USP [5,31]. Indeed, the absence of the recently published *USP Pharmacist's Pharmacopeia* [31] in a compounding pharmacy should certainly lead to caution regarding the sincerity of the compounding pharmacy in meeting the needs of the compounded product prescriber.

Expectations of Scientific Articles

As the profession seeks scientific validation of the use of compounded products in their patients, the number of peer-reviewed scientific reports should increase. Veterinarians should critique such references closely for evidence of validity of compounded products on which the study is based. The study should be supported by a detailed description of product preparation. Only USP or equivalent-grade drugs should be used; certificates of analysis should be verified for all ingredients. The source of all ingredients used to prepare the compounded product should be cited, and the product should be compounded from an approved finished drug or a bulk substance that meets federal standards. Accuracy and precision (if multiple batches) of each batch of product used should be verified, including evidence that the drug is distributed equally throughout the finished form used in the study so that accuracy of dosing is ensured. Storage conditions, including duration (from formulation to use), vials, temperature, and exposure to sunlight, should be described, and their impact on drug stability should be addressed. Stability of the active drug ingredient throughout the storage period of the product should be verified (eg, an aliquot of the preparation administered should be studied on formulation and then again immediately before drug administration). Studies on the drug preparation itself are only as good as the analytic procedure for the drug being tested. The methods of the report thus should describe the validation procedure for the analytic assay in the species of animal studied and in the vehicle in which the drug is being administered. Upper and lower limits of quantitation and accuracy and precision of the assay within the ranges of the concentrations reported should be documented. Conclusions drawn regarding the appropriateness of the product should be limited only to the conditions described in the study, and the publication should point out any aspects of the study that would be in conflict with the law should such practices be followed by a practicing veterinarian or pharmacist.

PHARMACOKINETICS OF COMPOUNDED PRODUCTS: FAILURE OF DRUG DELIVERY

Despite the implementation of an excellent quality control program and documentation of the accuracy in labeling of a compounded product, adverse events, particularly therapeutic failure, can occur because the method of delivery failed. Products are often compounded with the intent of improving the method of delivery to increase owner compliance. However, reformulation generates a new drug product with no guarantee of effective drug delivery. Compounding pharmacies may actively promote (to clients as well as to clinicians) the availability of "novel" drug delivery systems. Although promotion of such products by professionals would inherently imply evidence of efficacy, this simply, and unfortunately, is not always the case. Provision of standard of care should cause the veterinarian to assess the likelihood of a compounded product to deliver drug effectively; such critical assessment should include literature or other relevant source searches as well as discussion with the pharmacist regarding the efficacy of products. In the author's experience, when queried regarding the efficacy of a compounded product, pharmacists often site the lack of complaints directed toward their office or apparent clinical response as evidence of efficacy. However, evidence of efficacy is not actively sought. Issues, such as lack of an adverse event reporting system, placebo effects, and poor measurements of clinical response, generally are not taken into consideration. As with any therapeutic intervention, evidence of efficacy should be based, whenever possible, on well-designed, hypothesis-driven, placebo-controlled, blind studies.

Assuming that the active drug product is not substituted, because compounding alters only delivery of the drug and not the drug itself, absorption is the only aspect of drug disposition that should be altered by a compounded product. As such, the disposition of a drug intended for intravenous administration should not be altered by compounding. However, absorption of drugs that are not administered intravenously can be profoundly altered by compounding. Of these, oral drugs are most likely to be affected; however, disposition of topically applied drugs can also be affected, particularly if the drug is intended for systemic drug delivery, as can disposition of injectable drugs if the salt is changed.

ORAL PRODUCTS

Rate and extent of oral absorption are likely to be affected in a compounded finished drug compared with its approved version. The impact of reformulation on the pharmaceutics of orally administered drugs has been discussed;

their impact alters the amount of drug that is available for absorption in the product. Even if drug is available in the product, however, oral absorption may not occur. Many drugs are available commercially only as injectable preparations because they cannot be given orally for a variety of reasons. The availability of an oral version of the same drug should increase confidence that oral absorption is possible. Nevertheless, 100% bioavailability should not be assumed. In general, if an approved oral form of a drug is not available, prescribing a compounded oral product should be done only with reservations unless scientific information supports the specific formulation being compounded. For example, many drugs are not available orally, because they are destroyed by gastric acid (eg, many β-lactams, omeprazole). Others undergo first-pass metabolism (eg, opioids, many cardiac drugs) so extensive that the preparation cannot be physically made to allow a dose sufficiently high to compensate for the first-pass effect. Some drugs simply are not absorbable in the conditions of the gastrointestinal tract. Weakly basic drugs (aminoglycosides) and drugs that are extremely lipid (eg, cyclosporine, griseofulvin) or large in size (eg, amphotericin B) are not orally absorbed. Some of these drugs can be specifically formulated to facilitate oral absorption (eg, cyclosporine), but manipulations are often sufficiently sophisticated that they cannot be accurately reproduced by all compounding pharmacists. Selected prodrugs that require metabolism for activation are not absorbable in their parent drug form.

Selected commercial oral preparations have been formulated to alter (slow or facilitate) drug delivery, and reformulation of such products should be avoided. Compounding altered-release products from bulk substances requires sophisticated techniques not generally available through pharmacists. Enteric coated or spansule products should not be crushed. Although spansule products might be reformulated without crushing, the amount of drug in each spansule is not necessarily predictable and random distribution of drug content is likely to yield erratic dosing. Cyclosporine is a complex molecule characterized by poor oral bioavailability; oral absorption requires bile acids or special formulation as a microemulsion product. As such, it is an example of a drug for which compounding should be approached cautiously and supported by therapeutic drug monitoring. In the author's drug monitoring laboratory, cyclosporine blood concentrations were not detectable (two different samples 2 weeks apart) in one cat receiving a product compounded from an approved microemulsion human product. Following recommendations that the untampered animal-approved version be used at the same dose, concentrations expected at the administered dose were detected within 1 week of the change in the drug product.

TRANSDERMAL GELS

Compounded transdermal pluronic-lethicin organogels (PLOs) have become a popular method of drug delivery widely embraced by the veterinary profession, despite the lack of scientific evidence in support of this system. PLOs were developed by a compounding pharmacist as a practical alternative to traditional drug delivery systems. Descriptions of the gels cannot easily be found in the scientific literature and are largely limited to post-graduate class materials and other nonreferenced literature distributed to educators, such those distributed by the Professional Compounding Companies of America (PCCA).[1] The history of the creation of PLO gels has been reviewed [44].

The gels are composed of water-based compounds prepared in various organic solvents. The oil phase is composed of lecithin (generally of soy bean origin), which theoretically rearranges the stratum corneum, the major barrier to drug movement across the skin. Isopropyl palmitate acts as a solvent and penetration enhancer. The water phase is composed of purified water and a pluronic (poloxamer) gel composed of a surfactant (pluronic F127), which theoretically also contributes to disruption of the stratum corneum. Because lecithin promotes the growth of mold, potassium sorbate is included as a preservative [45]. The active drug ingredient is dissolved in the oil (lipid) or water phase, depending on its lipid solubility (Fig. 4). The amount of active drug added is based on the recommended dose; generally, the gel is designed so that the dose is delivered at a dose of 0.1 mL (cats and small dogs) to a dose of 0.5 to 1 mL (larger dogs). Lecithin and isopropyl palmitate (a ratio of 1:1) must comprise at least 24% of the system for micelles containing the drug to form properly. The remaining volume of a PLO is composed of the drug and the pluronic gel. Because manufactured drug preparations often are not available in concentrations sufficient to allow delivery of the calculated dose in the small volume of PLO, purified bulk powder (which may not be legal)

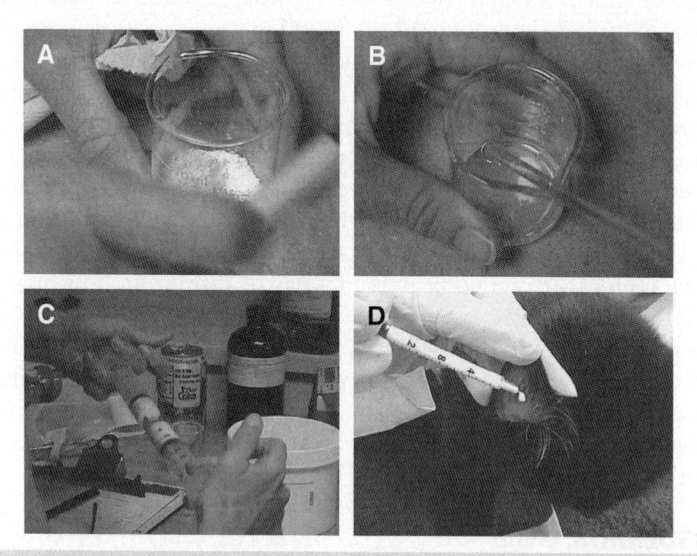

Fig. 4. The preparation of a transdermal PLO begins with mixing the drug (*A*) in the pluronic or lecithin phase (*B*), addition of the alternate phase plus excipients, and formation of drug-containing micelles by passage between two syringes (*C*). (*D*) Gel is generally transferred to a syringe and dispensed on the inside of the ear (in cats). Gloves should be worn with administration.

is preferred by compounding pharmacies formulating the gels. When subjected to proper shearing forces (generally accomplished by rapidly passing the mixture between a small-caliber catheter or two syringes; see Fig. 3), micelles containing the drug theoretically are formed. The micelles are believed to disorganize the stratum corneum slightly with minimal direct detrimental effects on the skin (based on light microscopy), although contact hypersensitivity or allergy to the lecithin component may occur [46,47]. The PLO seems to dissolve a variety of different chemicals, including lipophilic, hydrophilic, and amphoteric compounds. The gels can be easily and rapidly prepared and are theoretically stable in most clinical environments. Nevertheless, the gels are thermoreversible; at temperatures higher than 40°C, they are liquid, but they become high-viscosity gels after cooling to room temperature and remixing. At refrigerated temperatures, the gels again become liquid; accordingly, the gels should not be refrigerated. Thus, the PLO becomes more viscous at higher temperatures, rendering it more amenable to topical drug delivery.

At least two PLOs (ie, with the pluronic and oil phases already mixed) are commercially available: one is sold by the PCCA. This organization offers compounding training classes for pharmacists, including formulation of PLOs and recipes for the preparation of many different drug products as gels. The advent of PLOs as a method of systemic drug delivery and the formulation of the original PLO were generated through the PCCA Division of Research.[1] In addition to training, the PCCA sells validated ingredients to be used in compounding. Sale and compounding guidance is limited to PCCA members, however; membership at the time of publication of this article costs $20,000. The financial incentive for the PCCA to train pharmacists in the compounding of PLOs intended for veterinary use is problematic. Products for formulation of PLOs are also available through other companies (eg, Gallipot, Medota Heights, Minnesota, which sells a commercial PLO base as well as drugs, and chemical companies that sell pure drugs). The products that the PCCA offers for sale have drawn the attention of the FDA; a warning letter was sent in 2001 regarding their sale of bulk substances, including dipyrone and antibiotics (Fred Richman, Office of Compliance, Center for Drug Evaluation and Research, FDA, Rockville, Maryland, personal communication, 2005).

The availability of training in the preparation of PLOs and the level of promotion of gels by pharmacists suggest that this method of drug delivery has been validated scientifically. Yet, a review of the literature reveals little scientific support for the use of the PLO system and its ability to deliver drugs.

A review (based on an interview of the creator of the PLO gels) of the history of the creation of PLO gels offers some potential insight into the evidence (or lack thereof) for clinical efficacy of these preparations [43]. The review notes the gels to be an "exceptional based for transdermal preparations." Clinical evaluation of PLO was based on collaboration of the interviewee with "a few local physicians and their patients." Physicians were "willing to prescribe the PLO gel" as pharmacists suggested their use. Based on one hospice patient that responded to a transdermal medication, PLOs were subsequently presented at a PCCA seminar and their use encouraged for "problems or disease that were refractory to treatment" (probably the last situation in which a trial and error approach should be used for a patient). Interestingly, the initial response by the patient was recognized as an adverse event following an overdose of the PLO gel. When queried regarding drugs that might not be appropriate for use in PLO, the interviewee noted that "The use of antibiotics in PLO has not been well documented clinically in humans." Yet, a review of the literature indicates that no use of any drug has been well documented clinically in any human patient, and only methimazole in cats. Simply because a drug can be incorporated into a gel should not be interpreted to mean that delivery will accordingly be successful. Indeed, in a recent review of PLO gels [48], only a handful of systemic studies have been conducted by clinicians and most of these were studied by veterinarians in cats. The few studies that have been reported in humans have largely focused on local, rather than systemic, delivery of the analgesic diclofenac. In the review, the ideal drug for PLO administration is described as one that is potent, with the dose being only a few mg, the drug small in size, characterized by high lipid solubility, and non-irritating or sensitizing to the skin. Yet, a number of the drugs currently incorporated in PLO do not fit the ideal characteristics [48]. Further, she notes that the anecdotal efficacy attributed to transdermal delivery could have been a placebo effect.

Despite the lack of scientific validity, the number of compounding pharmacies offering compounding services, including the formulation of PLOs, is increasing as training in their preparation continues (eg, at the PCCA). Recipes for veterinary PLOs have been published in the *International Journal of Pharmaceutical Compounding*, a journal whose articles tend to focus on the sharing of compounding information rather than on the reporting of scientific studies. The list of PLO drug recipes for veterinary use is extensive and includes but is not limited to nonsteroidal anti-inflammatories, antimicrobials, anticonvulsants, prokinetic agents, anticancer drugs, behavior-modifying drugs, and hormones.[1]

Scientific data regarding the use of PLOs for systemic drug delivery are slowly becoming available in the veterinary literature. Methimazole is among the most common drugs formulated in a PLO for administration in cats and may be the most likely drug to be successfully delivered as a PLO because of its small MW of 115 (compared with MW >250 for most other drugs). Additionally, response to therapy can be monitored. A clinical abstract report (uncontrolled clinical trial) cited a response to methimazole administered as a PLO in 9 of 10 hyperthyroid cats based on decreased serum thyroxine (T_4) concentrations [49]. Yet, a subsequent experimental report in normal cats after single dose of methimazole as a PLO found that the drug reached detectable concentrations in only 2 of 6 cats but was not quantifiable in the remaining 4 cats [48]. A second abstract indicates that the efficacy of methimazole as a PLO requires 4 weeks of therapy and subsequent reports generally confirm the efficacy of methimazole administered as a PLO gel [50]. For other drugs, a number of studies have confirmed the failure of the PLO drug delivery system to predictably achieve therapeutic concentrations (concentrations often are non detectable) in cats after the administration of a single dose. These drugs include amikacin, enrofloxacin (non-detectable concentrations) (Fig. 5) and diazepam (with therapeutic concentrations being detected in some cats but not all) (Dawn Boothe, DVM, PhD, unpublished data, 2003), fentanyl or morphine (not predictably quantifiable) [51], diltiazem (not predictably quantifiable) [52], fluoxetine (multiple dosing yielding 10% bioavailability) [53], buspirone [54], amitriptyline (not quantifiable) [54], glipizide (some cats showing some response, but not predictably) [55], and dexamethasone (not quantifiable) [56]. As these reports become available, the pharmacy and veterinary professions are becoming educated regarding the applicability of PLO use to veterinary patients [57]. Clearly, the need for follow-up studies focusing on multiple dosing with PLOs is necessary; further, the use of the gels in situations in which an immediate drug response is necessary should be strictly limited to use validated by science or for drugs in which clinical response is clearly recognized by monitoring or the resolution of discreet and easily identifiable clinical signs.

There are other reasons why use of the PLOs (as with other novel delivery systems) should be based on demonstrated efficacy using properly controlled studies. The site of administration is likely to vary among species, and possibly among animals. Currently, PLOs are applied to the ear so that grooming by the animal does not remove the drug. Although the stratum corneum of the inner ear is the thinnest in cats, it is the site of the thickest stratum corneum in dogs [53,58]. The ability of a client to administer a drug repetitively at a dose of 0.1 mL accurately needs to be addressed; unreported studies by

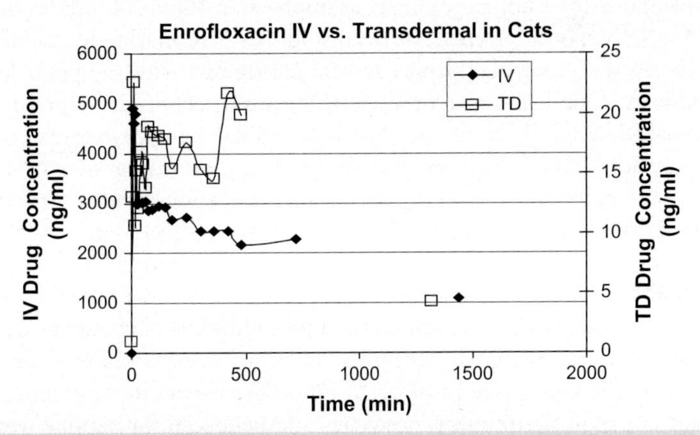

Fig. 5. Enrofloxacin administered at a dose of 5 mg/kg via a transdermal gel in normal healthy cats (n = 3) was essentially nondetectable (*open squares, right* y *axis*) compared with the same dose administered intravenously (*filled squares, left* y *axis*). IV, intravenous; min, minutes; TD, transdermal.

our laboratory using clients of the veterinary teaching hospital have found the actual volume administered by clients (using weighing paper) to range from 0.1 (the intended volume) to 1 mL. The vehicle for most of these topical formulations is a soy lecithin–based organic gel. Soy lecithin is a common allergen in people and has been reported to cause asthma and food allergies [26,27]. A suspected adverse (allergic) reaction to a topical formulation of methimazole has been reported (Katrina Mealey, Washington State University, personal communication, 2005) in a cat. A topical reaction has also been reported with multiple dosing after experimental use of the gel in cats [47]. The compounded PLO product also offers an example of increased risk of drug exposure to the veterinary client. Clients should wear nonpermeable gloves when administering the drug and be counseled regarding inappropriate exposure of the drug to children or other pets.

Design of dosing regimens using transdermal gels is complicated by the lack of knowledge regarding the impact of the stratum corneum on drug delivery. To assume that a transdermal drug is 100% bioavailable after transdermal delivery is optimistic at best; as such, however, transdermal doses probably should be increased compared with oral doses. This may also be true for drugs characterized by first-pass metabolism for three reasons. First, the skin can metabolize many drugs metabolized by the liver, although the extent of metabolism is likely to be less. Second, no study has yet to demonstrate greater than 10% bioavailability with a drug administered transdermally. As such, a drug characterized by a 50% first-pass metabolism might still be only 20% bioavailable after transdermal delivery. Finally, for many of the drugs, metabolites are equally or more active than the parent compound and first-pass metabolism may not affect efficacy. A final consideration regarding the use of compounded transdermal gels is the expiration date, which should be based on scientific evidence of maintained potency. As an example, a methimazole transdermal gel with a 6 month expiration date has been sold to a veterinarian for in-office use. A previuosly well controlled hyperthyroid cat treated with the gel failed therapy, exhibiting clinical signs of hyperthyoridism. The cat responded to a new preparation (Gigi Davidson, North Carolina State University, personal communication, 2006). This incident underscores the importance of scientific validation of extended expiration dates for any compounded product and the hazards of buying a compounded product for in-office use.

SUMMARY

The advent and growth of veterinary compounding and the increasing role of the pharmacist in drug dispensing, including compounding, should be embraced by the veterinary profession. For selected patients, extemporaneous compounding of prescriptions is necessary and beneficial for optimal treatment. By its nature, however, compounding is individualized and fraught with risks of failure. Pet owners should be informed of the risks associated with using a compounded product and consent to therapy based on disclosure that the use of the product may be scientifically unproven. The AVMA's Council on

Biologic and Therapeutic Agents has generated a position statement regarding the use of compounded products that offers sage advice. The position statement reminds veterinarians that although compounded products may have an important role in the treatment of veterinary patients, compounding may alter the ability of the product to deliver drug and should be reserved for those instances in which there is a legitimate need and, unless there is no alternative, for which evidence of efficacy or safety exists when the drug is administered as the compounded preparation. As the pharmacy profession increases its efforts to define and ensure its role in veterinary medicine, and as the regulatory agencies consider changes in the regulations that increase the flexibility of animal drug compounding, the veterinary profession must "step up to the plate" and implement actions that protect the patient and the public. Finally, although it is the responsibility of the pharmacist to ensure the integrity of any finished drug product dispensed to a patient, ultimately, it is the responsibility of the veterinarian to ensure the safety and therapy of any prescribed therapeutic intervention, and failure to do otherwise places the patient and pet owner as well as the veterinarian at risk.

Acknowledgments

The majority of the information presented in this manuscript was acquired by the author during her tenure as a member of the AVMA's Council on Biologic and Therapeutic Agents (COBTA). Accordingly, she would like to acknowledge COBTA and particularly, Dr. Elizabeth Curry Galvin, Director of the American Veterinary Medical Association (AVMA) Scientific Activities Division for their input into this manuscript. The author would also like to acknowledge Katrina Mealey, DVM, PhD, DACVIM, DACVCP, of Washington State University, and GiGi Davison, BS, DICVP of North Carolina State University, for their input.

References

[1] Available at: http://www.iacprx.org/index.html. Accessed July 15, 2004.
[2] Notices. Fed Regist 2006;71(63):16593–6.
[3] Bender GA. History of pharmacy. College of Pharmacy. Available at: www.pharmacy.wsu.edu/history. Accessed August 17, 2006.
[4] Thompson J. The United States Pharmacopeia. A leader in protection and promotion of health. Journal of the Pharmacy Society of Wisconsin 2002;34–8.
[5] United States Pharmacopeia. The United States pharmacopeia/national formulary (USP 27-NF 22). Rockville (MD): United States Pharmacopeia; 2004.
[6] Allen L. Compounding. Presented at the USP Stakeholders Meeting. Baltimore, August 2002.
[7] Bradley EW. Improving profitability with veterinary compounding. International Journal of Pharmaceutical Compounding 1999;3:180–1.
[8] Davis J. Compounding for creatures: what works. International Journal of Pharmaceutical Compounding 1999;3:182–5.
[9] Paoletti J. Veterinary flavor suggestions. International Journal of Pharmaceutical Compounding 1999;3:186.
[10] Yoakum J. Compounded injectables for veterinary use. International Journal of Pharmaceutical Compounding 2001;5:107.
[11] Hudson S. Call of the wild: compounding for zoos and exotics. International Journal of Pharmaceutical Compounding 1999;3:176–9.

[12] Swann JP. History of the FDA. FDA history office. Available at: www.fda.gov/oc/history/historyoffda. Accessed August 17, 2006.
[13] Seigner AW. When is compounding for animals legal? International Journal of Pharmaceutical Compounding 1999;3:188–92.
[14] Chan DS. Regulatory issues for the use of bulk drugs in veterinary compounding. International Journal of Pharmaceutical Compounding 2001;5:97–100.
[15] US Food and Drug Administration. Animal Medicinal Drug Use Clarification Act of 1994. Available at: http://www.fda.gov/cvm/amducatoc.htm. Accessed August 29, 2006.
[16] American Veterinary Medical Association. Extra label drug use algorithm. Available at: http://www.avma.org/scienact/amduca/amduca2.asp. Accessed August 17, 2006.
[17] Anonymous. The top 10 veterinary compounded products. International Journal of Pharmaceutical Compounding 1999;3:183.
[18] International Academy of Compounding Pharmacists. Available at: www.iacprx.org/vetissue.htm.
[19] Anonymous. DEA revokes pharmacy's registration. Available at: http://www.avma.org/onlnews/javma/jun06/060601i.asp. Accessed August 17, 2006.
[20] Anonymous. When can a veterinarian import a foreign durg? Available at: http://www.avma.org/onlnews/javma/aug05/050815f.asp. Accessed August 17, 2006.
[21] National Association of Board of Pharmacies. Available at: www.nabp.net. Accessed August 17, 2006.
[22] American Veterinary Medical Association. Available at: http://www.avma.org/issues/drugs/compounding/default.asp. Accessed August 17, 2006.
[23] Professional Compounding Accreditation Board. Available at: http://www.pcab.info. Accessed August 17, 2006.
[24] Davidson G. To benzoate or not to benzoate: Cats are the question. International Journal of Pharmaceutical Compounding 2001;5:89–90.
[25] Connors KA, Amidon GL, Stella VJ. Chemical stability of pharmaceuticals. New York: John Wiley; 1986.
[26] Allen L. Secondum artem. Current and practical compounding information for the pharmacist. Minneapolis (MN): Paddock Laboratories; 2004. p. 1–3.
[27] Nieto JE, Spier S, Pipers FS, et al. Comparison of paste and suspension formulations of omeprazole in the healing of gastric ulcers in racehorses in active training. J Am Vet Med Assoc 2002;221(8):1139–43.
[28] Kukamich B, Papich M. Fluorinated quinolone stability in vehicles for oral administration [abstract]. In: Proceedings of the American College of Veterinary Internal Medicine. Charlotte (NC), 2003. p. 285.
[29] Mistry B, Samuel L, Bowden S, et al. Simplifying oral drug therapy for patients with swallowing difficulties. Pharm J 1995;254:808–9.
[30] Canadian Society of Hospital Pharmacists. Extemporaneous oral liquid dosage preparations. Toronto: Canadian Society of Hospital Pharmacists; 1988.
[31] USP pharmacist's pharmacopeia. Rockville (MD): US Pharmacopeia; 2005.
[32] Bedford PGC, Clarke MA. Suspected benzoic acid poisoning in the cat. Vet Rec 1971;88:599–601.
[33] Flynn EA, Pearson RE, Barker KN. Observational study of accuracy in compounding i.v. admixtures at five hospitals. Am J Health Syst Pharm 1997;54:904–12.
[34] Buerger DK. Parenteral nutrition safe practices: a new roadmap for improved patient care. American Society of Consultant Pharmacists. Available at: www.ascp.com/public/pubs/tcp/1998/nov/roadmap.shtml. Accessed August 17, 2006.
[35] Stanley DS, Thomasy MS, Skinner W. Comparison for pharmaceutical equivalence of FDA-approved products and compounded preparations of ketoprofen, amikacin, and boldenone In: Proceedings of the 49th Annual Convention of the American Association of Equine Practitioners. New Orleans (LA); 2003.
[36] Gennaro AR, editor. Remington: the science and practice of pharmacy. 20th edition. Easton (PA): Mack Publishing Company; 2000.

[37] Trissel LA. Stability of compounded formulations. Washington (DC): American Pharmaceutical Association; 1996.
[38] Trissel LA. Handbook on injectable drugs. 8th edition. Bethesda (MD): American Society of Hospital Pharmacists; 2000.
[39] King's guide to parenteral admixtures. Pacemarq, Inc. St. Louis (MO).
[40] Woods DJ. Formulation in pharmacy practice. Dunedin (New Zealand): Healthcare Otago; 1993.
[41] American Society of Hospital Pharmacists. Committee on Extemporaneous Formulations. Handbook on extemporaneous formulations. Bethesda (MD): American Society of Hospital Pharmacists; 1987.
[42] Nahata MC, Hipple TF. Pediatric drug formulations. Cincinnati (OH): Harvey Whitney; 1990.
[43] Harvey A. Equipment for large-volume aseptic veterinary compounding. International Journal of Pharmaceutical Compounding 2001;5:106.
[44] Anonymous. The history of Marty Jones. Intern J Pharmaceut Compound 2003;7:180–3.
[45] Willimann H, Walde P, Luisi PL, et al. Lecithin organogel as matrix for transdermal transport of drugs. J Pharm Sci 1992;81:871–4.
[46] Lavaud F, Perdu D, Prvost A, et al. Baker's asthma related to soybean lecithin exposure. Allergy 1994;49:159–62.
[47] Palm M, Moneret-Vautrin DA, Kanny G, et al. Food allergy to egg and soy lecithins. Allergy 1999;54:1116–7.
[48] Hoffman SB, Yoder AR, Trepanier LA. Bioavailability of transdermal methimazole in a pluronic lecithin organogel (PLO) in healthy cats. J Vet Pharmacol Ther 2002;25(3): 189–93.
[49] Hoffmann G, Marks SL, Taboada J, et al. Transdermal methimazole treatment in cats with hyperthyroidism. J Feline Med Surg 2003;5(2):77–82.
[50] Sartor LL, Trepanier LA, Kroll M, et al. Clinical efficacy of transdermal methimazole in cats with hyperthyroidism [abstract]. In: Proceedings of the American College of Veterinary Internal Medicine. 2003. p. 21.
[51] Krotscheck U, Boothe DM, Boothe HW. Evaluation of a pluronic lecithin organogel for transdermal delivery of fentanyl and morphine in dogs [abstract]. In: Proceedings of the American College of Veterinary Internal Medicine Annual Forum, Charlotte (NC); 2003. p. 21.
[52] DeFrancesco TC. Transdermal cardiac therapy in cats: the NCSU experience. In: Proceedings of the American College of Veterinary Internal Medicine Annual Forum, Denver (CO); 2004. p. 22.
[53] Ciribassi J, Luescher A, Pasloske KS. Comparative bioavailability of fluoxetine after transdermal and oral administration to healthy cats. Am J Vet Res 2003;64(8):994–8.
[54] Mealey KM, Peck KE, Bennett BS, et al. Systemic absorption of amitriptyline and buspirone after oral and transdermal administration to healthy cats. J Vet Intern Med 2004;18(1): 43–6.
[55] Bennett N, Papich MG, Hoenig M, et al. Evaluation of transdermal application of glipizide in a pluronic lecithin gel to healthy cats. Am J Vet Res 2005;66(4):581–8.
[56] Willis-Goulet HS, Schmidt BA, Nicklin CF, et al. Comparison of serum dexamethasone concentrations in cats after oral or transdermal administration using pluronic lecithin organogel (PLO): pilot study. Veterinary Dermatology 2003;14:83–9.
[57] Davidson G. Veterinary transdermal medications: A to Z. International Journal of Pharmaceutical Compounding 2003;7:206–9.
[58] Riviere JE, Papich MG. Potential problems of developing transdermal patches for veterinary applications. Adv Drug Deliv Rev 2001;50:175–203.

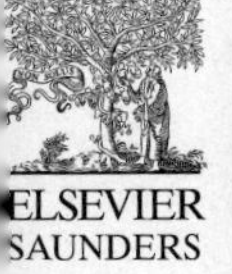

Vet Clin Small Anim 36 (2006) 1175–1181

VETERINARY CLINICS
SMALL ANIMAL PRACTICE

ELSEVIER
SAUNDERS

INDEX

A

Note: Page numbers of article titles are in **boldface** type.

0195-5616/06/$ – see front matter
doi:10.1016/S0195-5616(06)00093-3

vetsmall.theclinics.com

D

Moving?

Make sure your subscription moves with you!

To notify us of your new address, find your **Clinics Account Number** (located on your mailing label above your name), and contact customer service at:

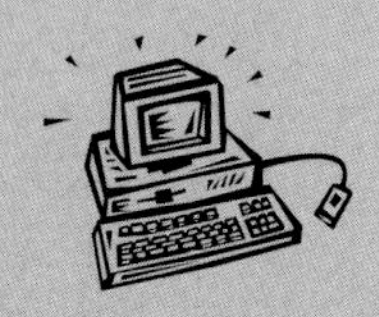

E-mail: elspcs@elsevier.com

800-654-2452 (subscribers in the U.S. & Canada)
407-345-4000 (subscribers outside of the U.S. & Canada)

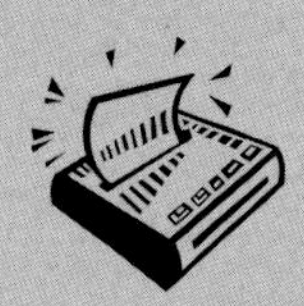

Fax number: 407-363-9661

Elsevier Periodicals Customer Service
6277 Sea Harbor Drive
Orlando, FL 32887-4800

*To ensure uninterrupted delivery of your subscription, please notify us at least 4 weeks in advance of move.

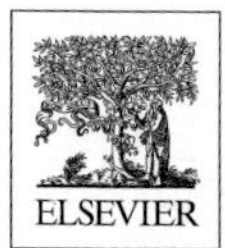